617.55

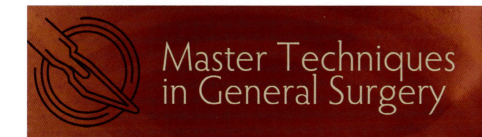

Master Techniques
in General Surgery

COLON AND RECTAL SURGERY: ANORECTAL OPERATIONS

Master Techniques in General Surgery

Also available in this series:

Master Techniques in Breast Surgery

December 2010
Kirby I. Bland, MD
V. Suzanne Klimberg, MD

Master Techniques in Colon and Rectal Surgery: Anorectal Operations

November 2011
Steven D. Wexner, MD
James W. Fleshman, MD

Coming Soon

Master Techniques in Hernia Surgery

September 2012
Daniel Jones, MD

Master Techniques in Stomach Surgery

September 2012
Michael S. Nussbaum, MD
Jeffrey H. Peters, MD

Master Techniques in Hepatobiliary and Pancreatic Surgery

December 2012
Keith Lillemoe, MD
William Jarnagin, MD

Master Techniques in Esophageal Surgery

March 2013
James Luketich

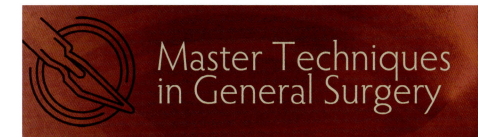

Master Techniques in General Surgery

COLON AND RECTAL SURGERY: ANORECTAL OPERATIONS

Edited by

Steven D. Wexner, MD, FACS, FRCS, FRCS(Ed)

Chairman, Department of Colorectal Surgery
Chief Academic Officer and Emeritus Chief of Staff,
   Cleveland Clinic Florida
Weston, Florida

Professor and Associate Dean for Academic Affairs
Florida Atlantic University, Boca Raton, Florida

Professor and Assistant Dean for Clinical Education
Florida International University College of Medicine
Miami, Florida

Professor of Surgery, Ohio State University
Columbus, Ohio
Affiliate Professor
Department of Surgery, Division of General Surgery
University of South Florida College of Medicine
Tampa, Florida

Affiliate Professor of Surgery
University of Miami, Miller School of Medicine

James W. Fleshman, MD

Professor of Surgery at Washington University in
   St. Louis
Chief of Colon and Rectal Surgery
Chief of Surgery
Barnes Jewish West County Hospital
St. Louis, Missouri

Series Editor

Josef E. Fischer, MD

William V. McDermott Professor of Surgery
Harvard Medical School
Chairman of Surgery, Emeritus
Beth Israel Deaconess Hospital
Boston, Massachusetts

Chairman of Surgery
Christian R. Holmes Professor of Surgery Emeritus
University of Cincinnati College of Medicine
Cincinnati, Ohio

Illustrations by: BodyScientific International, LLC.

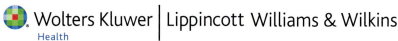

Wolters Kluwer | Lippincott Williams & Wilkins
Health

Philadelphia • Baltimore • New York • London
Buenos Aires • Hong Kong • Sydney • Tokyo

Acquisitions Editor: Brian Brown
Product Manager: Brendan Huffman
Production Manager: Bridgett Dougherty
Senior Manufacturing Manager: Benjamin Rivera
Marketing Manager: Lisa Lawrence
Design Coordinator: Doug Smock
Production Service: Aptara, Inc.

© 2012 by LIPPINCOTT WILLIAMS & WILKINS, a WOLTERS KLUWER business
Two Commerce Square
2001 Market Street
Philadelphia, PA 19103 USA
LWW.com

Printed in China

Library of Congress Cataloging-in-Publication Data

Colon and rectal surgery : anorectal operations / edited by Steven D. Wexner, James Fleshman.
   p. ; cm. – (Master techniques in general surgery)
  Includes bibliographical references and index.
  ISBN 978-1-60547-644-5 (hardback : alk. paper)
  I. Wexner, Steven D. II. Fleshman, James. III. Series: Master techniques in general surgery.
  [DNLM: 1. Rectal Diseases–surgery. 2. Anal Canal–surgery. 3. Colon–surgery. 4. Rectum–surgery. WI 650]
  617.5′55–dc23

2011040556

Care has been taken to confirm the accuracy of the information presented and to describe generally accepted practices. However, the authors, editors, and publisher are not responsible for errors or omissions or for any consequences from application of the information in this book and make no warranty, expressed or implied, with respect to the currency, completeness, or accuracy of the contents of the publication. Application of the information in a particular situation remains the professional responsibility of the practitioner.

   The authors, editors, and publisher have exerted every effort to ensure that drug selection and dosage set forth in this text are in accordance with current recommendations and practice at the time of publication. However, in view of ongoing research, changes in government regulations, and the constant flow of information relating to drug therapy and drug reactions, the reader is urged to check the package insert for each drug for any change in indications and dosage and for added warnings and precautions. This is particularly important when the recommended agent is a new or infrequently employed drug.

   Some drugs and medical devices presented in the publication have Food and Drug Administration (FDA) clearance for limited use in restricted research settings. It is the responsibility of the health care providers to ascertain the FDA status of each drug or device planned for use in their clinical practice.

   To purchase additional copies of this book, call our customer service department at (800) 638-3030 or fax orders to (301) 223-2320. International customers should call (301) 223-2300.

   Visit Lippincott Williams & Wilkins on the Internet: at LWW.com. Lippincott Williams & Wilkins customer service representatives are available from 8:30 am to 6:00 pm, EST.

10 9 8 7 6 5 4 3 2 1

Since books are tools by which teaching occurs, I dedicate this book to my loving sons, Wesley and Trevor who certainly taught me at least as many things as I have taught them. This book is also dedicated to that very special person who taught me the true meaning of life.

Steven D. Wexner

Maher A. Abbas, MD, FACS, FASCRS
Chief, Colon and Rectal Surgery
Chair, Center for Minimally Invasive Surgery
Kaiser Permanente Los Angeles
Assistant Professor of Surgery
University of California, Los Angeles
Los Angeles, California

Herand Abcarian, MD, FACS
Chairman
Division of Colon and Rectal Surgery
John H. Stroger Hospital of Cook County
Professor of Surgery
University of Illinois at Chicago
Chicago, Illinois

Jason W. Allen, MD
Colon & Rectal Surgery Resident
Cook County Colon & Rectal Surgery
Residency Training Program
University of Illinois at Chicago Medical Center
Chicago, Illinois

S. Alva, MD
Clinical Assistant Professor
Division of Colon and Rectal Surgery
UMDNJ—Robert Wood Johnson Medical School,
    New Brunswick
Edison, New Jersey

David N. Armstrong, MD, FRCS, FACS, FASCRS
Program Director
Georgia Colon and Rectal Surgical Clinic
Atlanta, Georgia

Cornelius Baeten, MD, PhD
Professor of Colorectal Surgery
Academic Hospital Maastricht
The Netherlands

Joshua I.S. Bleier, MD
Assistant Professor of Surgery
Division of Colon and Rectal Surgery
University of Pennsylvania
Hospital of the University of Pennsylvania
Philadelphia, Pennsylvania

S. O. Breukink, MD
Colorectal Surgeon
Academic Hospital Maastricht
The Netherlands

Federica Cadeddu, MD
Assistant Professor
Department of Surgery
Division of General Surgery
Tor Vergata University Hospital
Rome, Italy

Bertram Chinn, MD
Clinical Associate Professor
Program Director, Colon and Rectal Surgery Fellowship
Division of Colon and Rectal Surgery
UMDNJ—Robert Wood Johnson Medical School,
    New Brunswick
Edison, New Jersey

G. Willy Davila, MD
Chairman, Department of Gynecology
Head, Section of Urogynecology and Reconstructive Pelvic
    Surgery
Cleveland Clinic Florida
Weston, Florida

Kurt G. Davis, MD
Chief, General and Colon and Rectal Surgery
Department of Surgery
William Beaumont Army Medical Center
El Paso, Texas

C. Neal Ellis, MD
Professor of Surgery
Chief of Colon and Rectal Surgery
University of South Alabama
Mobile, Alabama

James W. Fleshman, MD
Professor of Surgery at Washington University in St. Louis
Chief of Colon and Rectal Surgery
Chief of Surgery
Barnes Jewish West County Hospital
St. Louis, Missouri

Robert D. Fry, MD
Emilie and Roland deHellebranth Professor of Surgery
Chief, Department of Surgery, Pennsylvania Hospital
Chair, Division of Colon and Rectal Surgery University of
    Pennsylvania Health System
Pennsylvania Hospital
Philadelphia, PA

Stanley M. Goldberg, MD
University of Minnesota
Division of Colon and Rectal Surgery
Minneapolis, Minnesota

Brooke Gurland, MD, FACS
Cleveland Clinic
Department of Colorectal Surgery
Cleveland, Ohio

Daniel O. Herzig, MD, FACS, FASCRS
Assistant Professor
Department of Surgery
Division of General Surgery
Oregon Health & Science University Hospital
Portland, Oregon

Tracy Hull, MD, FACS
Department of Colorectal Surgery
Cleveland Clinic
Cleveland, Ohio

Steven R. Hunt
Assistant Professor of Surgery
Section of Colon and Rectal Surgery
Department of Surgery
Washington University
St. Louis, Missouri

David Jayne, BSc, MBBCh, FRCS, MD
Senior Lecturer & Consultant Surgeon
John Goligher Colorectal Unit
Leeds Teaching Hospitals NHS Trust
St. James University Hospital
Leeds, United Kingdom

Hermann Kessler, MD, PhD
Professor of Surgery
Department of Surgery
University of Erlangen
Erlangen, Germany

Ira J. Kodner, MD
Solon & Bettie Gershman Professor, Surgery
Division of General Surgery
Section of Colon and Rectal Surgery
Director, Center for Colorectal and Pelvic Floor Disorders (COPE)
Washington University School of Medicine
St. Louis, MO

Jorge A. Lagares-Garcia, MD, FACS, FASCRS
Program Director, Colorectal Surgery Residency Program
Clinical Assistant Professor of Surgery
Warren Alpert Brown University School of Medicine
Providence, Rhode Island
Clinical Instructor of Surgery
Boston University
Boston, Massachusetts
R.I. Colorectal Clinic, LLC
Pawtucket, Rhode Island

Paul Antoine LeHur, MD
Head of the Department of Digestive and Endocrine Surgery
Clinique de Chirurgie Digestive et Endocrinienne (CCDE)
Institut des Maladies de l'Appareil Digestif (IMAD)
Professor of Digestive Surgery
School of Medicine of Nantes
Nantes, France

Antonio Longo, MD
Colorectal Surgeon
Department of Coloproctology
St. Elizabeth Hospital
Wien, Austria

Ann C. Lowry, MD, FASCRS, FACS
Clinical Professor of Surgery
Division of Colon and Rectal Surgery
Department of Surgery
University of Minnesota
Minneapolis, Minnesota

Kim C. Lu, MD, FACS, FASCRS
Assistant Professor
Department of Surgery
Division of General Surgery
Oregon Health & Science University Hospital
Portland, Oregon

Najjia N. Mahmoud, MD
Associate Professor of Surgery
University of Pennsylvania
Division of Colon and Rectal Surgery
Philadelphia, PA

David J. Maron, MD, MBA
Assistant Professor of Surgery
University of Pennsylvania
Division of Colon and Rectal Surgery
Penn Presbyterian Medical Center
Philadelphia, Pennsylvania

Klaus E. Matzel, MD
Head Section Coloproctology
Department of Surgery
University Erlangen
Erlangen, Germany

Giovanni Milito, MD
Associate Professor
Department of Surgery
Division of General Surgery
Tor Vergata University Hospital
Rome, Italy

Husein Moloo, MD
University of Ottawa
The Ottawa Hospital
Ottawa, Ontario, Canada

Sthela M. Murad-Regadas, MD, PhD
Adjunct Professor
Department of Surgery
School of Medicine of the Federal University of Head of the
    Anorectal Physiology Unit
Clinic Hospital
Ceara, Brazil

Abdel Rahman A. Omer, MBBS, MS, PhD, FRCS (Eng), FICS, MASCRS, FISUCRS, FRCS (Gen)
Lead Consultant Colorectal, Laparoscopic and General
    Surgery
Colorectal Surgical Unit
The Ipswich Hospital NHS Trust
Ipswich, United Kingdom

Pablo E. Piccinini, MD, MAAC, MSACP
Staff Colorectal Surgeon
Professor in Surgery
Department of Surgery
Hospital Universitario CEMIC
Buenos Aires, Argentina

Rodrigo A. Pinto, MD
Surgical Associate
Division of Colorectal Surgery
Department of Gastroenterology
University of Sao Paulo, School of Medicine
Sao Paulo, Brazil

Fabio M. Potenti, MD, FACS, FASCRS
Affiliate Associate Professor of Clinical Biomedical Sciences
Charles Schmidt College of Medicine
Florida Atlantic University
Affiliate Associate Professor
Herbert Werthein College of Medicine
Florida International University

F. Sergio P. Regadas, MD, PhD
Titular Professor of Digestive Surgery
School of Medicine of the Federal University of Ceara
Vice President of the Brazilian Society of Coloproctology
Ceara, Brazil

Bruce W. Robb, MD
Assistant Professor
Department of Surgery
Indiana University School of Medicine
Indianapolis, Indiana

Guillermo Rosato, MD, MAAC, MSACP, FASCRS
Staff Colorectal Surgeon
Professor in Surgery
Department of Surgery
Hospital Universitario Austral
Buenos Aires, Argentina

David A. Rothenberger, M.D.
Deputy Chairman and Professor
Department of Surgery
University of Minnesota
Minneapolis, Minnesota

Theodore J. Saclarides, MD
Professor, Department of Surgery
Rush University Medical Center
Chicago, Illinois

Dana R. Sands, MD
Cleveland Clinic Florida
Weston, Florida

Oliver Schwandner, MD
Department of Surgery and Pelvic Floor Center
Caritas Krankenhaus St. Josef
Regensburg, Germany

Ian KH Scot, MChir, MD, FRCS
Emeritus Consultant Colorectal and General Surgery
Colorectal Surgical Unit
The Ipswich Hospital NHS Trust
Ipswich, United Kingdom

Anthony J. Senagore, MD, MS, MBA
Chief, Division of Colorectal Surgery
Skirball Chair of Colorectal Diseases
Keck School of Medicine at the University of Southern
    California
Los Angeles, California

Matthew J. Sherman, MD, MS, FACS, FASCRS
Colon & Rectal Surgeon
Kaiser Permanente Orange County
Assistant Professor of Surgery
University of California
Irvine, California

Marc A. Singer, MD
Clinical Assistant Professor
Section of Colon and Rectal Surgery
North Shore University Health System
Evanston, Illinois

Clifford Simmang, MD
Surgeon
University of Texas Colon and Rectal Surgeons
Dallas, TX

Michael Solomon, MBBCh, BAO, MSc, FRACS
Colorectal Surgeon
Head, Surgical Outcome Research Centre
The Royal Prince Alfred Hospital
Clinical Professor
Discipline of Surgery
The University of Sydney
Sydney, Australia

Paul R. Sturrock, MD
Assistant Professor of Surgery
Department of Surgery
Division of Colon and Rectal Surgery
University of Massachusetts Medical School
Worcester, Massachusetts

T. Weidinger, MD
Department of Surgery
University of Erlangen
Erlangen, Germany

Steven D. Wexner, MD, FACS, FRCS, FRCS(Ed)
Chairman, Department of Colorectal Surgery
Chief Academic Officer
Emeritus Chief of Staff
Cleveland Clinic Florida
Weston, Florida
Professor and Associate Dean for Academic Affairs
Florida Atlantic University
Boca Raton, Florida
Professor and Assistant Dean for Clinical Education
Florida International University College of Medicine
Miami, Florida
Professor of Surgery
Ohio State University
Columbus, Ohio
Affiliate Professor
Department of Surgery, Division of General Surgery
University of South Florida College of Medicine
Tampa, Florida
Affiliate Professor of Surgery
University of Miami, Miller School of Medicine
Miami, Florida

Caroline Wright, MBBS, MS, FRACS
Colorectal Surgeon
The Royal Prince Alfred Hospital
Senior Lecturer
Discipline of Surgery
The University of Sydney
Sydney, Australia

Andrew P. Zbar, MD (Lond), FRCS (Ed), FRACS
Conjoint Professor of Surgery
Universities of New England and Newcastle
New South Wales, Australia

Oded Zmora, MD
Colon and Rectal Surgery
Department of Surgery and Transplantation
Sheba Medical Center
Tel Hashomer, Israel
Sakler School of Medicine
Tel Aviv University
Tel Aviv, Israel

We live in a high technology world where the "miracles" of modern surgery make headline news around the globe. It is no longer surprising to hear of yet another start-up medical technology company that promises a new surgical device that will save countless lives, improve outcomes, and significantly decrease pain and suffering. People find themselves mesmerized by watching "key hole surgery" broadcast in high definition to their home television and find it surprisingly elegant and bloodless compared to their prior mental picture of surgeons at work. So it is perhaps understandable that many patients today go online to find surgeons and institutions offering the newest approaches and latest technology. It seems as though the modern surgeon armed with high tech devices and digitalized equipment should be invincible. Indeed, it is easy for surgeons to be inappropriately swept up by the siren song of technical innovation.

In this kind of world, one might question the utility of yet another surgical textbook, especially one devoted to operative technique. Fortunately, editors Steven Wexner and James Fleshman have created a unique publication that is a far cry from the traditional textbook of the past. The list of contributing authors includes seasoned master surgeons schooled in traditional techniques and highly innovative researchers and entrepreneurs who are exploring new frontiers of surgical technology. Over the course of their busy clinical careers, the editors themselves have successfully bridged both perspectives. Their unique experiences are apparent in this new, tightly edited and highly practical textbook that emphasizes tried and true open techniques and new, less invasive techniques.

Drs. Wexner and Fleshman understand that surgical outcomes are dependent on many factors including clinical acumen and mature judgment to guide individualized decision-making. But they also know that surgeons must master basic operative skills and develop a full reservoir of different techniques that can be used to fit the demands of the case at hand. As importantly, they know that no matter how revolutionary or exciting, technology has its limits. Innovation is providing new tools but it is the surgeon's skill in deciding what tools to use and the way in which they are used that determines the surgical outcome. Operative technique remains critical to minimize patient morbidity, cure cancer and other life-threatening conditions, and preserve function and quality of life. All colon and rectal surgeons will find this book to be a valuable adjunct to their practice. The artist's color drawings are superb and anatomically correct. The text is easy to read, very focused, and useful for busy surgeons. I congratulate the editors for bringing this book to us.

David A. Rothenberger, MD
August 1, 2011

The Mastery of Colorectal Surgery textbook is a two volume compendium that demonstrates virtually all of the currently employed techniques for abdominal and anorectal surgery. All of the chapters have been written by internationally acclaimed experts, each of whom was given literary license to allow the book to be more creative and less rigorously formatted. Although some techniques are self-explanatory and the authors therefore concentrated their verbiage upon results and controversies surrounding a particular technique, other procedures are described in a more algorithmic manner. Specifically, some techniques require a much more heavily weighted description of preoperative and/or postoperative parameters rather than intraoperative variables. The matching of illustrations and videos has also been tailored to suit the needs of each chapter. Because of the quantity of material, the book is divided into two volumes: one that includes the abdominal and one that includes anorectal procedures. While many textbooks vie for the attention of surgeons in training and surgeons in practice, the Mastery series, edited by Dr. Josef Fischer, has established itself as the resource for expert management of each theme. Therefore, this book was deliberately crafted to augment rather than to replace several other excellent recently published textbooks. It is our hope that these volumes be used in that context so that the reader can learn the fundamentals and basics using many other excellent source materials and then rely upon the Mastery of Colorectal Surgery books for more clarity in terms of review of very specific procedures. In that same manner, these books perform a ready preoperative resource before embarking upon individual procedures.

We wish to thank Josef Fischer with having entrusted us with this latest of his literary offspring. The project took a considerable amount of time and effort and we certainly thank him for his patience. In addition, we thank our respective staff in Weston and in Saint Louis, especially Liz Nordike, Heather Dean, Dr. Fabio Potenti, and Debbie Holton for their extensive efforts as well as Nicole Dernoski at Wolters Kluwer. We wish to express our sincerest and deepest gratitude to each and every contributor for their time, attention, expertise, and commitment to the project. Without our individual chapter authors, this work would not exist. We know that each of them has many significant competing obligations for their limited time and thank them for having participated to such an important degree in this project. Last, our appreciation goes to our families for their love and support as it is always time away from them that allows us to produce these type of books. In particular, appreciation goes to Linda Fleshman and to Wesley and Trevor Wexner.

PART I: HEMORRHOIDECTOMY

PART II: ANAL FISTULA

PART III: RECTOVAGINAL FISTULA

1 Ferguson

Anthony J. Senagore

 ## INDICATIONS/CONTRAINDICATIONS

The most frequent symptoms leading to surgical intervention for hemorrhoidal suffers are bleeding, protrusion, and anorectal discomfort and pain.

1. Bleeding typically bright red blood on the toilet paper or dripping into commode.
2. Occasionally massive bleeding with very large internal hemorrhoids.
3. Hemorrhoidal prolapse usually with bowel movements that may spontaneously reduce, require manual reduction, or be irreducible depending on stage.
4. Severe, constant pain is usually related to acute thromboses of internal or external hemorrhoids and associated with a palpable perianal mass.

Examination of the patient with hematochezia requires inspection of the perianal area including anoscopy and either rigid proctoscopy or flexible sigmoidoscopy. Colonoscopy can be undertaken based on patient's history, age, or suspicious symptomatology. The author prefers examination in the modified Sims' position (left lateral decubitus with knees drawn toward the chest and the lower legs extended). This position approach allows relative patient comfort, while allowing the clinician to perform all components of the anorectal examination.

1. A careful digital examination of the anal canal and distal rectum and prostate
2. Anoscopy to clearly inspect the hemorrhoidal tissue and anal canal with assessment of size, degree of prolapse, and any fragility or bleeding
3. Proctoscopy or flexible sigmoidoscopy to exclude neoplasia or inflammation
4. Assessment of the three standard columns (right anterior, right posterior, and left lateral)

 ## PREOPERATIVE PLANNING

The decision to proceed to excisional hemorrhoidectomy requires a mutual decision by the physician and patient that medical and nonexcisional options have either failed or are inappropriate. Surgery is typically employed when the primary symptom is significant, intractable hemorrhoidal prolapse, or alternatively large external skin tags that impair anal hygiene. Preoperative preparation is generally minimal as the patient population is generally healthy and the procedure is typically ambulatory. If the patient is on therapeutic anticoagulation, this should be managed in conjunction with the managing physician to control the risk of hemorrhage postoperatively

1. The procedures are usually performed in the operating theater following preoperative sodium phosphate enemas to clear the distal rectum of stool.
2. The modified Sims' position is the preferred position by the author for all excisional procedures except for procedure for prolapsing hemorrhoid (PPH) that is optimally performed in lithotomy position.
3. Anesthetic selection is usually left to the anesthesiologist and patient; however, local anesthesia supplemented by the administration of intravenous narcotics and propofol is highly effective and short acting.
4. Avoid spinal anesthesia due to risk of urinary retention.
5. Restrict intraoperative fluids.
6. Administer preemptive analgesia with nonsteroidal anti-inflammatory drugs (NSAIDs) in operating room.

SELECTION OF EXCISIONAL TOOL

Surgery

Options for excisional hemorrhoidectomy include the following techniques:

Milligan-Morgan hemorrhoidectomy
1. This technique resects the entire enlarged internal hemorrhoid complex; in conjunction with ligation of the arterial pedicle correctly performed the intervening anoderm is preserved, while the distal anoderm and external skin are left open to heal by secondary intention.

Ferguson closed hemorrhoidectomy
2. Proposed as an alternative to the Milligan-Morgan technique with similar experience and efficacy. The technique employs an hourglass-shaped excision of the entire internal/external hemorrhoidal complex centered at the midportion of the anoderm with preservation of the intervening anoderm. Unlike the Milligan-Morgan, the rectal mucosa, anoderm, and perianal skin are closed primarily with an absorbable suture.

Whitehead hemorrhoidectomy
3. This technique employs a circumferential excision of the enlarged hemorrhoids with relocation of the prolapsed dentate line to its normal anatomic location in the anal canal. The procedure is effective but given the complexity and the high risk of mucosal ectropion and anal stricture it has largely been abandoned.

Procedure for prolapsing hemorrhoids
4. The technique involves transanal placement of a circular purse-string suture placed 1–2 cm rostral to the hemorrhoidal pedicle. A specially designed anoscope is used to reduce the hemorrhoids and protect the anoderm during the procedure. A 31-mm stapler is placed transanally to perform a circumferential excision of rectal mucosa just rostral to the hemorrhoidal columns. The purse-string suture is tied securely around the rod of the stapler and then threaded back through the barrel of the device to draw the rectal mucosa into the barrel and allow for repositioning of both the anoderm and hemorrhoidal columns prior to closing and firing the device.

Transanal hemorrhoidal dearterialization
5. This is a technique that involves Doppler-guided hemorrhoidal artery ligation, or transanal hemorrhoidal dearterialization (THD). While not truly an excisional technique, the guided reduction in arterial blood flow coupled with a suture fixation of the mucosa to correct the mucosal prolapse. A specifically designed proctoscope

with an attached Doppler transducer is inserted to allow identification of the feeding hemorrhoidal artery and via a small window the rectal mucosa 2–3 cm above the dentate line is transfixed so that the signal is ablated. A suture mucosopexy is almost always required to lift, pexy, and ultimately ablate the hemorrhoidal complex. The combination of dearterialization, replacement of the hemorrhoidal tissue, and tissue destruction work in concert to correct the hemorrhoidal symptoms.

Instrumentation for Excisional Hemorrhoidectomy

The classic instrument of performance of an excisional hemorrhoidectomy has been a scalpel or scissors. This approach is highly effective and of low cost compared to other devices. A variety of energy devices have been used with varying claims of superior speed, reduced bleeding, and less pain. The data remain highly debated and the authors' preference is to use. These instruments:

1. Nd-Yag laser—Although capable of excising hemorrhoidal tissue, the device was found to be slower, more costly, and actually delayed healing of the wound leading to increased pain.
2. Monopolar electrocautery—The device is an effective excisional tool capable of improved hemostasis compared to scalpel. It can allow transection of the hemorrhoidal pedicle without suture ligation, at the expense of greater tissue trauma because of lateral thermal spread.
3. LigaSure—A bipolar cautery device capable of simultaneous tissue division and blood vessel coagulation. It has been compared to other excisional tools and has been associated with faster operative times and allows for a sutureless technique.
4. Harmonic Scalpel—The device employs a rapidly reciprocating blade to generate heat for coagulation and tissue transection. The device is relatively expensive and has not demonstrated significant clinical advantages to offset that cost, primarily because of the associated thermal tissue injury.

 # POSTOPERATIVE MANAGEMENT

Pain remains the most challenging component of postoperative care following excisional hemorrhoidectomy, especially from the patient's perspective. The optimal analgesic regimen should begin with the accurate infiltration of bupivacaine into the wounds and perianal skin although its use has been variably successful in long-term pain reduction. NSAID, especially ketorolac, has been very efficacious in managing post-hemorrhoidectomy pain. The patient can then be transitioned to a less expensive oral NSAID for ambulatory analgesia in combination with oral narcotic supplements. The administration of narcotics either by patch or subcutaneous pump has been advocated for post-hemorrhoidectomy pain; however, these delivery systems are risky in the ambulatory setting respiratory depression.

Urinary retention is another frequent post-hemorrhoidectomy (1–52%) complication. Agents such as parasympathomimetics or α-adrenergic blocking agents may be beneficial. However, the use of sitz baths for comfort and the limitations of perioperative fluid administration to 250 ml may be a more effective approach.

Early postoperative bleeding (<24 hours) occurs rarely and almost always is associated with failure of primary surgical hemostasis and therefore is best managed by resuturing the bleeding site. Delayed hemorrhage following excisional hemorrhoidectomy occurs at 5–10 days postoperatively and in less than 5% of cases. The cause of late bleeding is usually the result of early separation of the thrombus in the ligated pedicle. The bleeding can be massive and almost always requires resuturing. Bladder catheter tamponade or anal packing may be temporizing.

The circular-stapled hemorrhoidopexy has been associated with a risk of perirectal sepsis because of the rectal perforation. This complication is clearly related to surgical technique and should be avoided with accurate suture placement and stapler application.

✳ CONCLUSIONS

Excisional hemorrhoidectomy provides a highly effective and safe therapy for advanced hemorrhoidal disease that cannot be treated by office procedures. The various methods described above represent variants on a theme, which includes resection of redundant distal rectal mucosa coupled with resuspension of the prolapsing rectal mucosa and anoderm. The long-term complications are rare in skilled hands and the patient's satisfaction is generally high with respect to symptom relief.

Suggested Readings

Armstrong DN, Frankum C, Schertzer ME, Ambroze WL, Orangio GR. Harmonic scalpel hemorrhoidectomy: five hundred consecutive cases. *Dis Colon Rectum* 2002;45(3):354–9.

Boccasanta P, Venturi M, Orio A, et al. Circular hemorrhoidectomy in advanced hemorrhoidal disease. *Hepatogastroenterology* 1998;45(22):969–72.

Chester JF, Stanford J, Gazet JC. Analgesic benefit of locally injected Bupivacaine after hemorrhoidectomy. *Dis Colon Rectum* 1990; 33:487–9.

Chung YC, Wu HJ. Clinical experience of sutureless closed hemorrhoidectomy with LigaSure. *Dis Colon Rectum* 2003;46(1):87–92.

Franklin EJ, Seetharam S, Lowney J, Horgan PG. Randomized, clinical trial of Ligasure vs conventional diathermy in hemorrhoidectomy. *Dis Colon Rectum* 2003;46(10):1380–3.

Ganchrow MJ, Mazier WP, Friend WG, Ferguson JA. Hemorrhoidectomy revisited: a computer analysis of 2,038 cases. *Dis Colon Rectum* 1971;14:128–33.

Giordano P, Overton J, Madeddu F, Zaman S, Gravante G. Transanal hemorrhoidal dearterialization: a systematic review. *Dis Colon Rectum* 2009;52(9):1665–71.

Hoff SD, Bailey HR, Butts DR, et al. Ambulatory Surgical Hemorrhoidectomy—A Solution to Postoperative Urinary Retention? *Dis Colon Rectum* 1994;37:1242–4.

Hussein MK, Taha AM, Haddad FF, Bassim YR. Bupivacaine Local Injection in Anorectal Surgery. *Int Surg* 1998;83:56–7.

Khubchandani M. Results of Whitehead operation. *Dis Colon Rectum* 1984;27:730–2.

Molloy RG, Kingsmore D. Life threatening pelvic sepsis after stapled hemorrhoidectomy. *Lancet* 2000;355:810.

Muldoon JP. The completely closed hemorrhoidectomy: a reliable and trusted friend for 25 years. *Dis Colon Rectum* 1981;24(3): 211–14.

Petros JG, Bradley TM. Factors influencing postoperative urinary retention in patients undergoing surgery for benign anorectal disease. *Am J Surg* 1990;159:374–6.

Quah HM, Seow-Choen F. Prospective, randomized trial comparing diathermy excision and diathermy coagulation for symptomatic, prolapsed hemorrhoids. *Dis Colon Rectum* 2004;47(3): 367–70.

Senagore A, Mazier WP, Luchtefeld MA, MacKeigan JM, Wengert T. Treatment of advanced hemorrhoidal disease: a prospective, randomized comparison of cold scalpel vs. contact Nd:YAG laser. *Dis Colon Rectum* 1993;36(11):1042–9.

Senagore AJ, Singer MS, Abcarian H, et al. A prospective, randomized, controlled multicenter trial comparing stapled hemorrhoidopexy and Ferguson hemorrhoidectomy: Perioperative and one-year results. *Dis Colon Rectum* 2004; 47:1824–36.

Tajana A. Hemorrhoidectomy according to Milligan-Morgan: ligature and excision technique. *Int Surg* 1989;74:158–61.

Wolff BG, Culp CE. The Whitehead hemorrhoidectomy. *Dis Colon Rectum* 1988;31(8):587–90.

2 LigaSure™

Giovanni Milito and Federica Cadeddu

Hemorrhoidectomy is the most effective and definitive treatment for grade 3 or 4 hemorrhoids. A variety of instruments, including the LigaSure vessel sealing system™, have been used in an attempt to reduce postoperative pain and blood loss and to allow fast wound healing and a quick return to work.

INDICATIONS/CONTRAINDICATIONS

Prior to selecting LigaSure™ hemorrhoidectomy, the following factors have to be considered:

Grade of Hemorrhoids

Traditional excisional hemorrhoidectomy is indicated for third or fourth degree hemorrhoids. In a recent study of the Association of Coloproctology of Great Britain and Ireland (ACPGBI) and the Association of Surgeons of Great Britain and Ireland (ASGBI), among 889 surgeons interviewed by a questionnaire on hemorrhoidectomy techniques and indications, the commonest indication was persistent grade III and grade IV hemorrhoids after failure of conservative management. There was no consensus regarding emergency hemorrhoidectomy for thrombosed or strangulated hemorrhoids—undertaken routinely by 20% of ACPGBI and 18% of ASGBI respondents. The majority (59% ACPGBI and 46% ASGBI) of the respondents occasionally performed emergency hemorrhoidectomy (1).

Type of Patient

In rare cases of large hemorrhoids in young patients, especially in female patients after pregnancy, the hemorrhoids may recur. For this reason, hemorrhoidectomy should not be performed on pregnant women and should be postponed until the age of 30–35 years.

Preexisting Medical Conditions

Inflammatory bowel diseases such as Crohn's disease and immune deficiency due to AIDS are both contraindications to this procedure. Moreover, cancer is also a contraindication to this procedure, as live cancer cells can be implanted in open wounds.

PREOPERATIVE PLANNING

Prior to hospital admission, the patient should be advised to take the appropriate steps to ensure healthy bowel habits and the passage of soft stool. Usually, a phosphate enema is performed 12 hours before surgery and 500 mg of metronidazole is given intravenously at the beginning of surgery. In the ACPGBI/ASGBI trial (1), preoperative bowel preparation was often used, with enema being used in 61% of ACPGBI group cases and 43% of ASGBI group and suppository being used in 13% ACPGBI group cases and 16% of ASGBI group. A significant number of surgeons prefer no bowel preparation (19% ACPGBI and 21% ASGBI).

SURGERY

According to the operative protocol of most centers, patients are operated under general anesthesia as a day-case procedure or short-term surgery.

Day-case hemorrhoidectomy (DCH) has become increasingly popular, possibly stimulated by bed reductions and spending constraints. In the ACPGBI/ASGBI trial, significantly more ACPGBI (20%) than ASGBI (48, 7%; $P < 0.01$) members performed DCH in 50% or more cases (1).

Vessel Sealing Technology

The term "radiosurgery" has been used to indicate utilization of high frequencies, allowing a considerable improvement of several surgical techniques, including proctologic ones.

The LigaSure vessel sealing system ™ is a bipolar electrothermal device that seals blood vessels through an optimized combination of pressure and radiofrequency.

After providing pressure on the tissues by the LigaSure™ forceps application, the Force Triad energy platform™ generates energy tailored to the tissue impedance, reducing fusion cycle time and tissue desiccation with consistently controlled tissue effect. The completion of coagulation is signalled by the feedback sensors and the tissue can be excised along the line of coagulum.

LigaSure™ is different from conventional bipolar systems by using low voltage and high current and works at lower temperatures (50–80°C) than the electric scalpel (600°C).

LigaSure™ preserves the patient's own collagen and uses it to form a permanent autologous seal that is strong enough to withstand up to three times the normal systolic (normal systolic: 120 mm/hg) on vessels or tissue bundles. This result makes LigaSure™ comparable to the mechanical methods of vessel occlusion; it ensures complete coagulation of arteries and veins up to 7 mm in diameter with minimal surrounding thermal spread up to 2 mm in diameter and limited tissue charring. Thus, a decrease in thermal injury at the surgical site may reduce anal spasm and pain. In addition, healing time is considerably shorter than that in the traditional techniques (14.8 days with LigaSure™ vs. 25.6 days with conventional diathermy in our experience (2)) and tissue damage is limited to the dissection line. The risk of cicatrization-linked stricture may also be reduced.

The area of thermal spread after monopolar electrocoagulation depends on many factors: time of application, power of electrocoagulation, and number of applications. Thermal injury after monopolar electrocoagulation, LigaSure™, bipolar electrocoagulation, and ultracision has been evaluated in many experimental studies (3). Monopolar electrocoagulation results in poorer hemostasis and more side-thermal injury of the adjacent tissue.

Operative Position

Open hemorrhoidectomy can be performed either in the lithotomy or prone position. In the lithotomy position, the buttocks are raised by a firm pad to project over the

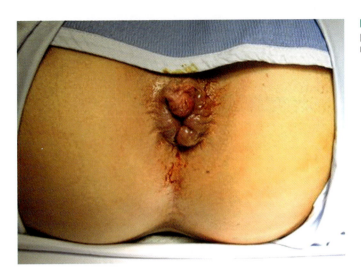

Figure 2.1 A patient in lithotomy position with IV degree hemorrhoids.

edge of the table. In the prone position, the patient lies face down, hips on a 6-inch gel ridge, with the buttocks projecting upward. Although the prone position may help reduce venous circulation from the anorectal area, extra care should be taken to prevent restriction of breathing and ensure proper lung inflation during surgery. In both the positions, the buttocks are strapped back with an adhesive tape to facilitate access, especially for obese patients. Most surgeons perform LigaSure™ hemorrhoidectomy using an Eisenhammer retractor with the patient in the lithotomy position (Fig. 2.1).

Operative Technique

Hemorrhoid Exposure

The main hemorrhoidal masses are identified and delineated, usually in the "classical" locations corresponding to the sites of inferior hemorrhoidal vessels—left lateral right posterolateral, right anterior quadrants. The hemorrhoids are prolapsed out from the anal canal with an Allis clamp or forceps. Tension should be applied in order to visualize the mucocutaneous junction.

Dissection and Hemorrhoid Removal

A small V-shaped anodermal seal is formed by applying the precise LigaSure™ forceps close to the outer edge of the internal hemorrhoid (Fig. 2.2). The seal is then transected with scissors along the line of coagulum. Care should be taken in order to limit the

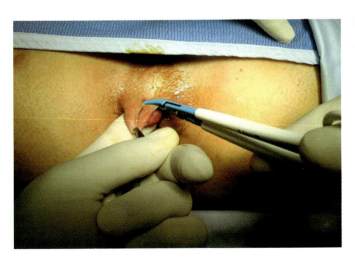

Figure 2.2 LigaSure™ hemorrhoidectomy is performed by applying the precise LigaSure™ forceps close to the edge of each pile. Completion of coagulation is signalled by the feedback sensors.

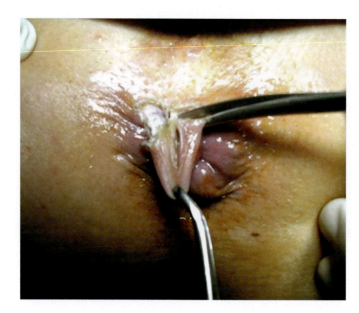

Figure 2.3 The tissue is excised along the line of coagulum.

amount of tissue removed to minimize the risk of stricture (Fig. 2.3). Repeated applications of the device are performed and the excision is continued into the anal canal, lifting the pile from the internal anal sphincter (Fig. 2.4). The vascular pedicle is finally sealed by LigaSure™ and divided (Fig. 2.5).

Final Control

The area is inspected with the Eisenhammer retractor to ensure hemostasis. The operation is terminated by placing a hemostatic absorbable gelatin sponge in the anal canal (Fig. 2.6). At the end of the operation, a single layer of nonadhesive gauze is used to dress the wounds. Finally, a large surgical dressing is applied to the buttocks and held in place with a bandage.

Treatment of Vascular Pedicles

In the LigaSure™ hemorrhoidectomy, pedicles are not transfixed, but sealed by LigaSure™ to avoid incorporation of the underlying sphincter in the ligatures.

Cheetham et al. recently randomized 31 patients to diathermy hemorrhoidectomy performed without pedicle legation or to stapled hemorrhoidectomy (4). Two cases of

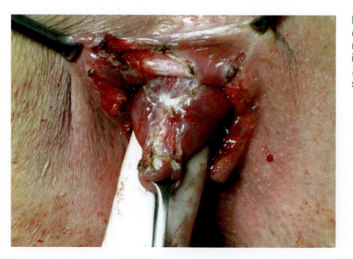

Figure 2.4 Repeated applications of the LigaSure precise are carried out to lift the pile from the internal anal sphincter (*black narrow*), taking care to avoid sphincter injuries.

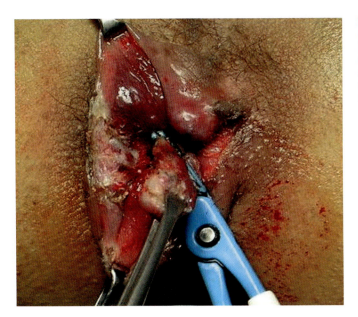

Figure 2.5 The vascular pedicle of the hemorrhoid is sealed by LigaSure precise and finally divided. The LigaSure vessel sealing system™ completes coagulation of arteries and veins up to 7 mm.

postoperative bleeding were observed, both in the stapled group. Mehigan et al. recently randomized 40 patients to diathermy or stapled procedure (5). In the diathermy group, the vascular pedicle was divided by diathermy without sutures. One case of postoperative bleeding was detected in the diathermy group and treated conservatively.

Vascular pedicle ligation might be a contributing factor to the development of ischemia and necrosis in the area where the sutures transfixing the vascular pedicles incorporate the sphincter muscle. The depth of these sutures, the bulk of incorporated muscle, and the subsequent necrosis might be the cause of acute postoperative pain, pedicle infection, and secondary bleeding. Pedicle ligation may also play a role in chronic ulceration in the late convalescence phase.

The preservation of intact anoderm and strips of mucosa between the excised, denuded areas is of paramount importance to prevent anal stenosis. These denuded strips, if too wide and deep, could play a role in the development of a rigid circular scarring at the anal verge. This scar tends to contract with time, and may lead

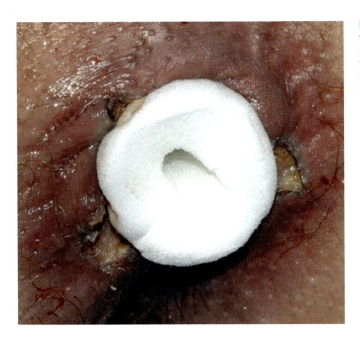

Figure 2.6 Final view. Excision of the three hemorrhoidal piles has been performed. The operation is terminated by placing a hemostatic absorbable gelatin sponge in the anal canal.

to severe stricture formation. Preservation of adequate anoderm between hemorrhoid excision lines also preserves the anal canal elasticity. Circumferential mucosal ischemia because of the excessive depth of vascular transfixation sutures at the apex of very large hemorrhoids and narrow mucosal bridges between the sutures often result in a circular mucosal scar. This complication should be promptly recognized by a simple digital examination 1 month after the operation. At this stage, a weekly digital dilatation throughout the healing process (approximately 3 months after the operation) usually results in an elastic anal canal with minimal functional disability.

 # POSTOPERATIVE MANAGEMENT

Postoperatively, patients receive lactulose (20 ml for day for 2 weeks), analgesics (ketorolac 10 mg on demand, never more than three times daily), topical 0.2% glyceryl trinitrate ointment three times a day after the first 24 hours, and metronidazole (500 mg three times daily for 1 week). The wound dressings are only inspected for bleeding during the first 24 hours. The dressings are then removed and the anal wounds are cleaned. The patient is encouraged to bathe to keep all wounds clean.

 # COMPLICATIONS

Early postoperative bleeding (within 48 hours) occurs in 1–2% of cases and is mainly secondary to inadequate hemostasis. Late postoperative hemorrhage occurs in 2.4% of cases, usually between 7–14 days after the operation and is mainly caused by pedicle infection, ischemia, and necrosis.

Several factors may contribute to the development of postoperative anal pain: sphincter fibers entrapped in the pedicle sutures, excessive excision of anal skin, wound infection, tissue charring with coagulation, edema of surrounding tissues, and retention of endoanal foreign material.

Late postoperative complications include anal stenosis and continence impairment.

An area of concern with anorectal surgery is the potential for anal sphincter injury causing fecal continence. In their study, Muzi et al. (2) found no cases of sphincter damage. Neither incontinence of flatus nor soiling was reported during the period of the study. One patient in each group (0.8%) developed late anal stenosis and was successfully treated using anal dilatators.

Jayne and coworkers also reported no case of sphincter injury, assessed by fecal incontinence score at 12-week follow-up (6). The same authors reported a better internal sphincter thickness and rectal urge sensation in the LigaSure™ group at 37 months.

Intraoperative sphincter stretching, which is minimized by using the LigaSure™ system, may play a role in impairment of fecal continence post hemorrhoidectomy.

It has been suggested that cauterizing with LigaSure™ could contribute to anal stenosis from thermal or electric injury. In a recent report, Gravante and Venditti described four cases of postoperative anal stenosis out of 203 patients who underwent the LigaSure™ procedure (2%) (7). The stricture was diagnosed at 2-month follow-up and successfully treated with anal dilatators. Additionally, Wang and colleagues reported one case of anal stenosis out of 42 patients treated with LigaSure™ (8). Ramcharan and Hunt suggested that the perianal skin should be retracted away from the bipolar blades to avoid any contact during diathermy of the hemorrhoid (9).

The results of the trials conducted by Sayfan et al. (10) and Palazzo et al. (11) described only one case (0.8%) of late anal stenosis in patients undergoing LigaSure™ hemorrhoidectomy. Late anal stenosis has been reported in 4–5% of patients after conventional hemorrhoidectomy.

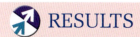 RESULTS

Postoperative Bleeding and Anal Pain

Muzi et al. prospectively compared the clinical outcomes of 250 patients with either grade 3 or grade 4 hemorrhoids randomized between LigaSure™ and conventional diathermy hemorrhoidectomy (2).

In their study, although not statistically significant, there was a difference between the two groups with respect to postoperative bleeding: postoperative hemorrhage in 3/125 in the LigaSure™ group and 7/125 in the diathermy group.

LigaSure™ hemorrhoidectomy has been shown to produce significantly less pain than conventional hemorrhoidectomy ($P = 0.01$) (2). Franklin and coworkers randomized 34 patients between LigaSure™ and diathermy hemorrhoidectomy and reported a reduction of postoperative pain in the LigaSure™ group, not only on day 1 and 14 after the operation, but also after the first evacuation (12).

Jayne and coworkers in a randomized trial of 40 patients showed that the LigaSure system™ reduces intraoperative blood loss (median value 0 ml in the LigaSure™ arm vs. 20 ml in the diathermy group), postoperative bleeding (no case of bleeding in the LigaSure™ group vs. two cases of postoperative continuous bleeding in the diathermy group), and facilitates same-day discharge (6).

In a randomized clinical trial of 34 patients, Palazzo et al. showed that LigaSure™ reduces blood loss and postoperative analgesic requirements compared to diathermy (11). However, there was no statistically significant difference between the two groups regarding postoperative pain scores.

Also Chung and Wu, in a larger series of patients (61 patients randomized to LigaSure™ ($N = 30$) or to the Ferguson procedure ($N = 31$)), demonstrated a significant reduction in postoperative pain on days 1 and 2 (13). The measurement of blood loss was not included in the study design, but the surgeons observed a reduction of postoperative bleeding using LigaSure™. Postoperative bleeding occurred in three patients in both groups.

Harmonic Scalpel™ hemorrhoidectomy has the same advantage as the LigaSure™ system of producing less thermal injury and less postoperative pain. However, it requires a longer operating time. Armstrong et al (14) and Khan et al. (8) reported operating time using Harmonic Scalpel to be even longer than conventional diathermy owing to the time-consuming hemostasis. In a recent randomized trial of LigaSure™ hemorrhoidectomy (24 patients) versus Harmonic Scalpel hemorrhoidectomy (25 patients), Kwok and colleagues showed that the LigaSure™ procedure is faster (median operating time values 11 vs. 18 minutes) and more effective in hemostatic control (15).

Wound Healing and Convalescence Period

Chung and Wu found no statistically significant difference between LigaSure™ ($N = 30$) and the Ferguson procedure ($N = 31$) in patients' return to work (13). However, Muzi et al. observed significantly faster wound healing and a faster return to normal daily activities in the LigaSure™ group in comparison to the diathermy group (2). Complete wound healing was achieved, in the LigaSure™ group, at an average of 14.8 days (10–21), and in the diathermy group, at an average of 25.6 days (14–40) ($P = 0.01$). Finally, the mean return to work was after 12 days (5–21) for LigaSure™ and 16 days (10–30) for diathermy hemorrhoidectomy, ($P = 0.01$).

Similarly, Sayfan and colleagues observed a significantly shorter convalescence period in patients treated with LigaSure™ (average convalescence period 7.4 days) as compared to diathermy procedure (mean convalescence period 18.6 days) (10) ($P < 0.001$).

Accordingly, Wang and coworkers, in a recent clinical trial on 84 patients, observed an earlier return to work after LigaSure™ than after the Ferguson procedure (8.8 vs. 13.7 days), as a consequence of the reduction of postoperative pain, analgesic requirements, and tissue injury (16).

Meta-Analyses of Randomized Controlled Trials

Several randomized trials comparing LigaSure™ and conventional hemorrhoidectomy showed that the LigaSure™ procedure is a safe and simple method to improve surgical outcomes and outlined the benefits of the LigaSure™ hemorrhoidectomy: effective hemostatic control with reduced bleeding and operative time, less tissue injury and postoperative anal pain, possibility of day-care procedure, reduction of wound healing time, and faster return to work and daily activities.

A recent meta-analysis of 11 randomized controlled trials (850 patients) comparing LigaSure™ versus conventional hemorrhoidectomy found that LigaSure™ hemorrhoidectomy had a significantly shorter duration of operation ($P < 0.001$) and reduced postoperative pain score ($P = 0.001$) (Classic fail safe $N > 35$) but no significant differences in healing rates ($P > 0.05$) (17). Another meta-analysis of nine randomized controlled trials found better outcomes in the LigaSure™ arm regarding operative time ($P < 0.001$), postoperative pain, and convalescence ($P < 0.001$) (18). A larger meta-analysis of 11 randomized controlled trials (1,046 patients) found a significant advantage in the LigaSure™ group regarding intraoperative and postoperative outcomes (postoperative pain [$P = 0.001$], wound healing time [$P = 0.004$], and convalescence [$P = 0.001$]) (19).

Finally, in the Cochrane Database System Review comparing LigaSure™ versus conventional surgery for hemorrhoid treatment, Nienhuijs meta-analyzed 12 randomized controlled trials (1,142 patients) and concluded that LigaSure™ technique resulted in significantly less immediate postoperative pain without any adverse effect on postoperative complications, convalescence, and incontinence rate. Thus, this technique was superior in terms of patient tolerance (20).

However, some limitations of the trials included in the above mentioned meta-analyses should be underlined: the limited sample size and the heterogeneity of the studies owing to the different operative protocols and outcome measures. Moreover, the limited follow-up of the studies, up to 6 months in several trials, affected the evaluation of long-term results in terms of continence impairment, anal stenosis, and relapses.

A large meta-analysis of trials based on commonly accepted operative protocols and end points with a long-term follow-up is warranted.

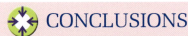 CONCLUSIONS

In summary, the benefits of the LigaSure vessel sealing system™ in performing hemorrhoidectomy include effective hemostatic control with reduced bleeding and operative time, less tissue injury and postoperative anal pain, possibility of day surgery procedure, and faster return to work and daily activities. However, one must be cognizant of the potential complications of any excisional procedure. Surgeons must assiduously avoid sphincter muscles and injury to the adjacent normal mucosa.

Recommended References and Readings

1. Beattie GC, Wilson RG, Loudon MA. The contemporary management of haemorrhoids. *Colorectal Dis* 2002;4:450–4.
2. Muzi MG, Milito G, Nigro C, et al. Randomized clinical trial of Ligasure and conventional diathermy haemorrhoidectomy. *Br J Surg* 2007;94:937–42.
3. Diamantis T, Kontos M, Arvelakis A, et al. Comparison of monopolar electrocoagulation, bipolar electrocoagulation, ultracision, and ligasure. *Surgery Today* 2006;36:908–13.
4. Cheetham MJ, Cohen CR, Kamm MA, Phillips RK. A randomized, controlled trial of diathermy hemorrhoidectomy vs. stapled hemorrhoidectomy in an intended day-care setting with longer-term follow-up. *Dis Colon Rectum* 2003;46:491–7.
5. Mehigan BJ, Monson JR, Hartley JE. Stapling procedure for haemorrhoids versus Milligan-Morgan haemorrhoidectomy; randomized controlled trial. *Lancet* 2000;355:782–5.
6. Jayne DG, Botterill I, Ambrose NS, Brennan TG, Guillou PJ, O'Riordain DS. Randomized clinical trial of Ligasure™ versus conventional diathermy for day-case haemorrhoidectomy. *Br J Surg* 2002;89:428–32.
7. Gravante G, Venditti D. Postoperative anal stenoses with Ligasure™ haemorrhoidectomy. *World J Surg* 2007;31:245.
8. Khan S, Pawlak SE, Eggenberger JC, et al. Surgical treatment of haemorrhoids: prospective, randomized trial comparing closed excisional haemorrhoidectomy and the Harmonic Scalpel technique of excisional haemorrhoidectomy. *Dis Colon Rectum* 2001;44:845–9.
9. Ramcharan KS, Hunt TM. Anal stenoses after Ligasure™ haemorrhoidectomy. *Dis Colon Rectum* 2005;48:1670–1.
10. Sayfan J, Becker A, Koltun L. Sutureless closed haemorrhoidectomy: a new technique. *Ann Surg* 2001;234:21–4.
11. Palazzo FF, Francis DL, Clifton MA. Randomized clinical trial of Ligasure™ versus open haemorrhoidectomy. *Br J Surg* 2002;89:154–7.

12. Franklin EJ, Seetharam S, Lowney J, Horgan PG. Randomised, clinical trial of Ligasure™ vs conventional diathermy in haemorrhoidectomy. *Dis Colon Rectum* 2003;46:1380–3.

13. Chung YC, Wu HJ. Clinical experience of sutureless closed haemorrhoidectomy with Ligasure™. *Dis Colon Rectum* 2003; 46:87–92.

14. Armstrong DN, Ambroze WL, Schertzer ME, Orangio GR. Harmonic Scalpel® vs. electrocautery haemorrhoidectomy: a prospective evaluation. *Dis Colon Rectum* 2001;44:558–64.

15. Kwok SY, Chung CC, Tsui KK, Li MKW. A double blind, randomized trial comparing Ligasure™ and Harmonic Scalpel haemorrhoidectomy. *Dis Colon Rectum* 2005;48:344–8.

16. Wang JY, Lu CY, Tsai HL, et al. Randomized controlled trial of Ligasure™ with submucosal dissection versus Ferguson haemorrhoidectomy for prolapsed haemorrhoids. *World J Surg* 2006; 30:462–6.

17. Milito G, Cadeddu F, Muzi MG, Nigro C, Farinon AM. Haemorrhoidectomy with Ligasure versus conventional excisional techniques: meta-analysis of randomized controlled trials. *Colorectal Dis* 2009; doi:10.1111/j.1463–1318.2009.01807.

18. Tan EK, Cornish J, Darzi AW, Papagrigoriadis S, Tekkis PP. Meta-analysis of short-term outcomes of randomized controlled trials of LigaSure vs conventional hemorrhoidectomy. *Arch Surg* 2007;142:1209–18.

19. Mastakov MY, Buettner PG, Ho YH. Updated meta-analysis of randomized controlled trials comparing conventional excisional haemorrhoidectomy with LigaSure for haemorrhoids. *Tech Coloproctol* 2008;12:229–39.

20. Nienhuijs S, de Hingh I. Conventional versus LigaSure hemorrhoidectomy for patients with symptomatic hemorrhoids. *Cochrane Database Syst Rev* 2009; 21:CD006761.

Part I: Hemorrhoidectomy

3 Harmonic Scalpel®

David N. Armstrong and Kurt G. Davis

 ## INDICATIONS/CONTRAINDICATIONS

The advantages of Harmonic Scalpel® hemorrhoidectomy over the more traditional use of electrocautery lie in the Harmonic Scalpel's® improved hemostasis, resulting in an almost "bloodless" hemorrhoidectomy (1,2). In addition, postoperative pain is reduced, as a result of the reduced lateral thermal injury, compared to electrocautery.

Harmonic scalpel® hemorrhoidectomy should be reserved for patients with large external hemorrhoids, or for large, prolapsing internal hemorrhoids, that are too large for successful rubber-band ligation.

The presence of large external hemorrhoids precludes successful rubber-band ligation, for two reasons: First, the external components may become engorged, edematous, and painful after ligation because of the redirection of blood flow; second, the external components are the most obvious source of patient's discomfort, irritation and hygiene problems, and therefore require surgical removal for patient's satisfaction alone. Excision of the internal components is an integral and important part of standard Harmonic Scalpel® hemorrhoidectomy.

The standard classification of internal hemorrhoids (Grade 1: No prolapse; Grade 2: Prolapse with spontaneous reduction; Grade 3: Prolapse with manual reduction, and Grade 4: Irreducible prolapse) is not particularly useful when choosing patients for Harmonic Scalpel® hemorrhoidectomy, since these relate only to internal hemorrhoids. For this reason, it is often difficult to determine the contribution of internal versus external components by history alone, and the decision to perform Harmonic Scalpel® hemorrhoidectomy is determined by the examination of the perianal region and anal canal.

The anatomic distribution of internal and external hemorrhoids generally conform to the classic "3, 7, and 11 o'clock" (right anterior, right posterior, and left midlateral) formula. In many cases, this may not be immediately obvious, but careful intraoperative examination with a Pratt speculum usually clarifies and confirms the standard and accepted locations. Smaller components located at intervening locations are usually extensions from the main components, or simply skin tags.

Having removed the three main components, the surgeon should avoid the temptation to excise any more tissue, since such removal may result in anal stenosis. If the patient remains concerned about the residual skin tags after the procedure, these tags can be excised under a local anesthetic in the office setting after healing has taken place. Nonetheless, such excision should only be performed on obvious protruding skin tags and only after explaining to the patient that a perfectly smooth wrinkle-free perianal region is rarely, if ever achievable.

The presence of a concomitant fissure is not a contraindication to Harmonic Scalpel® hemorrhoidectomy, as fissure debridement or internal sphincterotomy can be performed at the same time. Performing an internal sphincterotomy has never been demonstrated to reduce pain after hemorrhoidectomy, and should never be routinely performed unless in the presence of a very rigid anal stenosis.

Contraindications include any coagulopathy, use of anticoagulants, or profound immunosuppression. Apirin or other nonsteroidals are discontinued for 10 days before and 10 days after the procedure. If anticoagulants cannot be safely discontinued (e.g., mechanical heart valves), the oral anticoagulant is converted to a short-acting heparin analogue for 5 days preoperatively, and 7–10 days postoperatively. The reason for the longer postoperative hold is posthemorrhoidectomy hemorrhage that typically occurs between 5–10 days after surgery.

Patients with known anorectal Crohn's disease should generally not undergo any form of hemorrhoidectomy. If the surgery is performed, the postoperative period is characterized by severe anorectal pain, discharge, and nonhealing incisions.

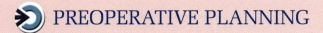 PREOPERATIVE PLANNING

Colonoscopy

If the patient requires colonoscopy for any of the standard indications, it can most conveniently be performed on the morning of the surgery. Colonoscopy can exclude any serious pathology within the colon and can confirm that any rectal bleeding is indeed from the hemorrhoids and not from a second unrecognized source.

Bowel Preparation

Although mechanical bowel preparation does not rise to "standard of care" prior to a Harmonic Scalpel® hemorrhoidectomy, it may be a sensible and safe precaution. First, the mechanical bowel preparation effectively prevents the constant oozing of stool into the surgical field during the surgery itself. Suctioning and irrigation stool out of the surgical field simply adds additional time to the procedure, and is an unpleasant inconvenience. Second, the mechanical bowel preparation postpones the patient's first bowel movement for a few days, allowing some degree of healing to occur before this sentinel event.

Consent

The patient should be thoroughly informed of the risks of Harmonic Scalpel® hemorrhoidectomy. These risks include anorectal incontinence; postoperative bleeding; persistent pain/discomfort; posthemorrhoidectomy fissure or fistula.

Lab Work

Aside from preanesthetic requirements, a complete blood count usually suffices to exclude a dangerously low hemoglobin and hematocrit from prolonged severe hemorrhoidal bleeding or a dangerously low white blood count from an unrecognized immunosuppression. Both of these conditions require correction prior to an elective Harmonic Scalpel® hemorrhoidectomy.

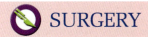

SURGERY

The Harmonic Scalpel® Instrument

The Harmonic Scalpel® consists of cutting shears that vibrate at 55,500 Hz, at amplitudes of 60–100 microns. The vibratory energy results in disruption of hydrogen bonds that cause denaturing of intracellular proteins. This mechanism results in shearing of the coapted tissue and creation of a sticky coagulum that further assists in hemostasis.

The principles of cutting tissue lie in two main modalities:

Pressure results from compression (coaptation) of the "active" blade onto a "pressure pad" on the opposite blade of the shears. The pressure pad focuses pressure and vibratory energy to optimize cutting of the coapted tissue.

The hemostatic coagulum is formed from denatures intracellular proteins. Because of these nonthermal modalities, the tissue is divided at a lower temperature than electrocautery, and lateral thermal injury is minimized.

The reduction in lateral thermal injury results in less postoperative pain after Harmonic Scalpel® hemorrhoidectomy compared to electrocautery (1). Furthermore, the hemostatic coagulum, and coapting hemostatic properties result in minimal, if any, blood loss during hemorrhoidectomy.

The Harmonic Scalpel® generator transmits energy to the hand piece at energy levels of 1–5. The lower the setting, the less the excursion of the blades and conversely, higher settings increase blade excursion.

The hand piece has two available energy settings: MIN and MAX. The MIN setting (1–4) results in more effective hemostasis, and is therefore used to divide the proximal pedicle of the internal hemorrhoid, ensuring complete hemostasis of the internal hemorrhoidal arteries. The MAX setting (defaults to level 5) results in more effective and faster cutting, and is therefore used on the tougher and less vascular external hemorrhoidal tissue.

Anesthesia

Harmonic Scalpel® hemorrhoidectomy is most conveniently performed in the prone-jackknife position, and under these circumstances, maintenance of the patient's airway is the most immediate and primary concern. Harmonic Scalpel® hemorrhoidectomy may be performed under local monitored anesthesia care (MAC) (usually propofol (3)), but requires very close coordination and cooperation between the surgeon and anesthetic team. Oversedation may easily compromise the patient's airway, especially in obese individuals.

A useful and successful compromise between local MAC anesthesia and general anesthesia with endotracheal intubation is general anesthesia using laryngeal mask anesthesia (LMA) technique (4). This technique allows the patient to be positioned awake in prone position. The LMA is inserted whilst still prone, and the table is then positioned in jackknife prior to starting the surgery (Figs. 3.1 and 3.2). After the procedure, the table is flattened, the patient rolled supine onto a stretcher, and the LMA removed from the airway. This technique avoids having to perform endotracheal intubation, avoids having to "roll" the patient from supine to prone prior to the surgery, but still maintains a safe and secure airway.

Positioning

As described above, Harmonic Scalpel® hemorrhoidectomy is most conveniently performed in the prone-jackknife position (Fig. 3.1). Exceptions to this are obese individuals. These patients are difficult to maneuver into prone position in the operating room (OR), and it is difficult to maintain a safe airway. Modified lithotomy is a safer and more convenient position under these circumstances.

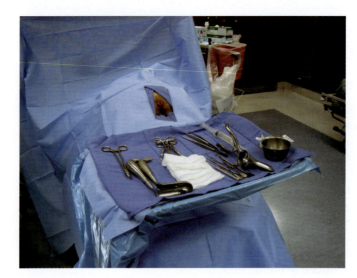

Figure 3.1 The patient is placed in prone-jackknife position for Harmonic Scalpel® hemorrhoidectomy. A Mayo table positioned at the foot of the bed serves as a convenient and accessible instrument stand.

Technique

Using a Pratt speculum, the three hemorrhoidal complexes are examined to ensure they conform to the standard right anterior, right posterior, and left lateral configuration (Fig. 3.3). The external component is grasped with a hemostat and placed on gentle traction in order to "tent-up" the apex of the external hemorrhoid (Fig. 3.4). Using the MAX setting on the Harmonic Scalpel® handpiece, the apex of the external hemorrhoid is divided using the Harmonic Scalpel® blades, and excision progresses toward the internal component (Fig. 3.5).

The Harmonic Scalpel® blades straddle the entire external hemorrhoid, and are excised "skin to skin" rather than individually excising the lateral skin margins. This method avoids inserting one of the blades into the substance of the hemorrhoid itself (which causes bleeding) and eliminates the possibility of excising too much tissue from the perianal skin. However, one must be careful not to injure or excise any of the external and sphincter muscle.

The internal component is then addressed. Again, the blades of the Harmonic Scalpel® straddle the internal component, to avoid excising too much tissue from the anal canal (Fig. 3.6). The fibers of the internal sphincter can be easily identified and preserved (Fig. 3.7). The entire internal component is excised off the underlying internal sphincter, until the nonhemorrhoidal-bearing rectal mucosa in encountered (Fig. 3.8). The apex of

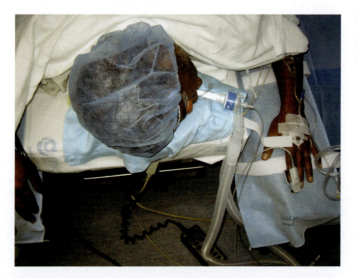

Figure 3.2 A laryngeal mask airway is easy to insert in prone position, and protects the airway during the procedure.

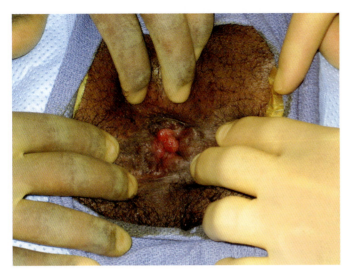

Figure 3.3 Large external hemorrhoids and prolapsing internal components are located at the classic right anterior, right posterior, and left lateral locations.

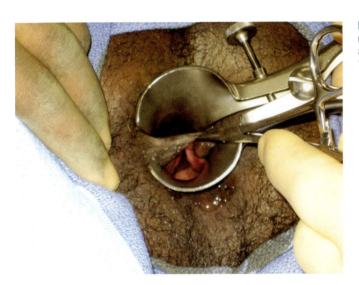

Figure 3.4 The external hemorrhoid is grasped with a hemostat and placed on gentle traction to "tent up" the external component.

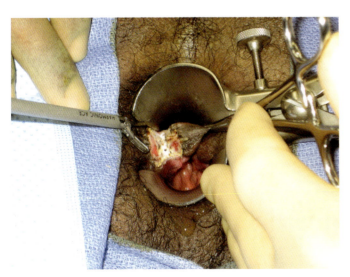

Figure 3.5 Using the MAX setting on the Harmonic Scalpel®, the external component is excised to the level of the external sphincter, which is identified and preserved.

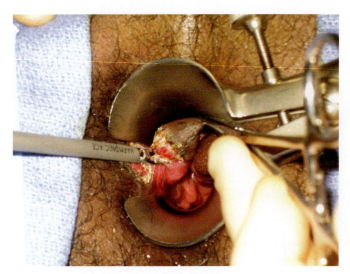

Figure 3.6 The excision is continued toward the internal component, which is excised from the underlying internal sphincter. By placing the internal sphincter on stretch using a Pratt speculum, and by "straddling" the hemorrhoid, damage to the internal sphincter is avoided.

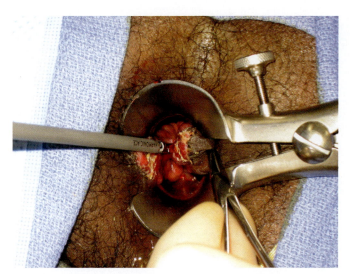

Figure 3.7 Once the normal appearing rectal mucosa is reached, the dissection angles toward the surface of the anorectal mucosa. This avoids the common pitfall of leaving residual internal hemorrhoid, which can result in persistent bleeding.

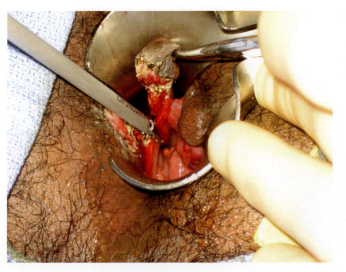

Figure 3.8 The internal hemorrhoidal artery and vein course through the apex of the internal hemorrhoid. To maintain perfect hemostasis, and to adequately coagulate the vessels, the MIN setting is used on the Harmonic Scalpel®.

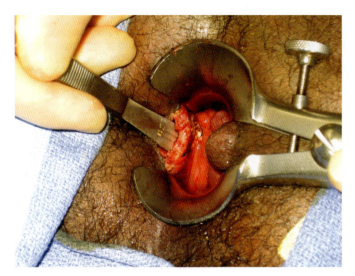

Figure 3.9 The internal sphincter can be easily identified after the internal hemorrhoid has been completely excised. At this point, the defect can be left open, or closed using a running locking 3-0 chromic suture.

the internal hemorrhoid is excised using the MIN setting on the Harmonic Scalpel® handpiece that results in a safer and more secure hemostasis of the internal hemorrhoidal vessels (Fig. 3.9). Because hemostasis is excellent after Harmonic Scalpel® hemorrhoidectomy, the defect can be left open, or closed using a running locking suture.

The defect is closed by inserting a deep figure-of-eight suture (3-0 chromic suture on a SH needle) at the apex of the defect. This is tied to secure the vessel-bearing apex or pedicle of the hemorrhoidectomy site. Using the same 3-0 chromic suture, the defect is closed in a running locking suture to the anal verge.

At the anal verge, the Pratt speculum is removed and the skin defect is placed on traction, to form a linear defect. The same 3-0 chromic suture is continued along the skin defect to the end of the incision. The same technique is repeated for all three hemorrhoids.

The use of a Pratt speculum and the "straddling" technique ensures that excess removal of skin and mucosa between the pedicles is avoided to prevent anal stenosis.

Local anesthesia (Marcaine [bupivicaine] 0.25% with epinephrine 1:100,000 μ) is injected into each surgical site (approx. 5 cc per site) to ensure adequate postoperative analgesia.

A cigarette-shaped roll of gelfoam is inserted into the anal canal and topical 10% metronidazole cream applied to the perianal area.

POSTOPERATIVE MANAGEMENT

Patients are monitored in the post anesthesia care unit (PACU) for a minimum of 1 hour, to ensure they are fully awake, comfortable, and have a stable airway. Patients are offered clear liquids after the surgery to moisten their mouths after oropharyngeal intubation, but also to ensure they can adequately protect their airways.

Care is taken to ensure that patients can adequately void after the procedure. If necessary additional intravenous or oral fluids are given to fill the bladder and facilitate maturation, an ultrasonic "Bladder Scan®" can be used to exclude incipient urinary retention (Figs. 3.10 and 3.11). If urinary retention develops, the patient may be straight-cathed, and try to void again. Alternatively, an indwelling bladder catheter may be inserted and left in place for 24 hours.

There is also data to suggest that limiting intraoperative fluid intake reduces the incidence of urinary retention.

The majority of Harmonic Scalpel® hemorrhoidectomy patients are discharged the same day. Elderly patients, patients who develop urinary retention, or those individuals with multiple comorbidities are admitted overnight for observation.

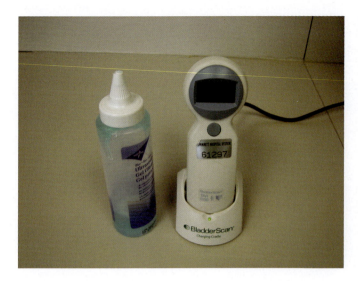

Figure 3.10 It is important to ensure the patient can void adequately before discharge. The Bladder Scan® is a useful tool to determine whether the bladder is empty (requiring more fluids) or full (requiring catheterization).

Patients are instructed to perform Sitz bath soaks 2–3 times daily, and apply topical 10% metronidazole ointment (9–11) as desired.

A psyllium fiber supplement such as Konsyl® is taken twice a day, as is 30 cc mineral oil twice daily, and copious fluids taken by mouth, all to try to prevent constipation.

A narcotic analgesic (hydrocodone 5–10 mg) is taken by mouth every 4–6 hours as needed.

Patients are instructed to call in the event they experience bleeding, fever, excessive pain, or any other worrisome symptom. Patients are reviewed in the office 2–3 weeks after surgery.

COMPLICATIONS

The most common postoperative complication is delayed healing and persistent discomfort. The focus is to ensure patients are taking adequate fiber supplements, copious fluids by mouth; adequate perineal hygiene (Sitz baths), and topical 10% metronidazole cream tid. Fissures are unusual after Harmonic Scalpel® hemorrhoidectomy, but the management is the same as idiopathic fissure in anorectal region. Surgery is reserved for persistent and severe symptoms in spite of maximum conservative therapy.

Urinary retention occurs in approximately 2% of patients after Harmonic Scalpel® hemorrhoidectomy. This problem can be avoided by limiting perioperative fluid

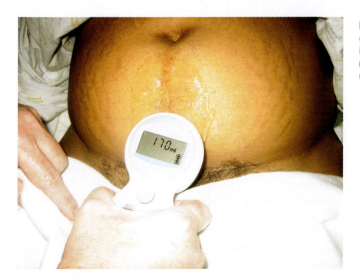

Figure 3.11 The Bladder Scan® determines the volume of urine in the bladder and simplifies management of postoperative urinary issues.

administration to no more than 1,000 cc. Use of the "bladder scan" has been discussed above (2).

Postoperative bleeding occurs in 0.6% of patients and is usually attributable to postoperative use of aspirin, or nonsteroidal anti-inflammatory agents (2). Bleeding generally occurs between 5–10 days postoperatively. Optimal treatment for severe and persistent bleeding is immediate return to the OR for oversewing of bleeding sites. Quite commonly, no active bleeding site is identified at the time of surgery and these patients should be kept under close observation for the next few days to ensure they do not rebleed. Other rarer causes of postoperative bleeding are platelet dysfunction (von Willebrand disease) and connective tissue disorder (Ehrers Danlos syndrome) (2).

Anorectal incontinence occurs in 0.2% of patients after Harmonic Scalpel® hemorrhoidectomy (2). This problem usually occurs in patients with some degree of pre-existing impairment in sphincter function. Added to these issues, excessive tissue removal or internal sphincter damage can result in overt incontinence. Lateral thermal injury is minimized after Harmonic Scalpel® hemorrhoidectomy, but in patients with borderline continence, even minimal thermal injury or thinning of the internal sphincter may lead to symptomatic incontinence. Both of these potential complications (excessive tissue removal and internal sphincter damage) can be avoided by using the "straddle" technique wherein the shears are placed around the entire hemorrhoid, rather than dividing each lateral aspect individually. This optimizes coaption of the tissue; avoids excising too much tissue, and protects the underlying internal sphincter from thermal and surgical injury.

Postoperative sepsis (abscess/fistula) (0.8%) or fissure (1.0%) is rare after Harmonic Scalpel® hemorrhoidectomy.

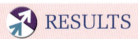 ## RESULTS

Although hemorrhoidectomy by any method is associated with significant anorectal discomfort, Harmonic Scalpel® hemorrhoidectomy results in less postoperative discomfort and faster recovery than conventional hemorrhoidectomy (1,2,6–8). Recovery is further accelerated by the use of topical 10% metronidazole applied tid to the perianal region (9–11).

If an adequate three-quadrant Harmonic Scalpel® hemorrhoidectomy is performed, the incidence of "recurrent hemorrhoids" should approach zero.

If the entire internal hemorrhoidal component is not carefully excised off the internal sphincter all the way to its apex, some residual internal component may persist. These patients may experience recurrent bleeding, but this can usually be controlled by rubber-band ligation of the residual hemorrhoid.

CONCLUSIONS

Harmonic Scalpel® hemorrhoidectomy provides an excellent means of performing an almost "bloodless" hemorrhoidectomy. The tissue can be divided at lower temperatures compared to electrocautery, and this translates into reduced postoperative pain.

Harmonic Scalpel® hemorrhoidectomy should be reserved for patients with symptomatic external hemorrhoids, or with large internal components too large for ligation. The management of anticoagulants is an important aspect of preoperative management, and avoiding these in the postoperative period reduces the risks of posthemorrhoidectomy bleeding.

The use of LMA protects the patient's airway whilst in prone-jackknife position, and minimizes excessive patient positioning before and after surgery.

Use of topical 10% metronidazole accelerates postoperative healing and reduces postoperative discomfort.

Harmonic Scalpel® hemorrhoidectomy is a safe and effective modality that simplifies performing hemorrhoidectomy, and optimizes postoperative results.

Recommended References and Readings

1. Armstrong DN, Ambroze WL, Schertzer ME, et al. Harmonic scalpel hemorrhoidectomy: five hundred cases. *Dis Colon Rect* 2002;45(3):354–9.
2. Armstrong DN, Frankum C, Ambroze W, Schertzer ME, Orangio GR. Harmonic scalpel hemorrhoidectomy: five hundred consecutive cases. *Dis Colon Rect* 2001;44(4):558–64.
3. Haveran LA, Sturrock PR, Sun MY, et al. Simple harmonic scalpel hemorrhoidectomy utilizing local anesthesia combined with intravenous sedation: a safe and rapid alternative to conventional hemorrhoidectomy. *Int J Colorectal Dis* 2007;22(7):801–6.
4. Kisli E, Agargun MY, Tekin M, Selvi Y, Karaayvaz M. Effects of spinal anesthesia and laryngeal mask anesthesia on mood states during hemorrhoidectomy. *Adv Ther* 2007;24(1):171–7.
5. Sohn VY, Martin MJ, Mullenix PS, Cuadrado DG, Place RJ, Steele SR. Comparison of open versus closed techniques using the harmonic scalpel in outpatient hemorrhoid surgery. *Mil Med* 2008;173(7):689–92.
6. Ramadan E, Vishne T, Dreznik Z. Harmonic scalpel hemorrhoidectomy: preliminary results of a new alternative method. *Tech Coloproctol* 2002;6(2):89–92.
7. Ozer MT, Yigit T, Uzar AI, et al. A comparison of different hemorrhoidectomy procedures. *Saudi Med J* 2008;29(9):1264–9.
8. Chung CC, Ha JP, Tai YP, Tsang WW, Li MK. Double-blind, randomized trial comparing harmonic scalpel hemorrhoidectomy, bipolar scissors hemorrhoidectomy, and scissors excision: ligation technique. *Dis Colon Rectum* 2002;45(6):789–94.
9. Nicholson TJ, Armstrong D. Topical metronidazole (10 percent) decreases posthemorrhoidectomy pain and improves healing. *Dis Colon Rectum* 2004;47(5):711–16.
10. Carapeti EA, Kamm MA, McDonald PJ, Phillips RK. Double-blind randomised controlled trial of effect of metronidazole on pain after day-case haemorrhoidectomy. *Lancet* 1998;351(9097):169–72.
11. Ala S, Saeedi M, Eshghi F, Mirzabeygi P. Topical metronidazole can reduce pain after surgery and pain on defecation in postoperative hemorrhoidectomy. *Dis Colon Rectum* 2008;51(2):235–8.

4 Procedure for Prolapse and Hemorrhoids (PPH; Stapled Hemorrhoidopexy)

Oliver Schwandner

 ## INDICATIONS/CONTRAINDICATIONS

Stapled hemorrhoidopexy or "procedure for prolapse and hemorrhoids" (PPH) for the treatment of hemorrhoidal disease was introduced in the last decade. In contrast to conventional hemorrhoidectomy that includes submucosal excision of prolapsing hemorrhoidal tissue, stapled hemorrhoidopexy introduced by Antonio Longo in 1998 involves simultaneous circumferential resection of excess hemorrhoidal mass with mucosal anastomosis, and residual hemorrhoidal tissue that plays a major role for continence is returned to its original position (1).

According to Goligher's classification, PPH is ideally indicated in patients with grade III hemorrhoidal prolapse (2). As outlined in Table 4.1, PPH can also be performed in prolapsed second-degree hemorrhoids that have not responded to nonsurgical interventions (e.g., rubber band ligation) or in grade II hemorrhoids with full circumferential involvement (3). PPH is also suitable for patients with hemorrhoids-associated rectal mucosal prolapse.

The use of PPH in grade IV hemorrhoidal prolapse is more controversial (4,5). A prerequisite to its use is that the hemorrhoidal prolapse should be reducible under anesthesia. However, reflecting to the authors' experience, PPH is not recommended for grade IV, fixed and nonreducible hemorrhoidal prolapse. Only in a minority of patients suffering from hemorrhoidal prolapse grade IV for whom residual external prolapse or skin tags would not be a significant concern, the application of PPH can be discussed individually if performed by an experienced surgeon. Alternatively, PPH can be combined with segmental excisional hemorrhoidectomy or excision of skin tags.

In general, there are a few contraindications to perform PPH, which were documented in a 2003 consensus paper produced by an international working party (6). Absolute contraindications for stapled hemorrhoidopexy include anal stenosis, presence of coexistent anorectal infection (perianal sepsis, complex anorectal fistula, or abscess), anal or rectal cancer, previous coloanal anastomosis, previous sphincter recon-

TABLE 4.1	Indications for Procedure for Prolapse and Hemorrhoids

Grade III hemorrhoidal disease
Grade II hemorrhoids with circumferential involvement
Grade II hemorrhoids associated with rectal mucosal prolapse
Grade II hemorrhoids nonresponding to ligation therapy

struction, intra-anal condylomata, coexistent proctitis (Crohn's disease, radiation induced), and presence of anorectal sexually transmitted diseases (Table 4.2).

Derived from this consensus position paper, experience with anorectal surgery, understanding of anorectal anatomy, and experience with circular stapling devices have been defined as prerequisites to perform transanal stapling procedures (6). In the era of transanal stapling procedures for hemorrhoidal prolapse, the majority of procedures can be performed by transanal stapling techniques if strict criteria of indication and patient selection are respected (7). However, although strict selection criteria for a transanal stapling approach are respected, there is a minority of patients in whom a stapling procedure is not possible or appropriate (Table 4.3); in a personal series, a 4.6% rate of "conversion" to conventional hemorrhoidectomy was documented because of anatomical, clinical, and technical factors (8). Obviously, this fact has an impact on informed consent. Therefore, every patient should be informed about anatomical and technical reasons that can make a stapling approach difficult or lead to conversion to a conventional treatment option. Consequently, experience in patient selection and alternative procedures without a stapling device is mandatory.

PREOPERATIVE PLANNING

Focusing on patient selection, it is crucial that hemorrhoidal prolapse is reducible. Moreover, patients suffering from large external hemorrhoids or skin tags must be informed that these tags will not be routinely excised with the stapled approach. Informed consent must be obtained considering potential risks, benefits of PPH in the short term, the risk of prolapse recurrence in the long-term course, and alternative treatments (conventional excisional hemorrhoidectomy). Finally, patients must be suitable for either general or regional anesthesia.

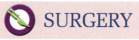 SURGERY

Patient Preparation

In general, no specific preparation is necessary. However, it is a general practice to preoperatively administer one or two phosphate rectal enemas. Although no evidence

TABLE 4.2	Contraindications for Procedure for Prolapse and Hemorrhoids	
Absolute		**Relative**
Anal stenosis		Grade IV hemorrhoids
Coincidence of anal sepsis, abscess, or complex fistula		Previous major rectal surgery (e.g., low rectal or coloanal anastomosis)
Anal or rectal cancer		Previous sphincter reconstruction
Coexistent proctitis (e.g., Crohn's disease, radiation induced)		Patients practicing receptive anal intercourse
Anorectal sexually transmitted disease		

TABLE 4.3	**Potential Reasons for Conversion in Procedure for Prolapse and Hemorrhoids**	
Reasons for conversion		
Anatomical and technical	Deep anal canal Prominent os ischii Narrowed sphincter	
Morphological	Nonreducible hemorrhoidal prolapse	
Unexpected clinical findings	Proctitis Anorectal sepsis Full-thickness rectal prolapse	

derived from randomized studies exists, a single-shot antibiotic prophylaxis should be provided (e.g., cefotaxime and metronidazole). In high-risk patients, such as immuno-suppressed patients, antibiotic prophylaxis is mandatory.

Patient Positioning

The PPH procedure can be performed in either the prone jackknife or lithotomy position. In my personal experience, lithotomy position is preferred as it enables intraoperative transvaginal examination. Technically, it is important that the hips are completely flexed to expose the entire perineum. Skin preparation and draping are routinely carried out.

Technique

Surgery is performed in a standardized technique and described using the commercially available PPH03® procedure set (Ethicon Endo-Surgery, Cincinnati, OH, USA). The PPH set is shown in Figure 4.1. As outlined in Figure 4.2, it is ideally suitable for grade III hemorrhoids.

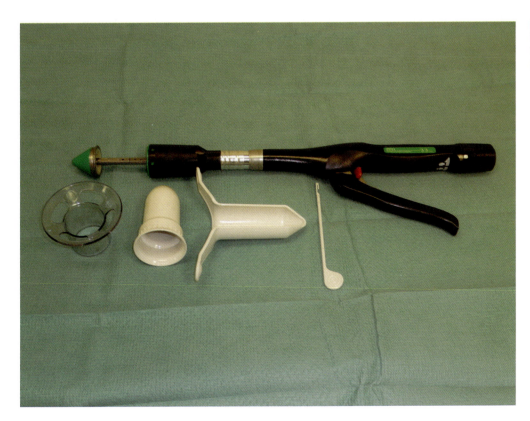

Figure 4.1 PPH03 procedure set including circular stapler, obturator, circular anal dilatator, and purse-string threading instrument.

Part I: Hemorrhoidectomy

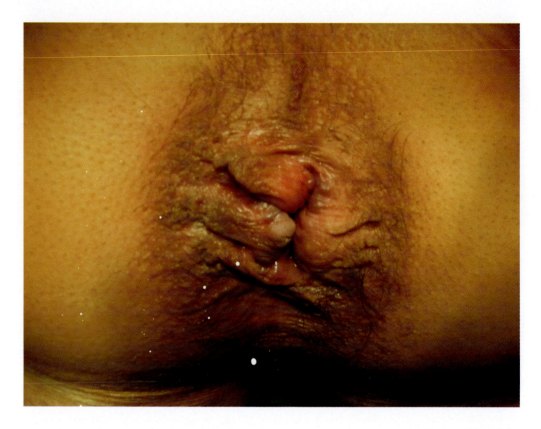

Circular Anal Dilatator Insertion

From the technical view, a transanal stapling procedure should be performed only if the circular anal dilatator (CAD) (with the corresponding obturator) specifically created for the procedure could be inserted without any tension. It is recommended to gently dilatate the anus before inserting the obturator (Fig. 4.3). For the PPH procedure, the CAD 33 (diameter 33 mm) is used and fixed with four quadrant sutures at the anal verge (Fig. 4.4). After placement of the CAD, a gauze swab can be inserted into the distal rectum and withdrawn to expose the extent of hemorrhoidal and/or rectal mucosal prolapse. It is important that the CAD is in correct position, which includes that the dentate line is the CAD (Fig. 4.5). In fact, the dentate line should be visible through the clear plastic of the CAD.

Purse-String Suture Placement

Using a specific anoscope, a purse-string suture (2/0 Prolene; Ethicon, Somerville, NJ, USA) is submucosally placed (not including rectal muscularis propria) in a circumferential and continuous way. It is crucial that the purse-string suture is positioned either 1–2 cm above the hemorrhoidal apex or 3–5 cm above the dentate line (Fig. 4.6). Of course, this step primarily depends on the volume of hemorrhoidal tissue, but it is important not to place the suture too low or too high. In the former circumstance, significant postoperative pain and incontinence due to sensory impairment may ensue. In the latter situation, insufficient reduction of the hemorrhoids symptom persistence may occur. It is the objective of PPH to reduce hemorrhoidal prolapse rather than to excise the hemorrhoidal tissue completely.

Stapler Insertion

Following circumferential placement of the purse-string suture, the circular stapler is inserted under direct vision into the distal rectum ensuring that the head is positioned above the purse string (Fig. 4.7). The purse string is then tied and the ends are pulled through the holes in the stapler device. The suture ends are then held to apply firm traction on the purse string and the stapler can be closed. While closing the PPH instrument, it is important to ensure correct alignment in the axis of the anal canal (Fig. 4.8).

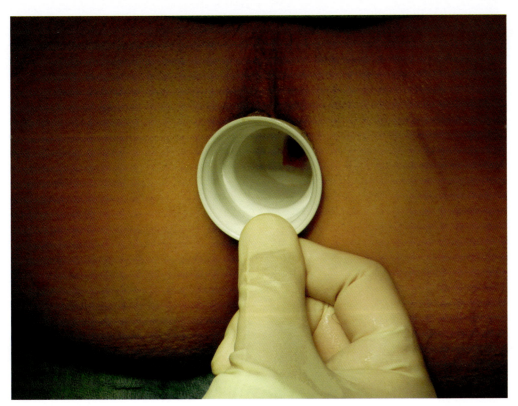

Figure 4.3 Insertion of anal obturator without tension.

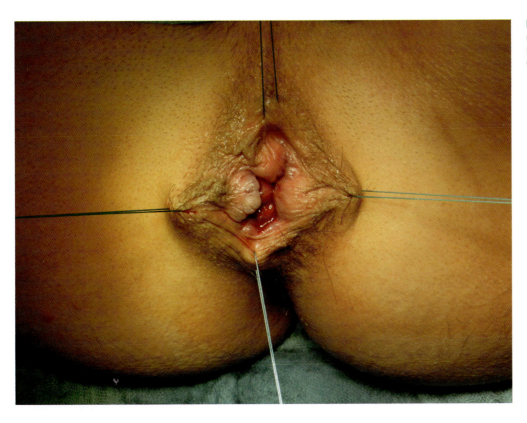

Figure 4.4 Placement of four quadrant sutures at the anal verge prior to placement of circular anal dilatator.

Figure 4.5 Circular anal dilatator in place.

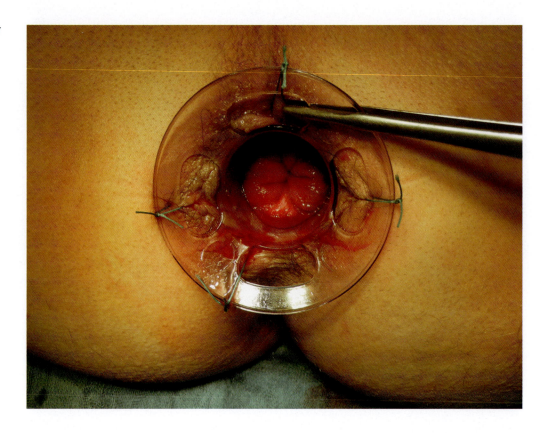

Figure 4.6 Placement of purse-string suture.

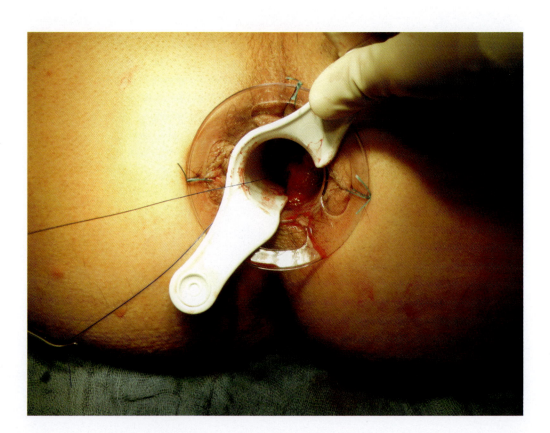

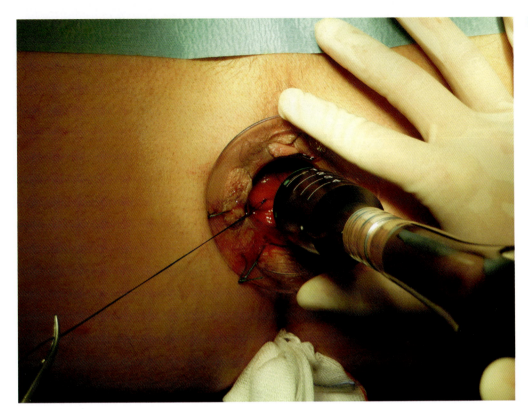

Figure 4.7 Insertion of stapler.

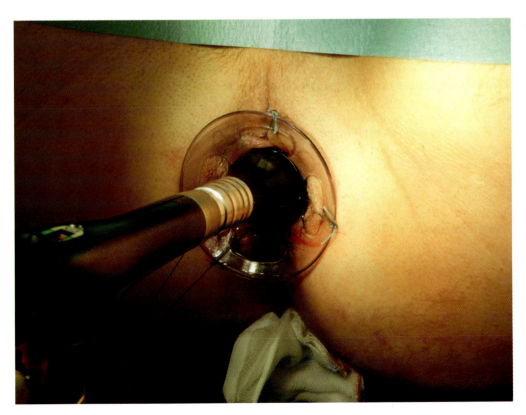

Figure 4.8 Closure of stapler.

Figure 4.9 Location of staple line above physiological hemorrhoidal plexus.

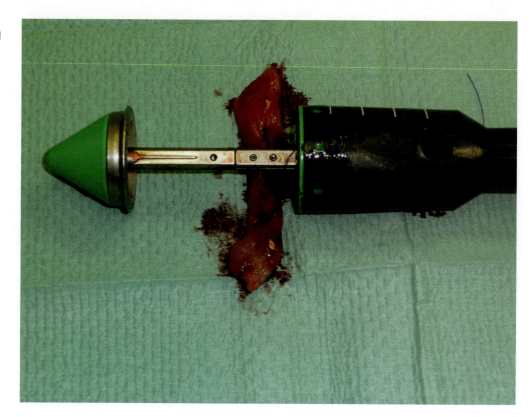

Furthermore, transvaginal examination is recommended to prevent accidental inclusion of the posterior vaginal wall. Finally, the stapler can be fired and carefully removed from the distal rectum.

Checking Staple Line and Resected Specimen
The staple line is regularly checked for completeness and for hemostasis. If bleeding from the staple line occurs, oversewing with absorbable sutures is mandatory (Vicryl 3/0; Ethicon). It is the surgical objective that the staple line is located above the physiological hemorrhoidal plexus (Fig. 4.9).

The resection specimen is removed from the stapling instrument and checked macroscopically (Fig. 4.10). The tissue ring is seldom a "pure" mucosectomy specimen, but usually includes muscular tissue, and histopathological examination is recommended. Finally, the CAD is removed and the procedure may be completed by insertion of a degradable sponge dressing or a hemostatic pad. From the surgical objective, PPH should provide complete reduction of hemorrhoidal prolapse with potential resuspension of the anoderm (Fig. 4.11).

POSTOPERATIVE MANAGEMENT

Postoperatively, patients receive oral administration of analgesics including nonsteroidal anti-inflammatory drugs combined with stool regulation treatment such as psyllium supplements and stool softeners for some days. Particularly in young males, intra-anal topical administration of diltiazem can lead to reduced pain related to a reduction of sphincter spasm. Routine postoperative administration of antibiotics is not unnecessary. Furthermore, no restriction in oral feeding is indicated. As urinary retention can occur particularly in males, patients should be informed prior to surgery; occasionally, a temporary placement of a urinary catheter can be necessary. Patients may be discharged on the day of surgery; however, discharge policy and financial reimbursement depend

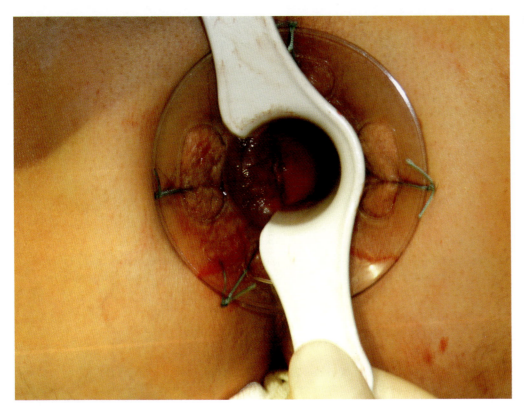

Figure 4.10 Resected specimen removed from the stapler.

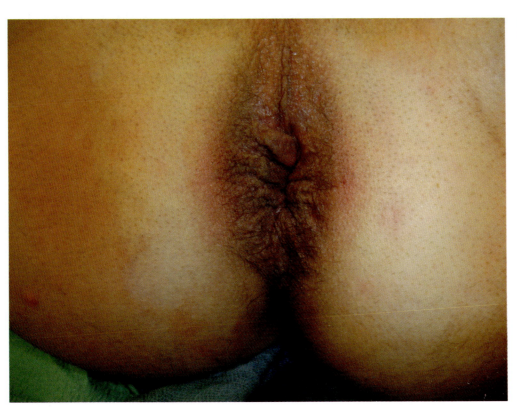

Figure 4.11 Status after procedure for prolapse and hemorrhoids.

TABLE 4.4	**Potential Complications Following Procedure for Prolapse and Hemorrhoids**	
Early onset		**Late onset**
Bleeding (major and minor, including retrorectal hematoma)		Recurrent prolapse
Urinary retention		Stenosis of staple line
Anal thrombosis and external thrombosed hemorrhoids		Fecal urgency
Staple line complications (dehiscence)		Fecal incontinence
Anorectal pain		
Fecal impaction		
Anal fissure		
Residual or persistent prolapse		
Anorectal sepsis		

on local factors. Patients should be informed to contact the surgeon if there is increasing anal pain, major bleeding, fever, or impaction of feces as these symptoms may be indications of postoperative infection.

 # COMPLICATIONS

There are no specific circumstances indicating a higher or different risk of complications after PPH for prolapsing hemorrhoids in comparison with conventional hemorrhoidectomy. Although the PPH procedure has been shown to be safe, there is always the risk of morbidity. Focusing on PPH, early- and late-onset symptoms can be differentiated (Table 4.4). In addition, complications can be directly related to surgery such as fissure and stenosis, and infection can result in significant symptoms indicating pain, bleeding, and urinary retention, and can have a great impact on function causing fecal urgency or fecal incontinence. It has been demonstrated that most common early and late complications after PPH are postoperative bleeding, persistent pain, and recurrent prolapse. If major bleeding occurs within the first 24 hours postoperatively, reexploration under anesthesia is advisable because direct bleeding from the staple line is probably the cause. In general, postoperative bleeding and pain are mainly related to anal fissure, thrombosed or persistent hemorrhoids, or troublesome retained staples. Although a primary course of conservative treatment including stool regulation, topical anesthetic ointment, and topical application of diltiazem, among others, may be successful. Early reintervention should be discussed as delayed reintervention may result in a chronicity of symptoms, which is more difficult to resolve.

Focusing on infectious or septic complications, some case reports on severe septic complications following PPH—including rectal perforation, retroperitoneal sepsis, and Fournier's gangrene—had a tremendous impact on the application of PPH (9,10). However, these septic complications have also been reported following injection sclerotherapy or rubber band ligation (11,12).

In summary, the majority of complications can be avoided by strict patient selection and meticulous surgical technique. The reports on adverse outcomes related to stapled hemorrhoidopexy in terms of morbidity, reinterventions, and poor functional outcome probably refer to poor patient selection as much as poor surgical technique including the learning curve (13–15).

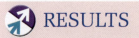 # RESULTS

Interpretation of the literature is made difficult by heterogeneity of published trials. Many studies have compared stapled hemorrhoidopexy with conventional hemorrhoidectomy including Milligan-Morgan open or Ferguson's closed hemorrhoidectomy. The majority of these studies have included patients with third- and fourth-degree hemorrhoids. However, other studies have included patients with second-degree hemorrhoids, or have restricted their investigation to patients with fourth-degree hemorrhoids. Moreover, in many studies there has been no clear definition related to patient selection and degree of hemorrhoidal prolapse. Furthermore, the majority of published randomized trials focus only on short-term outcome, whereas conclusions derived from controlled long-term data are limited (16). From this "melting pot" of data, comparative results of the PPH procedure versus conventional hemorrhoidectomy cannot be generally conclusive.

Randomized controlled data evidence limited to the HCS33 circular stapler device (PPH01 and PPH03; Ethicon Endo-Surgery). In 2007, the British National Institute for Health and Clinical Excellence published its updated guidance on stapled hemorrhoidopexy (3). It stated that "stapled haemorrhoidopexy, using a circular stapler specifically developed for haemorrhoidopexy, is recommended as an option for people in whom surgical intervention is considered appropriate for the treatment of prolapsed internal haemorrhoids" (3). However, this guidance did not provide any specific recommendations as to the indications or contraindications for stapled hemorrhoidopexy. It considered 27 randomized controlled trials comparing stapled hemorrhoidopexy with either Milligan-Morgan or Ferguson's hemorrhoidectomy. This collective included a mixed cohort of patients suffering from grade II internal hemorrhoids to grade IV hemorrhoidal prolapse. It is in the treatment of grade III hemorrhoids that stapled hemorrhoidopexy appears to be particularly beneficial, effective, and safe. The use of stapled hemorrhoidopexy in grade IV prolapse is more controversial. A prerequisite to its use is that the hemorrhoidal prolapse should be reducible under anesthesia. Following the National Institute for Health and Clinical Excellence report, PPH is safe and probably as effective as conventional hemorrhoidectomy in the short-term course (3).

A recently published meta-analysis including 27 randomized trials comparing PPH with conventional hemorrhoidectomy ($n = 2,279$) clearly demonstrated that the majority of studies reported less pain (95% of studies), shorter time of surgery (89%), a reduced hospitalization (88%), and a shorter convalescence time (93%) following PPH; no significant differences were documented in morbidity rates or postoperative bleeding (17). However, this meta-analysis also noted a higher risk of recurrent prolapse and the need for surgical reinterventions for prolapse after PPH in the long term (17). In general, short-term benefits of PPH also included better wound healing and a higher patient satisfaction (18). In terms of cost-effectiveness, there seems to be no fundamental difference between PPH and conventional hemorrhoidectomy, but this phenomenon depends on many economic variables and can be evaluated only within country levels (18).

According to a Cochrane review published in 2006 including all randomized studies comparing PPH and conventional hemorrhoidectomy (1998–2006) (19), PPH was associated with a higher long-term risk of hemorrhoid or prolapse recurrence and the symptom of prolapse; in addition, PPH was likely to be to associated with a higher likelihood of long-term symptom recurrence and the need for further surgical reinterventions compared with conventional hemorrhoidectomy (20).

Following a recent meta-analysis solely focusing on long-term outcome (15 randomized studies; $n = 1,201$; minimum follow-up of 12 months), a higher incidence of prolapse recurrence after PPH was also documented (21). Moreover, patients who had undergone PPH were more likely to undergo further treatment to correct recurrent prolapse compared with conventional hemorrhoidectomy (21).

Derived from these data, PPH is associated with various benefits in the short term; however, long-term follow-up reveals a higher likelihood of recurrent prolapse (Table 4.5). It would appear that the higher incidence of recurrent prolapse after PPH in comparison with conventional hemorrhoidectomy is related to insufficient prolapse resection produced by the stapler in "large-volume" hemorrhoidal disease and, finally, to poor patient selection. In addition, there is a considerable proportion of patients with hemorrhoidal prolapse (grade III) who have associated obstructed defecation syndromes—in a current series the incidence was 16% (22); in these patients diagnostic workup prior to any surgery is mandatory and PPH as primary procedure is not appropriate (22).

Part I: Hemorrhoidectomy

TABLE 4.5	Results of PPH versus Conventional Hemorrhoidectomy (CH) Provided by Evidence (16–21)
Variable	**PPH versus CH**
Operating time	Favors PPH
Hospital stay	Favors PPH
Postoperative pain	Favors PPH
Complications	No difference
Postoperative bleeding	No difference
Wound healing	Favors PPH
Time to work/normal activity	Favors PPH
Patient satisfaction	Favors PPH
Costs	No difference
Recurrent prolapse	Favors CH
Reinterventions for prolapse	Favors CH

PPH = procedure for prolapse and hemorrhoids.

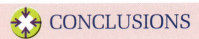 CONCLUSIONS

Over the past 12 years, PPH had gained popularity for the surgical treatment of hemorrhoids and/or rectal mucosal prolapse. Surgical technique, experience with anorectal surgery, understanding of anorectal anatomy, and experience with circular stapling devices are prerequisites to perform PPH. Formally, stapled hemorrhoidopexy aims to reduce the volume of prolapsing hemorrhoidal tissue and to restore it to its normal anatomical position within the anal canal. On the basis of common consensus that patient selection for PPH is the key to success and a strict adherence to various contraindications for a stapling procedure, there is the need for conversion to conventional hemorrhoidectomy in a minority of procedures in which a stapling procedure is planned but cannot be performed because of anatomical, clinical, or technical circumstances.

According to Goligher's classification, stapled hemorrhoidopexy is ideally indicated in patients with grade III hemorrhoidal prolapse (2). Moreover, PPH can be performed in prolapsed second-degree hemorrhoids that have not responded to nonsurgical interventions, with full circumferential involvement or with associated rectal mucosal prolapse. The use of PPH in grade IV hemorrhoidal prolapse is more controversial. In my personal view, PPH is not appropriate for grade IV hemorrhoidal prolapse. In these patients, conventional hemorrhoidectomy will lead to superior long-term results.

Outcome analysis of PPH has clearly shown short-term benefits including less pain, shorter hospitalization, and earlier return to work and to normal activity. Randomized trials with long-term follow-up have demonstrated that the risk of recurrent prolapse with the need for further surgical intervention is significantly higher after PPH in comparison with conventional hemorrhoidectomy.

In conclusion, the main goal of PPH is to provide symptom resolution and anatomical reposition of hemorrhoidal prolapse. It is ideally indicated in grade III hemorrhoids. For the surgeon, experience in both patient selection and alternative procedures without a stapling device is mandatory. Respecting the indications and contraindications with special attention to anatomical and technical variables of PPH can lead to excellent functional and anatomical results and can help to prevent some disappointing anatomical and functional results.

Recommended References and Readings

1. Longo A. Treatment of hemorrhoids disease by reduction of mucosa and haemorrhoidal prolapse with a circular suturing device: a new procedure. In: 6th World Congress of Endoscopic Surgery (IFSES); June 3–6, 1998; Rome.
2. Goligher JC. *Surgery of the Anus, Rectum and Colon.* 5th ed. London: Bailliere Tindall, 1984.
3. National Institute for Health and Clinical Excellence. Stapled haemorrhoidopexy for the treatment of haemorrhoids: NICE technology appraisal guidance 128. 2007.
4. Finco C, Sarzo G, Savastano S, Degregori S, Merigliano S. Stapled haemorrhoidopexy in fourth degree haemorrhoidal prolapse: is it worthwhile? *Colorectal Dis* 2006;8:130–4.
5. Mattana C, Coco C, Manno A, et al. Stapled hemorrhoidopexy and Milligan Morgan hemorrhoidectomy in the cure of fourth-

degree hemorrhoids: long-term evaluation and clinical results. *Dis Colon Rectum* 2007;50:1770–5.

6. Corman ML, Gravie JF, Hager T, et al. Stapled haemorrhoidopexy: a consensus position paper by an international working party—indications, contraindications and technique. *Colorectal Dis* 2003;5:304–10.

7. Schwandner O, Scherer R. Patient selection for stapled hemorrhoidopexy and STARR. In: Jayne D, Stuto A (eds.). *Transanal Stapling Techniques for Anorectal Prolapse.* 1st ed. London: Springer, 2009:59–69.

8. Schwandner O. Conversion in transanal stapling techniques for haemorrhoids and anorectal prolapse. *Colorectal Dis* 2011;13: 87–93.

9. Molloy RG, Kingmore D. Life threatening pelvic sepsis after stapled haemorrhoidectomy. *Lancet* 2000;355:810.

10. Bonner C, Prohm P, Storkel S. Fournier gangrene as a rare complication after stapled hemorrhoidectomy. Case report and review of the literature. *Chirurg* 2001;72:1464–70.

11. Barwell J, Watkins RM, Lloyd Davies E, Wilkins DC. Life-threatening retroperitoneal sepsis after hemorrhoid injection sclerotherapy: report of a case. *Dis Colon Rectum* 1999;42:421–3.

12. O'Hara VS. Fatal clostridial infection following hemorrhoidal banding. *Dis Colon Rectum* 1980;23:570–1.

13. Jongen J, Boch JU, Peleiks HG, Eberstein A, Pfister K. Complications and reoperations in stapled anopexy: learning by doing. *Int J Colorect Dis* 2006;21:166–71.

14. Brusciano L, Ayabaca SM, Pescatori M, et al. Reinterventions after complicated or failed stapled hemorrhoidopexy. *Dis Colon Rectum* 2004;47:1846–51.

15. Pescatori M, Gagliardi G. Postoperative complications after procedure for prolapsed hemorrhoids (PPH) and stapled transanal rectal resection (STARR) procedures. *Tech Coloproctol* 2008; 12:7–19.

16. Tjandra JJ, Chan MK. Systematic review on the procedure for prolapse and hemorrhoids (stapled hemorrhoidopexy). *Dis Colon Rectum* 2007;50:878–92.

17. Burch J, Epstein D, Baba-Akbari A, et al. Stapled haemorrhoidopexy for the treatment of haemorrhoids: a systematic review. *Colorectal Dis* 2009;11:233–44.

18. Burch J, Epstein D, Baba-Akbari A, et al. Stapled haemorrhoidectomy (haemorrhoidopexy) for the treatment of haemorrhoids: a systematic review and economic evaluation. *Health Technol Assess* 2008;12:1–193.

19. Jayaraman S, Colquhoun PH, Malthaner RA. Stapled versus conventional surgery for hemorrhoids. *Cochrane Database Syst Rev* 2006;18:CD005393.

20. Jayaraman S, Colquhoun PH, Malthaner RA. Stapled hemorrhoidopexy is associated with a higher long-term recurrence rate of internal hemorrhoids compared with conventional excisional hemorrhoid surgery. *Dis Colon Rectum* 2007;50:1297–305.

21. Giordano P, Gravante G, Sorge R, Ovens L, Nastro P. Long-term outcomes of stapled hemorrhoidopexy vs conventional hemorrhoidectomy: a meta-analysis of randomized controlled trials. *Arch Surg* 2009;144:266–72.

22. Schwandner O, Bruch HP. Significance of obstructed defecation in hemorrhoidal disease: results of a prospective study. *Coloproctology* 2006;28:13–20.

23. Senagore—Us Trial PPH.

Part I: Hemorrhoidectomy

5 Flaps (Excision and Closure, Mucosal, Skin)

M. Solomon and C. Wright

Introduction

The management of complicated anal fistula disease remains a challenge for surgeons and a frustrating problem for patients. Treatment is aimed at cure, with the drainage of associated sepsis and eradication of the fistula tract, while at the same time preserving the integrity of the anal sphincter and continence.

The majority of perianal sepsis is idiopathic or cryptoglandular in origin, and arises from the obstruction of the anal glands, leading to stasis of glandular secretions and, if secondarily infected, suppuration and abscess formation. The abscess typically forms in the intersphincteric space but can extend into the ischiorectal fossa or supralevator/suprasphincteric spaces. A fistula tract may subsequently form.

A minority of cases are secondary to an underlying disease process, including Crohn's disease, local radiation, malignancy, trauma, tuberculosis, HIV, hidradenitis suppurativa, lymphogranuloma venereum, perianal actinomycosis, and rectal duplication. Rectal and foreign body trauma should also be considered as possible etiological causes. In these situations, the fistula tract is often atypical.

All methods of fistula repair rely on the elimination of the internal opening to the anal gland.

INDICATIONS/CONTRAINDICATIONS

Fistulotomy remains the mainstay of treatment for those fistulas involving a small amount of sphincter muscle such as low transsphincteric and intersphincteric fistula tracts. The challenge lies in the treatment of complex fistula tracts. In this situation, a simple fistulotomy is precluded because the division of sphincter muscle would result in an unacceptably high rate of incontinence. As a result, techniques that preserve sphincter function have been developed. These include simple excision and closure of the internal opening, the ligation of intersphincteric fistula tract (LIFT) procedure, advancement flap repairs, and more recently, the use of biological materials to occlude the tract such as fibrin glue and fistula plugs.

Excision and Closure of the Internal Opening

Some authors have reported treating the tract by simply closing the internal fistula opening, without using an advancement flap. The argument for this type of repair is that in the presence of adequate perfusion and the absence of undue tension, at the coapted surfaces, simple appositional closure should suffice (1). The repair maintains the sphincter integrity. This procedure is not practiced at our institution, as it has been shown to appear to be inferior to the methods using flap reinforcement, and is generally now combined with either a flap advancement procedure and/or a fistulotomy. The more recently described modification, the LIFT procedure (discussed in detail in Chapter 9, pages 79–84), which involves ligating the intersphincteric fistula tract, may change this attitude.

Flaps

Advancement flap procedures may be considered in any patient in whom the fistula tract is complex and cannot be laid open. A complex tract is defined as a tract that crosses >30–50% of the external sphincter and includes those tracts which are high transsphincteric, suprasphincteric, and extrasphincteric; rectovaginal or rectourethral; anterior in female patients; multiple or recurrent; or the patient has preexisting sphincter compromise. In addition, the tract is complex if it is associated with an underlying disease process, as listed above, including Crohn's disease.

The flap may be mobilized from the rectum as either a mucosal, partial thickness or full thickness rectal advancement flap or from the perianal skin as an anocutaneous advancement flap.

Relative contraindications to performing a flap repair include:

- undrained sepsis
- a fistula of less than 4 weeks duration
- a malignant fistula
- a fistula arising in an irradiated field
- the presence of active proctitis, particularly Crohn's disease

An anorectal stricture would be a relative contraindication to performing a mucosal rectal advancement flap and an anocutaneous flap would be preferably used in this situation. An anocutaneous advancement flap is also used to repair keyhole deformities related to sphincter defects and scarring as a result of previous fistulotomies.

PREOPERATIVE PLANNING

Understanding the anatomy of the pathology is a prerequisite for successful treatment.

Preoperative evaluation and planning determines the course of the tract in relation to the sphincter complex with identification of the internal opening, the secondary or external opening, the primary tract, and any secondary extensions of the tract. Baseline sphincter function should also be assessed and any coexisting disease should be identified. Clinical assessment is aimed at identifying any symptoms which suggest coexisting disease and assessing a patient's baseline level of continence. A past history of previous anal surgery and an obstetric history is also sought.

Digital examination and rigid sigmoidoscopy remain an essential part of the preoperative assessment and are often the only investigations required for simple fistulae. The internal opening may be felt as a palpable defect and the course of the tract is indicated by induration of the perianal tissues. The site of the external opening is usually clear. Digital examination is also a guide to sphincter function. Prior to more invasive tests the anal resting tone and voluntary sphincter "squeeze" pressure are also assessed clinically. Sphincter defects may be palpable and, deformity of the anal canal due to anorectal sepsis or previous surgery, is noted.

The findings often influence the choice of operative procedure. In the presence of anorectal stenosis, and/or extensive scarring and rigidity of the rectal mucosa as a result of chronic suprasphincteric sepsis for example, an anocutaneous flap repair is preferred because of the potential difficulty in mobilizing a rectally based advancement flap in this situation.

It is the authors' practice to perform a colonoscopy or flexible sigmoidoscopy for complex or recurrent fistulae, to help exclude associated gastrointestinal disease. The choice of investigation usually depends on the patient's age and whether or not they have the associated abdominal symptoms. If Crohn's disease is suspected on symptoms, and a colonoscopy is normal, then an upper endoscopy, small bowel series, enteroclysis, small bowel enteroscopy, or small bowel capsule imaging may be indicated.

The complex fistula tract may be imaged by endoanal ultrasound (EAUS) or magnetic resonance imaging (MRI). Fistulography and computed tomography (CT) have little to offer in the assessment of the fistula tract. The choice of imaging is dependent on availability, local expertise, and the complexity of the fistula tract. It has been the authors' practice to assess recurrent and complex fistula tracts with 2D EAUS and, more recently, using 3D US reconstruction.

EAUS is able to differentiate between simple and complex fistulae, detect abscesses, delineate the internal and external openings, and categorize the type of tract. Hydrogen peroxide injected via the external opening can enhance visualization of the tract as it acts as an ultrasonic contrast medium by producing hyper reflective gas bubbles (2). Although the use of hydrogen peroxide has been shown to increase the accuracy of assessment from 68–98%, it has not been our practice to need or to use enhancement routinely. EAUS facilitates surgical planning as well as confirming previous sphincter damage as a result of the disease process and/or previous surgical attempts at eradication. An advantage of EAUS over MRI is that EAUS can be performed during surgery as an adjunct to digital examination and examination under anesthesia (EUA) as well as provide a dynamic preoperative assessment of sphincter integrity.

In Australia, currently, MRI has limited availability and remuneration; it is also more time consuming, expensive, and not available as an intraoperative resource. It is, however, considered as the gold standard for assessment of anal sepsis by some surgeons. MRI is more accurate than clinical assessment in detecting previously missed secondary extensions of the primary tract, and in the correct assessment of the level of the fistula with respect to the sphincter complex. The use of endocouple receivers increases tissue resolution in close proximity to the anal canal, providing superior anatomical detail. Pelvic phased array coils can be used to assess supralevator or more extensive sepsis.

Both, EAUS and MRI, are associated with a learning curve in the interpretation of the images.

The internal sphincter is particularly at risk in fistula surgery, and baseline anal manometry to measure the anal canal pressures can also influence the choice of surgical technique.

Prior to definitive repair surgery an EUA to further assess the tracts is sometimes useful. The authors prefer to use Lockhart Mummery probes (Fig. 5.1) to the smaller

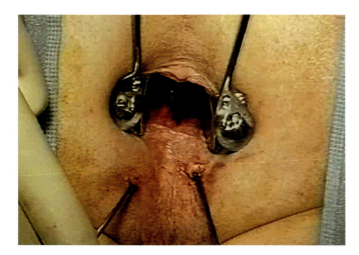

Figure 5.1 Confirmation of the course of the fistula tract using Lockhart Mummery probes.

Part II: Anal Fistula

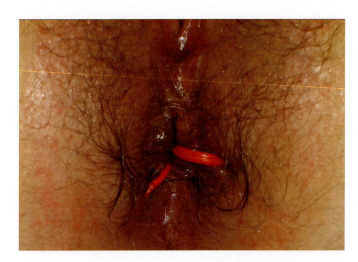

Figure 5.2 Two quiescent fistula tracts are demonstrated, with sepsis controlled following the placement of seton drains (vessel loops).

caliber lacrimal probes because of the greater risk of creating a false tract with the latter.

Definitive repair should only be undertaken after sepsis has been controlled, i.e. abscesses have been incised and drained and there has been a period of controlled drainage by placement of loose vessel loop seton drains (Fig. 5.2). Drainage from large chronic supralevator cavities is best controlled with small mushroom tip (de Pezzer) drains.

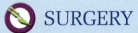 SURGERY

Perioperative Management

It is the authors' preference to use a sodium phosphate enema to clear the distal bowel. A full mechanical bowel preparation is rarely required.

Informed consent is obtained. The risks specific to fistula surgery that should be explained to the patient include:

- the risk of failure/recurrence (see results)
- inadvertent, or greater than expected, compromise of sphincter function and incontinence
- anorectal sepsis
- hematoma formation
- iatrogenic fistula formation including rectovaginal fistulae
- ectropion (following mucosal advancement flaps)

Positioning

In the operating theatre, consent and the procedure to be performed are checked by the operating surgeon prior to the commencement of the procedure. The patient's medical history is reviewed to check for any allergies to drugs that may be used. If the fistula tract is posterior or lateral then the patient is placed in the lithotomy position; some prefer the prone jackknife position for anterior tracts. The assistant is better positioned and more comfortable when the patient is prone.

The procedure is usually performed under general anesthesia using a laryngeal mask without muscle relaxation. Regional anesthesia with intravenous sedation is indicated on occasions because of patient morbidity. Antibiotic prophylaxis is routine, the authors' preference being the combination of gentamicin and metronidazole or a third generation cephalosporin and metronidazole. Thromboembolic prophylaxis is guided by the patient's age, weight and any associated comorbidities, and the estimated length of the procedure but subcutaneous heparin is used routinely.

The perineum, including the vagina and anal canal, is prepped with aqueous chlorhexidine and square draped. Fenestrated drapes should be avoided because they tend to shift and limit the access. Use of a headlight can optimize the view but is not usually necessary. When performing an anocutaneous flap the perianal buttock area is shaved if it is hirsute; an indwelling urethral catheter is not usually necessary.

Technique

A confirmatory EUA is performed and definitive repair is postponed if there is evidence of residual sepsis.

Retraction is important, so the buttocks are taped apart in the prone position. The Lone Star retractor alone, or together with either a Park's anal, bivalve retractor (Eisenhammer) or Hill-Ferguson retractor, provides adequate exposure.

Simple Excision and Appositional Closure

The authors do not practice this procedure but describe it for completeness. Thomson and Fowler used methylene blue to stain the tract's granulation tissue lining and enable close dissection around the opening of the tract. A narrow transverse ellipse is used to excise the internal opening and the defect is closed with two or three monofilament absorbable sutures. Athanasiadis et al, describe excising the internal opening and intersphincteric part of the fistula tract up to the intersphincteric plane, and then separately excising the external part of the tract and surrounding skin and fat up to the external sphincter (3). Closure is achieved using a three layer, non staggered technique; closing the mucosa and submucosa, internal sphincter, and external sphincter.

Flaps

Fundamental to the success of these procedures is being cognizant of the importance of the basic principles of flap surgery. They are

- the length: width ratio
- the thickness of the flap
- the absence of tension

Transanal/Endorectal Advancement Flap

This type of flap was first proposed by Noble (4) in 1902 for repair of a rectovaginal fistula and later modified by Elting (5) and Laird (6) in 1948 (1,7). The technique described here is a vertically incised or "tongue" flap. The term "mucosal" advancement flap (MAF) is a misnomer as these proximally based flaps invariably include the submucosa and at least the superficial fibers of, if not the entire, internal sphincter (video). A partial thickness flap does not impair incontinence but adds strength to the flap. This type of repair closes the internal opening and does not divide the external sphincter and, is therefore, associated with a lower risk of incontinence. It can be repeated and it avoids a keyhole deformity of the contour of the anal canal and healing is also quicker than after a fistulotomy. A Lone Star retractor is used to evert the anal verge, and a Parks' anal retractor or bivalve speculum is used for exposure within the anal canal. A broad based U flap is raised (Fig. 5.3). The apex should start 5–10 mm below the level of the internal opening and 10–15 mm on either side of the internal opening. The flap is raised with diathermy (Fig. 5.4). Often the most difficult part of the dissection is raising the apex of the flap, as in this area, the inflammatory changes around the internal opening as a result of previous sepsis make it difficult to develop the correct plane. If the dissection is started laterally, in virgin planes, then the correct dissection plane may be more easily identified.

The aim is to raise a broad based, tension free flap with an adequate blood supply.

The flap consists of mucosa, submucosa, and part of or occasionally the entire internal sphincter (Fig. 5.5, video) continuing proximally as the circular muscle fibers. Once the internal opening has been passed, the plane can be developed by infiltrating

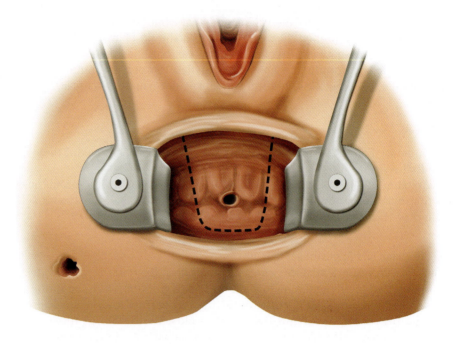

Figure 5.3 Line of incision for a broad based U endorectal advancement flap (schematic).

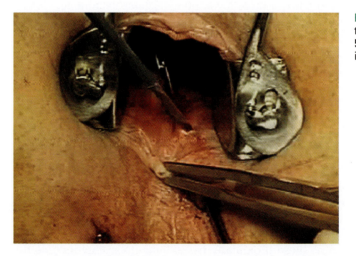

Figure 5.4 Incising the apex of the flap with diathermy, starting 5–10 mm below the level of the internal opening.

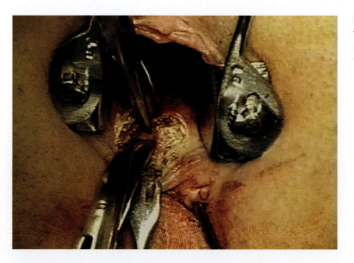

Figure 5.5 Developing the flap, in this case in the intersphincteric plane, raising a full thickness endorectal advancement flap.

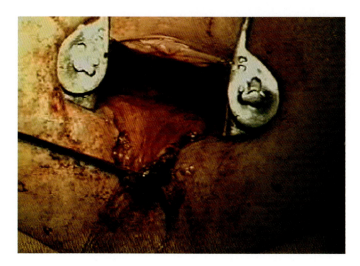

Figure 5.6 Fully mobilized flap prior to the excision of the internal opening.

with a saline solution; although this is often unnecessary. The authors avoid adrenaline containing solutions because their vasoconstrictive action may compromise the flap's blood supply.

The length of the flap should be such to allow a tension free closure (Fig. 5.6). In order to aid the retraction of the flap whilst mobilizing it, two holding sutures may be placed in its apex (Fig. 5.7). Tissue forceps, such as Alice forceps, may also be used but can obscure the view and get in the way.

Once the flap has been mobilized, the internal opening and the crypt-bearing tissue around the internal opening are excised and cored out. The apex of the flap is excised including the internal opening (Fig. 5.7). Meticulous hemostasis should be secured prior to closure of the flap to prevent hematoma formation which could lift the flap or predispose to recurrent sepsis. The internal opening is closed with a longitudinal line of interrupted absorbable monofilament sutures to help advance the flap down (Fig. 5.7). The flap is then secured to the "neo dentate" line covering the internal opening with interrupted absorbable braided sutures (Fig. 5.8). The authors' preference is 2/0–3/0 polyglactin.

If the external part of the tract is large then it is drained with a small mushroom tip catheter or left open and curetted.

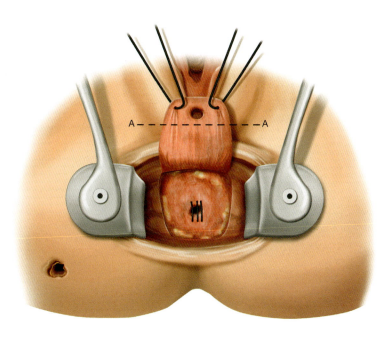

Figure 5.7 Fully mobilized flap retracted using two holding sutures. Internal opening excised along line A-A. Internal opening defect in the sphincter is closed with interrupted sutures (schematic).

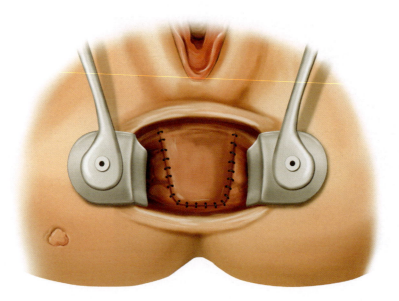

Anocutaneous Advancement Flap

The anocutaneous flap is a modification of a flap previously used in the management of anal stenosis. It is preferentially used in those patients who are not suitable for a rectal advancement flap procedure because of extensive scarring of the pararectal tissues as a result of chronic supralevator sepsis, or previous failed attempts at repair using a rectally based flap. In these cases, attempts to raise an adequate length flap are unlikely to be successful, or ectropion and keyhole deformities are present preoperatively, or are likely to be postoperative complications.

Technically this is a relatively easy procedure that does not carry the risk of ectropion and can help repair keyhole deformities resulting from multiple previous fistulotomies.

The authors prefer to use a 3–5 × 2–4 cm diamond shaped island flap comprising full thickness skin and subcutaneous fat. The flap outline is first marked on the non scarred buttock skin (Figs. 5.9 and 5.10A and B). The flap is elevated using diathermy, aiming to ensure that the edges slope out laterally in the subcutaneous tissue to give a broader base; this reduces the risk of the flap being devascularized when it is advanced into the anal canal.

The internal opening of the fistula is excised, including a small amount of the internal sphincter surrounding the internal opening, but the distal sphincter is not

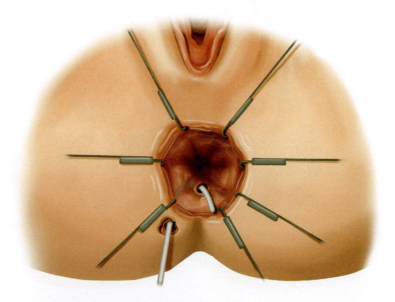

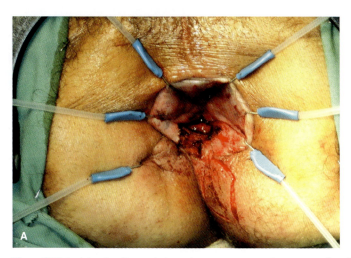 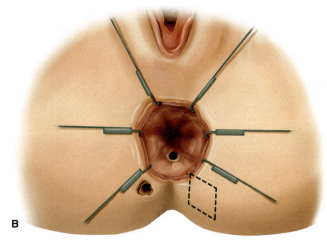

Figure 5.10 Incision for diamond shaped anocutaneous advancement flap **(A)** actual view **(B)** schematic.

divided. The internal opening is closed with a longitudinal line of interrupted absorbable monofilament sutures as above. The external component of the tract, extending from the external opening to the external sphincter, is also excised. The scar tissue between the internal and the external openings is also routinely incised, and if feasible, excised; or alternatively curetted.

It is very important to disconnect the leading edge of the flap from the subcutaneous tissues attached to the sphincter to give mobility. Once the flap is mobile it is advanced into the anal canal (Figs. 5.11A and B) and used to cover the internal opening. It is usually necessary to rotate the flap from the contralateral side to cover a defect because of ipsilateral scarring. The flap is sutured in situ using interrupted 2/0–3/0 absorbable braided sutures (polyglactin) (Figs. 5.12A and B). The buttock defect is also closed using 2/0 braided absorbable sutures. Braided absorbable sutures are used for patients' comfort. Previously, when more rigid monofilament sutures were used, patients complained of a "pricking discomfort" when sitting.

A small drain, such as a small de Pezzer or mushroom tip catheter, is placed into larger tracts via the external opening.

Note: Others prefer to use a broad based inverted U-shaped anocutaneous flap. The apex of the flap should be 2–2.5 cm in width and sited just proximal to the internal opening. It is marked out so that the base is approximately twice the width of the apex. Proximally, the flap should encompass the superficial fibers of the lower internal sphincter. The length should be such to allow a tension free closure. The distal part of the flap will include

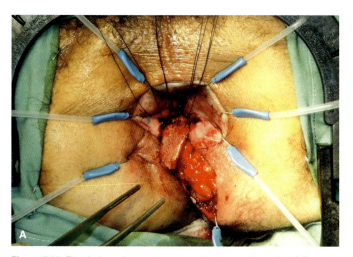 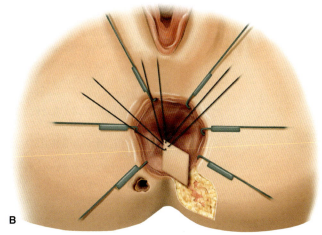

Figure 5.11 Flap being advanced to cover the internal opening **(A)** sctual view **(B)** schematic.

Part II: Anal Fistula

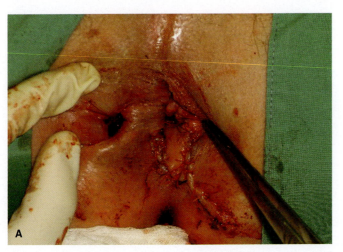
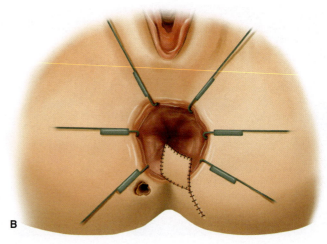

Figure 5.12 Sutured anocutaneous advancement flap **(A)** actual view, **(B)** schematic.

the skin and subcutaneous fat of the perianal region. Further advancement can be gained, if required, by excising Burrow's triangles of skin from the adjacent base. A disadvantage of these flaps is that they have limited length of mobility when compared with the island flaps which can be mobilized to above the anorectal junction when needed, for example, following a failed rectal advancement flap for a recurrent suprasphincteric fistula.

The use of local anesthetic is avoided in flap repairs to help prevent flap edema and/or ischemia. Stomas are only used if the patient has complex unresolved sepsis or there have been multiple previous attempts at repair.

POSTOPERATIVE MANAGEMENT

Oral analgesics are usually suffice as postoperative discomfort is minimal, in particular with the endorectal advancement flap, as there is no perineal wound. Patients are advised to shower gently. Sitz baths are avoided, particularly if an anocutaneous flap has been raised, to prevent the flap donor site becoming macerated. The wound should be dried thoroughly using a hairdryer and a dry dressing is applied only to separate the buttocks. The patient can have a normal diet but stool softeners are given. Low dose metronidazole can be continued in the postoperative period for 5 days for patients' comfort.

The patients are reviewed in the surgeon's office 4–6 weeks post discharge. The patients are advised to avoid vigorous exercise during this period. Patients are also advised not to be concerned if there is a partial dehiscence of the flap donor site wound (they are advised because this can occur in up to 50% of the patients). On an average it takes about 6 weeks for the perineal wound to heal completely. In our experience, patients tend to regularly check the appearance with a mirror and need reassurance about the appearance, particularly during the first couple of weeks.

COMPLICATIONS

Specific to the fistula repair. These include:

- failure/recurrence. It is important to reevaluate patients to assess the outcome as success rates decrease with time. Recurrence appears to be caused both by failure of the treatment and by recurrent patient disease
- flap breakdown
- sphincter compromise and incontinence (attributed to overstretching of the anal sphincters by the self retaining retractor, disruption of the sphincter complex by

inclusion of the internal sphincter fibers, and sensory disruption with advancement of rectal mucosa distally)
- anorectal sepsis
- hematoma formation
- iatrogenic fistula formation, including rectovaginal fistulae with anterior flap repairs
- ectropion (MAFs)

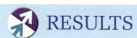 # RESULTS

Success rates relating to the different types of fistula repair vary widely in the published literature. There have been few randomized trials and most of the studies of the treatment of anal fistulae are small and heterogeneous with respect to the type of fistula included, surgical technique, and length of follow-up, making comparison difficult.

Simple Appositional Closure

The published literature includes only a few studies reporting excision and closure of the internal opening alone, without the use of a flap procedure. In 2004, Thomson and Fowler reported their experience in 44 patients of direct appositional closure of the internal opening without the use of a flap (1). Twenty six fistulae in 28 patients appeared healed at 2–5 months; with longer follow up, the repair failed in 41% of the patients. Athanasiadis et al, using a three layered closure reported a series of 90 patients having a total of 106 operations, and a follow-up time of between 6 months and 6 years (median 2.6 years) (3). The risk of recurrence was 18% (19 fistulae), with the predominant cause of failure being suture line dehiscence. Following repair, 94% of the patients were continent and 6% had minimal disordered continence.

Transanal/Endorectal Advancement Flaps

A wide range of success with this type of flap is reported in the literature ranging from 29-98%. More recent series, however with larger patient numbers, suggest success is in the order of 60-70%. The Cleveland Clinic, Ohio has published a primary success rate of 63.6% in 105 patients who underwent an endorectal advancement flap procedure, including 44% of the patients with Crohn's disease (8). The median follow up period was 17.1 (range 0.4–67) months.

Higher recurrence rates are associated with undrained sepsis, Crohn's disease, rectovaginal fistulae, and prior repair. In addition, the success rate decreases with time, and comparison of partial thickness with full thickness flaps suggests a lower rate of recurrence with the latter. Functional results following the endorectal advancement flap repair appear good, although in some series minor incontinence has been reported in up to 31%, and major incontinence, in up to 12% of patients; and incontinence increases with time after repeated attempts to close the fistula.

Anocutaneous Advancement Flaps

The authors' results using this technique in 16 patients with complex, recurrent or chronic suprasphincteric fistulae were published in 2005 (9). After a mean length of follow-up of 20 (range 1.5–43) months, complete healing was seen in 15 (94%) patients. A temporary defunctioning stoma was formed in two patients. 11 patients (almost 70%) reported improved incontinence, two patients reported no change in their level of incontinence, and three patients (19%) reported worse incontinence.

Other published studies report complete healing rates of 46-100% in non IBD patients. One of the largest studies by Nelson et al. included patients with both IBD and non IBD related fistula tracts (10). Seventy three dermal island flaps using a teardrop incision were performed in 65 patients. They reported a patient failure rate of 20% and a procedure failure rate of 23% after a mean follow-up of 28.4 (range 4–63) months.

✳ CONCLUSIONS

Good results are dependent on an understanding of the anatomy of the pathology, control of sepsis prior to a flap repair, and attention to detail to ensure a tension free, well vascularized flap. Despite these fundamental prerequisites, all colorectal surgeons are familiar with the challenges complex fistula disease pose and the frustration of failure and recurrence, and hence the informed consent must, therefore, include these limitations. Otherwise healthy young patients with complex fistulae also find the disease frustrating and often difficult to comprehend in terms of the need for staged repairs and potential need for multiple procedures. The use of long term seton's drainage should, therefore, always be included in the discussion of management of recurrent complex fistula disease; particularly, in those patients with suprasphincteric and extrasphincteric tracts.

Acknowledgement

To Professor A. Eyers for his kind permission to use his Endorectal Advancement Flap video in this publication.

Recommended References and Readings

1. Thomson WH, Fowler AL. Direct appositional (no flap) closure of deep anal fistula. *Colorectal Dis* 2004;6:32–6.
2. Cheong DMO, Nogueras JJ, Wexner S, Jagelman DG. Anal endosonography for recurrent anal fistulas: image enhancement with hydrogen peroxide. *Dis Colon Rectum* 1993;36:1158–60.
3. Athanasiadis S, Helmes C, Yazigi R, Köhler A. The direct closure of the internal fistula opening without advancement flap for transsphincteric fistulas-in-ano. *Dis Colon Rectum* 2004;47:1174–80.
4. Noble GH. New operation for complete laceration of the perineum designed for the purpose of eliminating infection from the rectum. *Trans Am Gynecol Soc* 1902;27:357–63.
5. Elting AW. The treatment of fistula-in-ano. *Ann Surg* 1912;56:744–52.
6. Laird DR. Procedures used in the treatment of complicated fistulas. *Am J Surg* 1948;76:701–8.
7. Golub RW, Wise WE Jr, Kerner BA, Khanduja KS, Aguilar PS. Endorectal mucosal advancement flap: the preferred method for complex cryptoglandular fistula-in-ano. *J Gastrointest Surg* 1997;1:487–91.
8. Sonoda T, Hull T, Piedmonte MR, Fazio VW. Outcomes of primary repair of anorectal and rectovaginal fistulas using the endorectal advancement flap. *Dis Colon Rectum* 2002;45:1622–8.
9. Hossack T, Solomon MJ, Young JM. Ano-cutaneous flap repair for complex and recurrent supra-sphincteric anal fistula. *Colorectal Dis* 2005;7:187–92.
10. Nelson RL, Cintron J, Abcarian H. Dermal island-flap anoplasty for transsphincteric fistula-in-ano: assessment of treatment failures. *Dis Colon Rectum* 2000;43:681–4.

Suggested Readings

Jun SH, Choi GS. Anocutaneous advancement flap closure of high anal fistulas. *Br J Surg* 1999;86:490–2.

Rickard MJ. Anal abscesses and fistulas. *ANZ J Surg* 2005;75:64–72.

Rieger N, Tjandra J, Solomon M. Endoanal and endorectal ultrasound: applications in colorectal surgery. *ANZ J Surg* 2004;74:671–5.

Solomon MJ, McLeod RS, Cohen EK, Cohen Z. Anal wall thickness under normal and inflammatory conditions of the anorectum as determined by endoluminal ultrasonography. *Am J Gastroenterol* 1995;90:574–8.

Whiteford MH, Kilkenny J 3rd, Hyman N, et al. Practice parameters for the treatment of perianal abscess and fistula-in-ano (revised). *Dis Colon Rectum* 2005;48:1337–42.

Williams JG, Farrands PA, Williams AB, et al. The treatment of anal fistula: ACPGBI position statement. *Colorectal Dis* 2007;9(4):18–50.

Wong S, Solomon M, Crowe P, Ooi K. Cure, continence and quality of life after treatment for fistula-in-ano. *ANZ J Surg* 2008;78:675–82.

6 Fistulotomy and Fistulectomy

H. Kessler and T. Weidinger

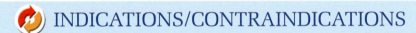

INDICATIONS/CONTRAINDICATIONS

The goals of fistula surgery are simple: to cure the fistula with the lowest possible recurrence rate, to minimize any alteration of continence, and to achieve a good result in the shortest period of time. To obtain this outcome, a number of principles have to be observed: the primary opening of the track has to be identified and also the relationship of the fistula to the puborectalis muscle; furthermore, the least amount of muscle should be divided to cure the fistula (4). The presence of a discharging opening in the perianal region, which is either persistent or recurrent is an indication for surgery. An anal fistula will rarely heal spontaneously. If left untreated, repeated abscesses with associated morbidity is probable to occur. Although nonoperative methods of therapy have been attempted, it is generally accepted that the only form of treatment affording reliable prospective cure is surgery.

An operation should be recommended unless there are specific medical contraindications to anesthesia. Patients with established compromised anal continence present a relative contraindication because the further division of muscle required when treating the fistula might render the patient totally incontinent. *It is important to know whether active Crohn's disease is present,* in which case a very thorough endoscopic investigation and magnetic resonance imaging (MRI) scan would be advisable. Control of active Crohn's disease should precede repair of an associated anal fistula. Under these circumstances, extensive fistula operations should be avoided.

It is controversial whether fistulotomy or fistulectomy is the more appropriate operative treatment for anal fistulas. There are several reasons, however, to prefer fistulotomy whenever possible. Fistulectomy means the complete removal of the fistulous track and adjacent scar tissue, which results in appreciably larger wounds. There is a larger separation of the ends of the sphincter after fistulectomy, which results in a greater chance of incontinence and a longer healing time. When a fistula crosses the sphincter muscle at a high level like a high transsphincteric or suprasphincteric fistula, there is always concern that division of the muscle below the track will impair continence. In these cases, the advancement rectal flap technique would be appealing with less sphincter muscle to be divided, avoidance of contour defects, less pain due to the absence of a perineal wound and faster healing (3) (Table 6.1).

TABLE 6.1	Overview of Recommendations for Surgery in Anal Fistula
Type of fistula	**Recommended therapy**
Subcutaneous, submucosal fistula	If uncomplicated: rarely conservative treatment
	If resistant to conservative therapy or recurrent: fistulotomy of mucosa and anal crypts
Intersphincteric anal fistula type I A of Parks	Fistulotomy
Intersphincteric anal fistula type I B of Parks	Fistulotomy with drainage of intersphincteric space
Intersphincteric anal fistula type I C of Parks	Fistulotomy with drainage of intersphincteric space, potentially closure of the rectal opening
Transsphincteric anal fistula type II A of Parks	Fistulotomy
Transsphincteric anal fistula type II B/C of Parks	Fistulectomy with flap technique
Suprasphincteric anal fistula	Fistulectomy, seton, advancement flap
Extrasphincteric anal fistula	Surgery of the rectal or extrarectal source
Primary pelvirectal fistula	Surgery depending on course of the fistula
Rectourethral fistula	Perineal or transanal closure
Anoperineal fistula	Fistulotomy
Rectovaginal fistula	Perineal access, flap technique
Submucosal anal fistula at Crohn's disease	Conservative treatment, unroofing of abscesses
Extensive fistulas at Crohn's disease	Conservative surgery

Source: Modified after Lange et al. (6).

 ## PREOPERATIVE PLANNING

Clinical Assessment

Localization of the internal opening in most cases enables the classification of perianal fistulas. The external opening of an intersphincteric fistula is almost always located near the anal verge, whereas the distance between the external opening of a transsphincteric fistula and the anal verge is several centimeters or more. In the past, Goodsall and Miles described several aspects regarding the relation between the external and the internal openings of perianal fistulas (Fig. 6.1). For many years, Goodsall's rule has been used in predicting the course of fistulous tracts. In a recent prospective study of 216 consecutive patients (1), Goodsall's rule was found, however, to be accurate in only 50% of these patients.

Surgical access depends upon accurate assessment, including a full medical history and proctosigmoidoscopy. It is necessary to exclude associated conditions. The classical

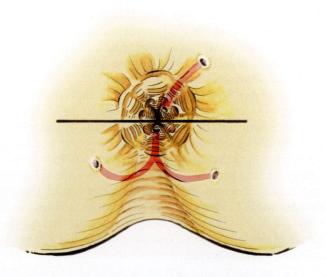

Figure 6.1 Illustration of Goodsall's rule.

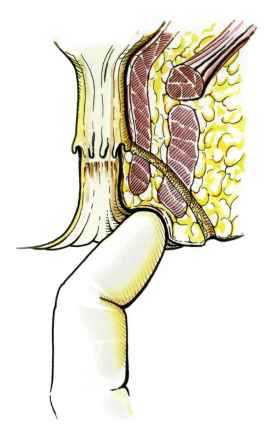

Figure 6.2 Assessment of the fistula track: superficial palpation.

five essentials of clinical assessment include identification of the internal opening, the external opening, the course of the primary track, the presence of secondary extensions, and the presence of other diseases complicating the fistula. The internal opening is the key to the assessment. The relative positions of external and internal openings indicate the likely course of the primary track. Palpable superficial induration suggests a relatively superficial track (Fig. 6.2), whereas supralevator induration suggests a track within the ischiorectal fossa or more likely a secondary extension (Fig. 6.3). The distance of the external opening from the anal verge may help differentiate an intersphincteric from a transsphincteric fistula; the greater the distance, the greater the likelihood of a complex cephalad extension. Exceptions from Goodsall's rule include anterior openings more than 3 cm from the anal verge, which may be anterior extensions of posterior horseshoe fistulas, or fistulas associated with other diseases, especially Crohn's disease and cancer.

The first component of preoperative assessment is to identify the site and level of the primary track. The second component is to determine the presence or absence of any secondary track (9).

Although advocated by some authors, it is questionable whether the internal opening of a perianal fistula can be localized accurately by digital examination. This method of examination is still important, however, since a tender palpable mass in the pelvis may reveal a supralevator abscess. It also provides some information regarding the quality of the anal sphincters by assessing the sphincter tone (10).

It is essential that the surgeon has an adequate choice of probes available. A soft, blunt-ended copper probe is preferable, which bends easily and does not break. A seton may be tied around its thickened end to thread it through the track if necessary. Probing, however, is not advocated on an outpatient basis, since it can be painful. Furthermore, there is a considerable risk of creating a false passage into the anal canal or into the rectum. It has also been suggested that injection of a diluted solution of methylene blue into the external opening enables the identification of the internal opening of a perianal fistula. A major drawback of this technique is staining of the surrounding

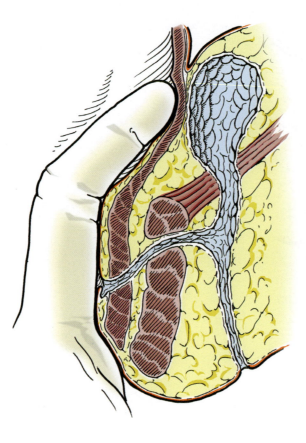

Figure 6.3 Palpation for deep induration originating from supralevatoric extension of a transsphincteric fistula.

tissues. An alternative is hydrogen peroxide, which does not stain the operative field (10) (Fig. 6.4).

At first glance, any external opening has to be identified (Fig. 6.5). The finger on the skin should feel for the direction of the track using a well-lubricated finger between the external opening and the anal orifice. An indurated track suggests a fairly superficial course: its direction will give a hint for the circumferential location of the internal

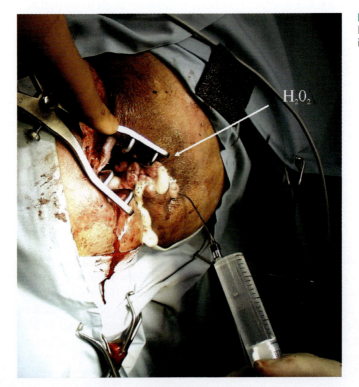

Figure 6.4 Hydrogen peroxide being applied to a perianal fistula in Crohn's disease.

H_2O_2

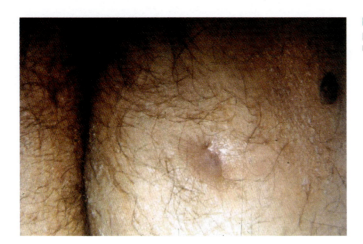

Figure 6.5 Inspection of the perianal region reveals the external fistula opening.

opening. Then, the internal opening has to be identified. This is the key to the surgical anatomy. The index finger should be used for feeling any induration within the anal canal. Counterpressure has to be applied on the perianal skin with the thumb. The internal opening is likely to be located at the level of the dentate line. There is often an enlarged papilla in the region of the internal opening and, with experience, the opening itself can be felt in most cases. The level of the internal opening in relation to the puborectalis muscle may be determined by asking the patient to contract the anal sphincter; it may be possible to feel how much functioning muscle would remain if the primary track had to be laid open.

Supralevator induration is normally a sign of primary track extension. A secondary track most usually arises from a transsphincteric primary track, extending upward to the apex of the ischiorectal fossa, or even through the levators. Alternatively, supralevator induration may arise from an upward extension of an intersphincteric track. Digital examination cannot distinguish between these two possibilities.

Examination under anesthesia should be routinely carried out under general anesthesia immediately before proceeding with surgery. This may identify features that are not easy to determine while the patient is awake. Probes should very rarely be used in the awake patient. Posterior retraction of the dentate line helps expose concealed openings; massage may release a bead of pus. Various agents injected along the track via the external opening have been used to locate the internal opening as described earlier. In most cases, with an anterior external opening, the internal opening will be located at the same circumferential point. Careful probing can delineate primary and secondary tracks. If the internal and external openings are easily detected, but the probe cannot easily traverse the path of the track, there may be a high extension. In this circumstance, a probe passed via each opening may then delineate the primary track. Persistence of granulation tissue after curettage indicates a continuing track (9).

Assessment by Imaging Techniques

For many years, fistulography was the only imaging technique for the preoperative assessment of perianal fistulas, including the localization of their internal opening. However, there are only few data regarding its accuracy. Based on limited and rather conflicting data, it is impossible to assess the exact role of fistulography in the preoperative imaging of perianal fistulas (10). Meanwhile, fistulography has been surpassed by endosonography and MRI. Advantages of both techniques are the direct visualization of the fistulous track and the imaging of the anal sphincters. Endosonography offers a 360° axial image. Installation of hydrogen peroxide improves the accuracy of the procedure. Most reports show an accuracy between 50% and 70% regarding the detection of the primary fistulous track (10). Besides, the presence of sepsis in the intersphincteric plane and sometimes in the deep postanal space may be detected. In addition, defects in the sphincters are identified, which may influence the management of anterior fistulas in women. Although some transsphincteric fistulas can be visualized, the perineal component of anal fistulas cannot be seen in most patients. Anal ultrasonography therefore gives more information about the sphincters than the anatomy of the fistula.

MRI is now regarded as the investigation of choice to define complex anorectal sepsis and fistulas. In the literature (5), it is claimed to provide 100% accuracy in defining the presence of a fistula and the site of extensions and is 85% accurate in locating the anatomy of the primary track. MRI scanning has proven particularly useful in patients with doubtful fistulas. It correctly identifies sepsis without fistulas, scar tissue alone, and blind tracks with no internal opening, thereby preventing unnecessary surgical exploration. MRI is also particularly useful in defining horseshoe fistulas but may miss internal openings because imaging of the intersphincteric space is not as good as with anal ultrasound. It may be useful to involve a single specialized radiologist to deal with this topic. Despite its excellent accuracy, MRI of perianal fistulas has several drawbacks as it is rather expensive and time-consuming and cannot be performed in patients with a metal implant or a pacemaker.

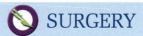

SURGERY

Principles

The principles of treatment are quite simple: to define the anatomy of the fistula track and its secondary extensions, to drain any coexisting pus, and then to provide definitive treatment by laying open, excision, or placement of a seton through the fistula track if it enters below the anorectal ring. If, on the other hand, the fistula lies outside the somatic cylinder and above the anorectal ring, the fistula track should be excised or defined with a seton and the defect in the gut may be closed.

Intersphincteric Fistulas

Intersphincteric fistulas can be readily treated with minimal morbidity or complication by merely laying open the fistula track into the anal canal. Only the distal part of the internal anal sphincter is divided. Subsequent incontinence for solid stool is rare, since the external anal sphincter remains intact. However, the permanent defect in the internal anal sphincter might result in soiling and incontinence for gas or liquid stool. The reported incidence for these "minor" continence disturbances varies between 8% and 50% (10). A simple low track fistula is also laid open or excised and in doing so, the internal sphincter is divided or partially excised. In case of a high blind track fistula, the internal sphincter is divided to the full height of the blind track. Failure to identify the upper extension may predispose to recurrence. A high track opening into the rectum is found by passing a probe along the fistula until an opening well above the anorectal ring becomes apparent. The complete fistula can be excised or laid open in the intersphincteric tract with impunity. High track fistulas with a perineal opening are quite uncommon. Pus emerges through the anal crypt and a probe usually only passes upward. The lower fibers of the internal sphincter should be opened in the line of the fistula. A failure to eradicate the glandular tissue at the level of the dentate line would predispose to recurrence. A track lying in the intersphincteric plane due to pelvic extrarectal disease should be treated by eradication by resection of the extrarectal disease and drainage of the pelvic sepsis. The intersphincteric fistula component merely requires gentle curettage and insertion of a drain.

Transsphincteric Fistula

The functional results after successful conventional fistula surgery for transsphincteric fistulas are inferior to those observed in patients with all other types of fistula, including the rare suprasphincteric and extrasphincteric fistulas, as well as the intersphincteric type. Soiling is more common. Recent evidence suggests that internal sphincter preservation is more important than was previously recognized (5). Four principal techniques are available for the management of mid or high transsphincteric fistula. The first is fistulotomy, still the most widely practiced technique. The track is merely laid open; since the fistula does not lie above the external sphincter or traverse the puborectalis, fecal incontinence is rare, but minor defects of control and soiling are reported in almost one-third of patients. The second method is seton fistulotomy. An inert material like a (doubled) vessel loop or a prolene thread is passed through the fistula and tied so that the sphincters are divided slowly over 1–4 weeks or even longer, in the belief that fibrosis occurs during division of the lower fibers of the sphincter, thereby preserving function. Recent results suggest rather low rates of recurrence and variable rates of impaired continence (5). The third approach is to excise the fistula track so that the lower part of the external sphincter, and if possible the internal sphincter, is preserved and the anal defect closed either directly or by an advancement flap of the anorectum. A fourth approach, used exclusively for high fistulas, has been laying open and total sphincter reconstruction, usually with a covering stoma. Fortunately, most transsphincteric fistulas cross at a low level so that laying open the fistula results in division of only the lower portion of the internal and external anal sphincters. If the track crosses at a higher level, the track itself may be excised, and the internal defect closed. Alternatively, a seton may be inserted. A high blind track fistula is potentially dangerous, particularly if complicated by a supralevator abscess fed by the high blind track. The abscess should never be opened into the rectum or else an extrasphincteric fistula will result. It is crucial, therefore, to identify the transsphincteric component. The primary and secondary tracks should be excised, or laid open. It is not always necessary to divide the lower fibers of the external sphincter, particularly if a seton is used for the primary track. The danger of this particular fistula is that probing may result in iatrogenic damage of the rectum.

Suprasphincteric Fistula

Fistulas of this type are usually due to an intersphincteric track with a blind upper component, complicated by an abscess, which bursts or, more commonly, is drained through the levator ani into the ischiorectal fossa. Once the track is correctly identified, the track lying lateral to the external sphincter is resected and the defect in the levator ani closed so that the fistula is converted into its original intersphincteric component. The residual fistula can then be laid open as a secondary procedure. The use of a seton is not generally advised for these fistulas. Another approach is to excise the track, using a mucosal advancement procedure to close the internal opening (5).

Extrasphincteric Fistula

Extrasphincteric fistulas may be iatrogenic, associated with rectal trauma, or occur as a complication of inflammatory bowel disease or secondary to pelvic sepsis. Most extrasphincteric fistulas not caused by Crohn's disease can be successfully treated by excision and closure of the rectal defect using an anorectal advancement flap. There is hardly any indication for mere fistulotomy or fistulectomy (5).

Horseshoe Fistula

Horseshoe fistula can be intersphincteric or transsphincteric. It is called so because it is composed of multiple external openings joined by a subcutaneous U- or horseshoe-shaped communication. The arms of the U are directed anteriorly, and the internal opening is in the posterior midline. Rarely, a horseshoe fistula presents with the opposite configuration; that is, the internal opening is in the anterior midline, and the arms of the U are directed posteriorly. Treatment of this condition has evolved to be much less radical than has often been described. The classic procedure required identification of the tracts and internal opening, and unroofing or excision of each of them (Figs. 6.6–6.10). This inevitably resulted in a huge, gaping wound, which required a prolonged healing time. Disability after this operation can last for many months. A conservative approach limiting the number and extent of incisions has been described. The internal opening is excised and adequate external drainage established. After the removal of the internal opening, the external openings will close. The deep postanal space must be entered, curetted, and irrigated if the fistula is transsphincteric. This involves incision of both

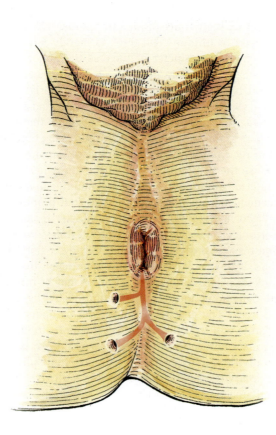

Figure 6.6 Horseshoe fistula, three external openings posterior to the anal verge.

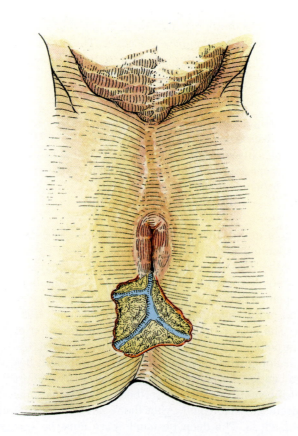

Figure 6.7 Laying open the fistula tracks with minimal damage of the sphincter muscles.

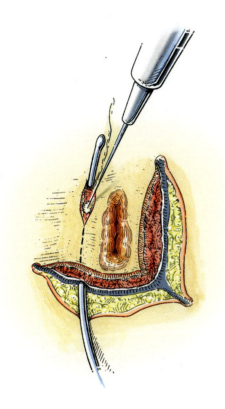

Figure 6.8 Laying open of a complex transsphincteric fistula over fistula probe; anterior horseshoe extension being laid open.

the internal sphincter and a portion of the external sphincter. It is then necessary only to unroof the external openings, curette the tracts, and drain the wound. Iodoform gauze may be used to pack the cut edges of the deep postanal space, and a dressing is applied. When the fistula is approached in this way, healing is rapid, and the risk of functional impairment to the anus from scarring and deformity is lessoned. Special care is necessary in the management of the rare anterior horseshoe fistula in women. There is no support from the puborectalis; there may have been previous anterior sphincter damage after deliveries, and division of the external sphincter will result in incontinence. Many authors therefore recommend the use of a seton for such lesions or the use of advancement flaps to preserve function.

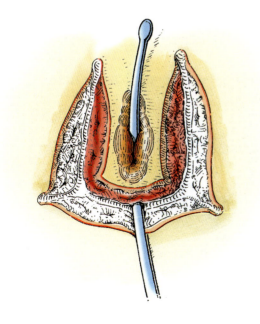

Figure 6.9 Identification of the internal opening of the horseshoe fistula.

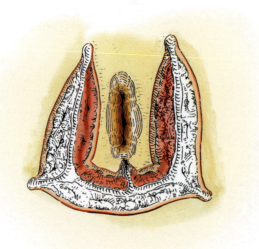

Figure 6.10 Internal opening being laid open with minimal division of sphincter muscles.

Principles of Surgery

Although it is quite impossible to assess an anal fistula with stool being present in the lower rectum, a full mechanical bowel preparation is rarely necessary. The patient may be admitted on the day of surgery, in an elective setting, and a special operating room (OR) designated for septic operations may be established. If done in the regular OR, cases like anal fistulas are placed toward the end of the operating list only after non-septic operations have been handled before. The patient is kept on clear liquids the day before surgery and a disposable enema is administered upon arrival in the hospital. General anesthesia is preferable since the duration of surgery is variable and extensive exploration may be needed to explore the track, also to facilitate accurate identification of the anorectal ring in relation to the fistula.

In our institution, a lithotomy position is routine. Especially for posterior fistulas, this position allows best access. In rare cases of anteriorly located fistulas, we have also used a prone jackknife position permitting an easier approach. A headlamp should at least be available in the OR, however, is not used in the majority of cases. A special little tray is placed under the buttocks for the placement of instruments. Hemostasis must be secured in each single case. Therefore, a weak adrenaline–saline solution may be used to infiltrate the submucosal and intersphincteric planes. A self-retaining intra-anal speculum and a wide selection of fistula probes should also be available (Figs. 6.11 and 6.12). If bleeding is encountered during excision of the fistula track, the cavity may be packed with a gauze swab soaked in adrenaline.

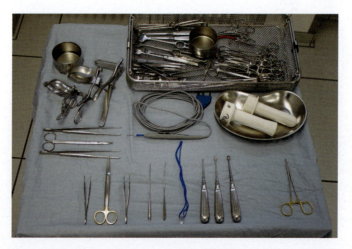

Figure 6.11 Set of instruments for initial operation of anal fistula in the operating room (OR) under general anesthesia.

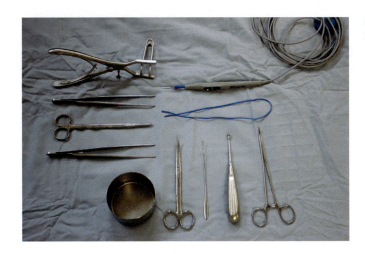

Figure 6.12 Set of instruments for revision in a staged procedure.

A fistula track should not always be identified and laid open at the time of draining an anorectal abscess. Primary fistulotomy, during drainage of an anorectal abscess, may lead to an increased functional disturbance compared with fistulotomy as a second-stage procedure. If easily feasible, it should be recognized if a fistula track is present at all, in cases with unclear involvement of the sphincter muscles, a seton may be placed. The patient will be readmitted to the hospital after 2 weeks for another staged exploration under anesthesia. Depending on the local situation, a fistulotomy may be performed then, or only after further revisional examinations in 2-weekly intervals until final fistulotomy. During the 2-weekly intervals, the patient is normally seen once in our proctologic outpatient unit.

Surgical Techniques

Fistulotomy

Laying open techniques are widely practiced for superficial fistulas entering deep through the anus and traversing only the lower fibers of the external sphincter muscles. Once the course of the fistula has been accurately located, a blunt bendable probe is passed along the track into the anus (Fig. 6.13). The roof of the track is laid open using a scalpel blade or a cutting diathermy current. Healthy granulating tissue should be present throughout the length of the fistula track. Normally, the fistula is curetted if there is any concern about the etiology, and material is sent for culture and histological examinations. The wound edges are excised to encourage healing in an inside-to-outside direction (Fig. 6.14). Hemostasis is secured and a dressing is applied to the wound.

Alternatively, the fistula track or parts of it may be excised after the track has been laid open. The disadvantages of this approach are that the wound is deeper, there is a greater risk of excising sphincter muscle, and healing may be delayed. Furthermore, the material obtained for histological examination is generally poor and blind tracks may be missed.

Fistulectomy

A careful preoperative assessment is required to determine the anatomy of the fistula, but the passage of probes is not mandatory. In fact, one of the arguments for performing fistulectomy is that false passages are not created by probing the track. The external opening is grasped with tissue forceps or stay sutures. It is advisable to commence the dissection posteriorly if the lithotomy position is used, since bleeding from anterior wounds may compromise assessment around a more posterior field. After dividing the skin around the external opening, the tissues around the fistula may be infiltrated with a weak adrenaline–saline solution to reduce bleeding. Homeostasis must be meticulous

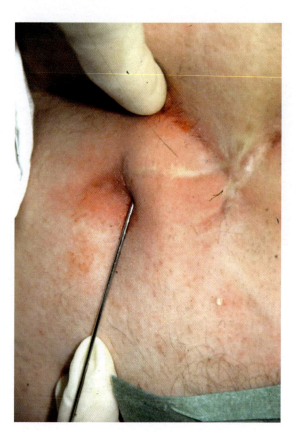

Figure 6.13 Probing of an anal fistula recurrence.

Figure 6.14 Fistulotomy of a low transsphincteric fistula.

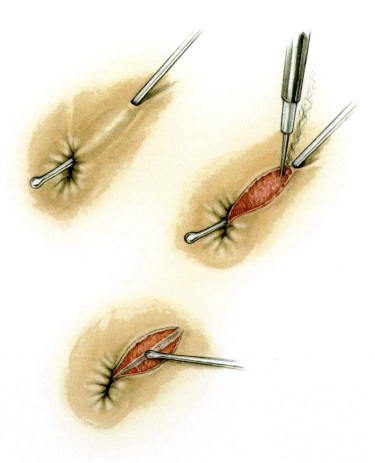

throughout the operation. Only in this way can the appearance of granulation tissue in the wound be transected with certainty, indicating that a side track, or the fistula itself, has been divided. After dividing the skin, fine scissors are used to core out the surrounding tissues, leaving the granulating track and its surrounding fibrous tissues, which is withdrawn by gentle traction. If a side track is inadvertently divided, it is advisable to trace the secondary extension before proceeding further with the main fistula. Blind tracks may extend up or even through the ischiorectal fossa and may be difficult to trace to their extremity unless an assistant retracts the surrounding tissues. In this way, the peripheral components of the fistula can be precisely defined and the granulation tissue excised. As the dissection proceeds toward the anus, sufficient overlying skin and fascia must be divided to gain access to the sphincter. This maneuver allows the precise relationship of the fistula to the sphincter to be identified. Before running any risk of sphincter damage, a decision can then be made as to how best to proceed, depending upon the course of the track and the site of the internal opening. If there is any uncertainty, a flap of mucosa and internal sphincter may be raised around the internal opening at the anal verge to display the anatomy and, if necessary, allow closure of the defect by advancement flap to preserve the muscles of continence. No striated muscle should be divided until the precise anatomy has been displayed. If the fistula occupies a low transsphincteric position, the overlying external anal sphincter may be divided without compromising continence. If a tunnel is left after coring out the fistula, this may be laid open once it has been established how much sphincter can safely be divided. If, on the other hand, it proves to be a mid or high transsphincteric fistula, or the patient is elderly, or there is a history of obstetric trauma, or preoperative manometry indicates poor anal function, the fistula track can merely be cored out from the muscle and then either rerouted into the intersphincteric plane, or excised, leaving the defect in the sphincter to heal by secondary intention; alternatively, it may be closed by suture or by raising an advancement flap (Figs. 6.15–6.18).

The coring out technique is particularly useful for suprasphincteric fistulas, the intersphincteric portion of which may be left in situ once the defect in the levator is closed. The fistula may then be removed or laid open as a secondary procedure. If the track is extrasphincteric, it may be completely excised, leaving only a small defect in the levator ani and rectal wall, which may be closed either by direct suture of the levator, rectal muscle, and mucosa, or obliquely, to prevent two suture lines from overlying each other, using the anorectal flap technique. If, on the other hand, the track is horseshoe in configuration, a rotating flap may be more convenient. One of the great advantages of fistulectomy is that no muscle is divided until the precise anatomical

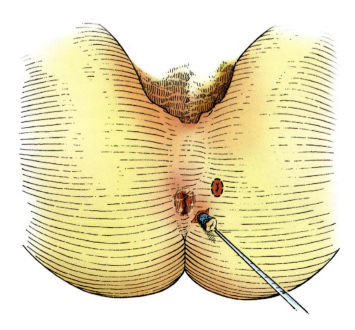

Figure 6.15 Fistulectomy. Two openings are seen, excision of a small skin area around the openings, which is pulled outside.

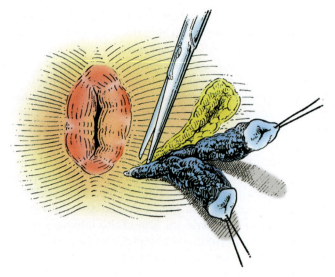

Figure 6.16 Dissection of both fistula tracks using scissors.

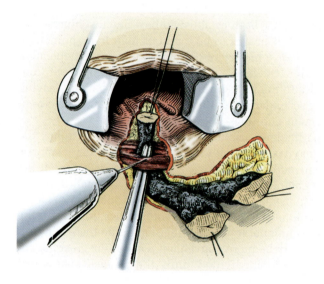

Figure 6.17 Identification of the internal opening and careful dissection and preservation of the external sphincter muscle.

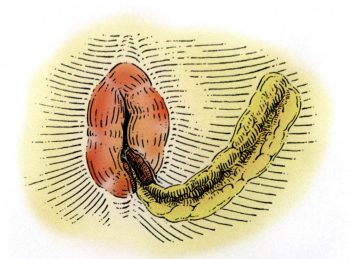

Figure 6.18 Completion of low-lying fistulectomy.

relationship of the track to the sphincters is ascertained with confidence. If doubt still exists, the fistula may be dissected out as it penetrates the muscle without jeopardizing the function. An additional advantage is that material is available for histology (5).

Use of Setons and Staged Fistulotomy

It is remarkable that, in the literature, setons have been used by surgeons for a large variety of purposes, such as to drain pus, to mark a fistula track, to allow staged division, or to deliberately cut through the sphincters (5).

Few would argue against the use of setons as a method of marking a fistula track—this is their first main use. They may therefore aid in identification of the track during excision. Indeed, during excision of a fistula, a single thread, with a bead on the end to act as a means of traction, may be passed along the track during excision of a transsphincteric fistula.

A second role of a seton is merely to act as a drain, in the belief that control of sepsis may sometimes achieve spontaneous healing. This is especially true in Crohn's disease where conventional surgical treatment may be contraindicated for fear of nonhealing or incontinence. Likewise, in cryptoglandular fistula, the loose seton may be used simply to drain pus prior to definitive treatment.

A third approach is to tie a seton loosely around the fistula track to stimulate fibrosis. It is thus argued that after 2, 4, or 6 weeks or even later, the intervening muscle can be divided without risk because the fibrous reaction prevents retraction of the cut ends. Staged fistulotomy is a simple option, but should be used only if there appears to be sufficient muscle above the level of the seton. After an interval of a few weeks, the primary track is laid open by division of muscle within the seton. At the same time, the wound should be shaped if necessary to allow any residual secondary tracks to heal. Careful analysis of the functional results has shown that there is no difference between delayed division of sphincter muscle after application of a seton compared with fistulotomy as an initial procedure. This approach may prolong therapy because of repeated operations and hospital admissions. In our own experience, this approach has been used frequently with very good results (Figs. 6.19–6.22).

Among female patients with a high anterior transsphincteric fistula, the use of a seton is regarded as optimum treatment. Some surgeons, however, will prefer fistulectomy and advancement flap or even a direct division and sphincter repair in this situation. A second situation where setons have been advised is for suprasphincteric or extrasphincteric fistulas (5).

Crohn's Disease

Lesions in patients with Crohn's disease tend to be chronic, indurated, and cyanotic, but are often painless unless an abscess is present. They do not stick to the regular anatomic spaces (Fig. 6.23). Skin irritation is frequently noted, which may be caused by diarrhea rather than by intrinsic disease of the anus. The fistula may be low-lying, with an internal opening at the level of the crypt. More commonly, however, the fistula is associated with a deep ulcer, and the internal opening may either be inapparent or found in a supralevator location.

The presence or absence of symptoms is the important criterion that determines therapy. Many individuals with fistulas are relatively asymptomatic; approximately 25% of patients in one series did not even require specific treatment. It has been suggested that metronidazole can produce symptomatic improvement in some patients with perianal disease, but no irrefutable proof indicates that fistulas are likely to close with continued therapy. When anal fistula occurs as a complication of the condition, it is important to distinguish between anal Crohn's disease with fistula, and Crohn's disease of the intestinal tract and a coincidental fistula-in-ano. This distinction is critical, because the fistula procedure can be performed with relative safety in a patient whose abdominal condition is quiescent. A definitive fistula operation that is undertaken in the presence of active inflammatory bowel disease, however, is hazardous. The resulting wound may be a greater management problem than was the original condition. Another

Figure 6.19 Insertion of a seton.

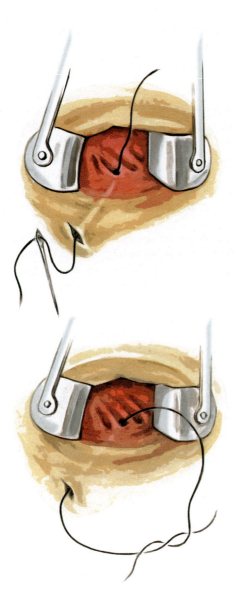

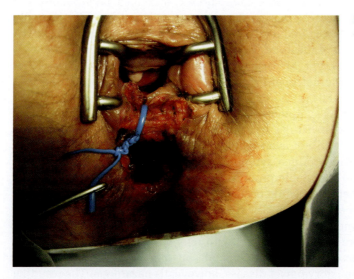

Figure 6.20 The seton being tied after fistulotomy.

COMPLICATIONS

Fistulotomy and fistulectomy are the most frequently used surgical techniques for anal fistula, also because of their low rates of complications and recurrences. In dependence on the amount of sphincter muscles transected, however, continence may be impaired, in a range from a slight transitory disorder to a permanent dysfunction (6). Patients with complicated fistulas, high openings, anterior openings, and fistula extensions have been found to be at higher risk. In the treatment of complicated fistulas and those with high openings, more muscle is divided, thus decreasing anal pressure. Some posterior fistula wounds have been associated with higher rates of incontinence because of their more circuitous routes. Drainage of extensions may accidentally damage small nerves and create more scar tissue around the anorectum. If the edges of the fistulotomy wound do not approximate precisely, the anus may be unable to close properly, resulting in intermittent leakage of gas and stool. In addition to these factors, impaired continence was associated with increasing age and female gender. Vaginal delivery may be a reason for the latter by anal sphincter disruption or traction injury to the pudendal nerves (11). Preexisting sphincter weakness, previous fistula surgery, surgery at multiple locations of the sphincter, scar formation, or even scar deformities are factors of high risk. Sphincter manometry before surgery is advisable in such cases. Functional problems are rare after isolated lesions of the internal sphincter or may at least not be realized by the patient. Typical signs would be temporary soiling or flatus. Symptoms like stress defecation in the consequence of impaired coordination of the rectal ampulla and the sphincter muscles are stated only when taking a detailed history of the patient.

Recurrences may be due to a failure to identify a primary opening or recognize lateral or upward extensions of a fistula. Inability to locate the primary opening may imply a circuitous tract, spontaneous closure of the primary opening, or a microscopic opening. Diligent postoperative care can also reduce recurrence rates by avoiding bridging and pocketing of the wound. Epithelialization of the fistula tract from internal or external openings rather than chronic infection of an anal gland has also been suggested as the cause of a persistent anal fistula.

Early postoperative complications that have been reported after fistula surgery include urinary retention, hemorrhage, fecal impaction, and thrombosed external hemorrhoids, which were found to occur in less than 6% of cases; later complications such as pain, bleeding, pruritus, and poor wound healing have been reported in 9% of patients. Anal stenosis may occur and is usually the result of loose stools allowing healing of the anal canal by scar contracture (11).

RESULTS

The three primary criteria for determining success or failure of fistula surgery are recurrence, delayed healing, and incontinence. If more sphincter is divided, it takes longer to heal, and the greater is the likelihood of recurrence and risk of fecal soiling (2). The internal opening has to be identified and adequately excised to avoid recurrence. Generally, recurrence rates vary from 4% to 10%, with missed internal openings at the initial surgery accounting for most such recurrences. When there is doubt regarding the competence of the sphincter, it is wise to divide it into stages at successive operations.

In a recent review of 21 randomized controlled trials (7) evaluating fistulotomy versus fistulectomy and other techniques, it was found that marsupialization after fistulotomy reduced bleeding and allowed for faster healing. Results from small trials suggested flap repair to be no worse than fistulotomy in terms of healing rates. Flap repair combined with fibrin glue treatment of fistulas increased failure rates.

In a systematic Cochrane review, Malik et al. (8) compared outcome after fistula surgery with drainage of perianal abscess with drainage alone. The primary outcomes were recurrent or persistent abscess/fistula, which may require repeat surgery and short-term and long-term incontinence. Secondary outcomes were duration of hospitalization, duration of wound healing, postoperative pain, and quality of life scores. For dichotomous variables, relative risks and their confidence intervals were calculated. Six trials were identified, involving 479 subjects. Meta-analysis showed a significant reduction in recurrence, persistent abscess/fistula, or repeat surgery in favor of fistula surgery at the time of abscess incision and drainage (RR = 0.13, 95% confidence interval of RR = 0.07–0.24). Transient manometric reduction in anal sphincter pressures, without clinical incontinence, occurred after treatment of low fistulae with abscess drainage. Incontinence at 1 year following drainage with fistula surgery was not statistically significant (pooled RR = 3.06, 95% confidence interval RR = 0.7–13.45) with heterogeneity demonstrable between the trials (P = 0.14). It was concluded that fistula surgery with abscess drainage significantly reduced the recurrence or persistence of abscess and fistula or the need for repeat surgery. There was no statistically significant evidence of incontinence following fistula surgery with abscess drainage.

 # CONCLUSIONS

A very thorough assessment of all anorectal fistulas and excision of almost all fistula tracks by primarily fistulotomy or secondarily fistulectomy is advisable. This way, also lateral extensions and high tracks may be identified more accurately. A potentially present extrasphincteric component of the fistula has to be removed; the site at which the track traverses or bypasses the sphincters needs to be explored. Intersphincteric fistulas are excised and the tracks laid open. Most transsphincteric fistulas and fistulas with unclear relation to the sphincter muscles at primary surgery are managed using a cutting seton. The patients are readmitted every 2 weeks until a staged fistulotomy is carried out.

References

1. Cirocco WC, Reilly JC. Challenging the predictive accuracy of Goodsall's rule for anal fistulas. *Dis Colon Rectum* 1992;35: 537–42.
2. Corman ML, Allison SI, Kuehne JP. Handbook of Colon and Rectal Surgery. Philadelphia: Lippincott, Williams & Wilkins, 2002:161–83.
3. Gordon PH. High anal fistula. In: Fielding LP, Goldberg SM (eds.). Surgery of the Colon, Rectum and Anus. Oxford: Butterworth-Heinemann, 1988:828–40.
4. Hawley PR. Low anal fistula. In: Fielding LP, Goldberg SM (eds.). Surgery of the Colon, Rectum and Anus. Oxford: Butterworth-Heinemann, 1988:814–27.
5. Keighley MRB, Williams NS. Surgery of the Anus, Rectum and Colon. London: WB Saunders, 1997:487–538.
6. Lange J, Mölle B, Girona J. Chirurgische Proktologie. Heidelberg: Springer, 2006:217–76.
7. Malik AI, Nelson RL. Surgical management of anal fistulae: a systematic review. *Colorectal Dis* 2008;5:420–30.
8. Malik AI, Nelson RL, Tou S. Incision and drainage of perianal abscess with or without treatment of anal fistula. *Cochrane Database Syst Rev* 2010;7, DOI:10.1002/14651858.CD006827. pub2.
9. Phillips RKS, Lunniss PJ. Anorectal sepsis. In: Nicholls RJ, Dozois RR (eds.). Surgery of the Colon and Rectum. New York: Churchill Livingstone, 1997:255–84.
10. Schouten WR. Abscess, Fistula. In: Herold A, Lehur PA, Matzel KE, O'Connell PR (eds.). *Coloproctology*. Berlin: Springer, 2008: 53–62.
11. Vasilevsky CA, Gordon PH. Benign anorectal: abscess and fistula. In: Wolff BG, Fleshman JW, Beck DE, Pemberton JH, Wexner SD (eds.). The ASCRS Textbook of Colon and Rectal Surgery. New York: Springer, 2007:192–14.

7 Anal Fistula Plug

Bruce W. Robb and Marc A. Singer

INDICATIONS/CONTRAINDICATIONS

Treatment of anal fistula can be a frustrating problem for both the patient and the surgeon. While simple fistulas are generally very effectively treated with fistulotomy, the treatment of complex fistula has proven more difficult. Fistulotomy or cutting seton is an effective treatment for fistula closure, but may cause fecal incontinence. The search for effective treatments that do not compromise continence has led to the use of fibrin glue, the ligation of the intersphincteric fistula tract (LIFT), endorectal advancement flaps, and the use of absorbable materials as anal fistula plugs. Initial use of anal fistula plugs was conceived and described by Brad Sklow. Inspired by a case report by Schultz and coworkers in the *Journal of the American College of Surgeons*, which described the use of a tightly rolled sheet of porcine small intestine submucosa placed in an enterocutaneous fistula tract as a plug. This technique was modified for anal fistula. Subsequently, a specially designed plug was fashioned by Cook Medical Inc. (Surgisis® Anal Fistula Plug™). Conceptually simple, anal fistula plugs provide a matrix upon which tissue growth may occur leading to fistula closure with no theoretical risk to continence.

Indications

1. Transsphincteric fistula
2. Intersphincteric fistula (when fistulotomy is contraindicated)

Contraindications

1. Persistent abscess or infection
2. Intersphincteric fistula (when no contraindication to fistulotomy exists)
3. Inability to identify the internal and external openings
4. Allergy to plug material

Currently, there are two commercially available fistula plugs approved by the FDA: Cook Surgisis® AFP™ Anal Fistula Plug (Cook Surgical Inc., Bloomington, IN) and the Gore® Bio-A® Fistula Plug (a new product from W.L. Gore Corporation, Newark, DE). They vary in both design and material from which they are constructed.

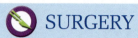 PREOPERATIVE PLANNING

Patients should have undergone previous surgical drainage of the perirectal abscess and have had a draining seton placed 6–12 weeks in advance of fistula plug placement. A plug may be placed primarily only in those patients who have no evidence of infection and a well-formed fistula tract. A single dose of a broad-spectrum preoperative antibiotic is recommended. No consensus about bowel preparation exists, with some authors advocating complete mechanical preparations and others simply administering an enema on the morning of the procedure. It should be stressed that there should be no active infection present at the time of surgery and the patients have a well-formed tract.

SURGERY

The anal fistula plug has been widely adopted for complex anal fistula surgery because of its favorable safety profile with regards to continence and purported technical ease. There have been wide variations in published outcomes with those authors who are most successful attributing the differences to patient selection and technical details. In 2007, a group of surgeons experienced in the use of the Surgisis® Anal Fistula Plug™ met and issued a set of recommendations for its most effective use.

Positioning

Patient positioning and anesthesia can be performed according to the surgeon's preference for anorectal procedures. Positioning is generally easily accomplished with patients sedated in the prone jack-knife position with either a pudendal nerve block or a spinal anesthetic. However, many published series employ general anesthesia and the lithotomy position.

Technique

The previously placed draining seton is noted (Fig. 7.1). The perineum and anal canal are again inspected to confirm that all internal and external openings have been identified. A thorough inspection should also verify that there is no active infection prior to preparing the fistula plug. A 2-0 suture is secured to the seton. The seton is then cut and pulled out of the fistula so that the suture now crosses the fistula leaving the needle on the "internal opening" side of the fistula (Fig. 7.2). The fistula tract is then irrigated with dilute hydrogen peroxide using an angiocatheter or gently debrided with a cytobrush or small curettes (Figs. 7.3 and 7.4). Finally, the tract is irrigated with saline. The plugs require rehydration fully submerged in sterile saline for no more than 2 minutes. Placement of a surgical instrument such a hemostat over the plug in a bowel of saline will keep the material submerged. The previously placed suture is secured to the plug material on the "external opening" side of the plug. The suture is then used to draw the plug material through the fistula tract. The plug is then secured at the internal opening. The plug is secured with an absorbable suture such as a 2-0 coated polyglycolic acid, anchoring it to the sphincter complex and covering the plug. Two sutures placed at right angles to one another are recommended. These sutures are placed through the sphincter muscle and then separately through the plug so as to "bury" the plug. If necessary, the plug is trimmed at this time. Some surgeons choose to create small mucosal flaps to better cover the plug at the internal opening. The Gore® Bio-A® Fistula Plug is designed to be sized to the fistula tract with removable limbs attached to a central disk. Placement is similar to that of the Surgisis® Anal Fistula Plug™ in that the seton is used to bring a suture through the tract, which is then secured to the "sized" plug that has been previously wetted. The suture should be placed approximately 3 mm from the ends of the plug so as to have enough strength to pull the plug into the tract but not to fold over too much and make it difficult to pull into the tract (Figs. 7.5 and 7.6). It is easier to draw the material through the tract if the limbs are

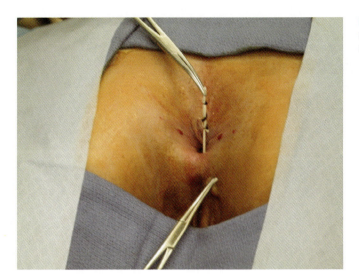

Figure 7.1 The previously placed seton is cut. Careful inspection shows no inflammation or infection.

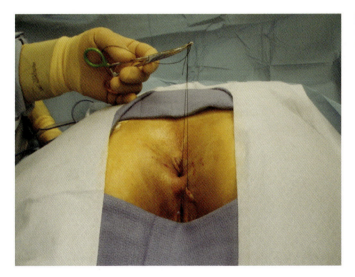

Figure 7.2 The suture material is now passed through the fistula tract.

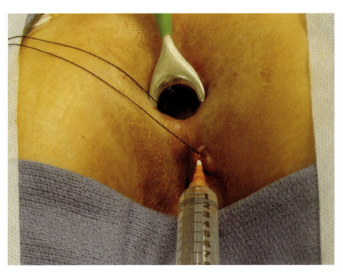

Figure 7.3 The tract is irrigated with hydrogen peroxide.

Part II: Anal Fistula

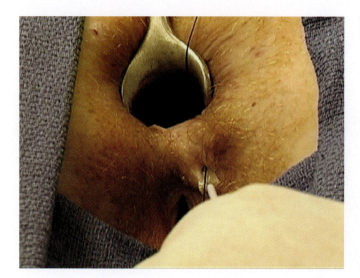

Figure 7.4 The tract is gently debrided with a soft brush.

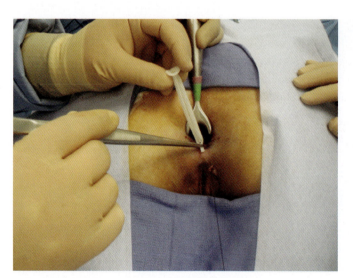

Figure 7.5 The "sized" plug is passed from the internal to the external opening.

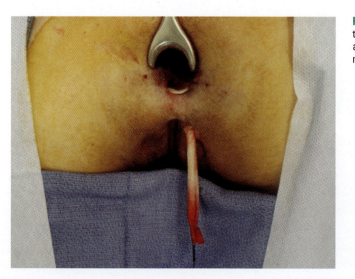

Figure 7.6 The plug is pulled through the fistula so that the attached disc sits flat on the mucosa or in a mucosal "pocket."

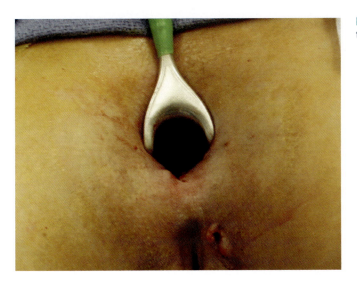

Figure 7.7 The disc is secured and the external opening left open.

gently twisted. The Gore® Bio-A® Fistula Plug is secured with a 2-0 coated polyglycolic acid suture on a UR needle using the attached disk with a minimum of three sutures to the surrounding tissues. The disk can be buried in a mucosal pocket or simply sutured securely to the surrounding tissue per the surgeon's preference. The excess material is trimmed at the skin. In both cases, the external opening is either left open or loosely closed without fixing the plug at the external opening (Fig. 7.7).

Identify internal and external openings.
Confirm absence of active infection.
Gently debride the tract.
Place the plug within the tract.
Secure the plug to the internal opening.
Leave external opening wide open to allow for drainage

 POSTOPERATIVE MANAGEMENT

Postoperative care is in the outpatient setting. Patients are encouraged to avoid any strenuous activity for 2 weeks. Many surgeons use 10% metronidazole ointment. Metronidazole ointment is available as a commercial preparation, but can be easily and economically compounded by most hospital pharmacies in white petrolatum and supplied to the patient. Patients should be counseled that they may have persistent drainage for several months after the procedure. They should also be told to expect that there may be plug material extrusion. The consensus statement recommended no dietary restrictions or bowel regimen other than the prevention of constipation. Failure is defined as technical if there is extrusion of the plug material within 1 week of surgery. A minimum of 3 months is suggested prior to considering the fistula plug attempt to be a failure.

 COMPLICATIONS

Complications of anal fistula plug surgery encompass the full range of complications for anorectal surgery, but are thankfully rare. The most frequent complication other than failure to close the fistula tract is abscess. The incidence of which has been highly variable but generally infrequent. Infectious complications are managed with antibiotics or may at times require drainage procedures either in the office or in the operating room. This may require replacement of the seton or simple drainage of the external opening with either packing or a drainage catheter. Pain is generally minimal and easily managed

TABLE 7.1	Published Results for the Use of Anal Fistula Plug		
Author	**Total patients (*n*)**	**Fistula closure (%)**	**Follow-up (mo)**
Champagne et al.	46	83	12
O'Connor et al.	20	80	10
van Koperen et al.	17	41	7
Lawes et al.	17	24	7
Ky et al.	37	55	12
Christoforidis et al.	47	43	5
Safar et al.	35	14	4
Wang et al.	29	34	9
Schwander et al.	60	62	12
Ellis et al.	63	81	>12
van Koperen et al.	31	29	11

with oral narcotics. Plug extrusion or fall out has frequently been listed among the complications or technical failures of these procedures.

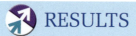 RESULTS

The published success of fistula plug surgery has been highly variable among different groups (see Table 7.1). While initial enthusiasm has subsequently been tempered, and initial success rates have not been duplicated, anorectal fistula plugs do appear to be effective in some individuals. The great variation in results is in part due to variations in patient selection. Some series have included patients who have had multiple prior attempts at closure and some only first attempts. Some series have had extrusion as a more frequent complication, which is more likely a technical failure or related to post-operative management. Infectious complications have been seen in up to one quarter of procedures in one series with expected poor overall results. Fistula tract length is not accounted for in most early studies and has been shown by McGee et al. to be predictive of successful closure by anal fistula plugs (see Table 7.2).

Most data have come from studies of the Surgisis® Anal Fistula Plug™. The only study to compare the two commercially available plugs by Buchberg et al. showed an improved procedural success rate for the Gore® Bio-A® Fistula Plug (54.5% vs. 12.5%) with the Surgisis® Anal Fistula Plug™. Longer-term studies of the Gore® Bio-A® Fistula Plug are in progress.

The anal fistula plug has been shown in one analysis by Adamina et al. to be cost-effective when compared with endorectal advancement flap even when conservative estimates of anal fistula plug effectiveness are employed with generous estimates of advancement flap of efficacy. This coupled with its low morbidity in almost all investigators use will likely ensure the continued use of anal fistula plugs for complex anal fistula.

TABLE 7.2	Longer Fistula Tract Length Predicts Closure with Anal Fistula Plug		
Author	**Total patients**	**Tract length (cm)**	**Fistula closure (%)**	**Follow-up (mo)**
McGee et al.	23	>4	61	24
	19	<4	21	24

CONCLUSIONS

Treatment of complex fistulas can be extremely frustrating for both patients and surgeons. Anal fistula plugs have been an extremely popular option because of their ease of use and good safety profiles. Although there is great variability among different groups in the published efficacy for the treatment of fistulas, their safety is generally not questioned. Anal fistula plugs provide one more option to surgeons for the treatment of complex anal fistulas.

Suggested Readings

Adamina M, Hoch JS, Burnstein MJ. To plug or not to plug: a cost-effectiveness analysis for complex anal fistula. *Surgery* 2010; 147:72–8.

Buchberg B, Masoomi H, Choi J, et al. A tale of two (Anal fistula) plugs: is there a difference in short-term outcomes? *Am Surg* 2010;76:1150–3.

Champagne BJ, O'Connor LM, Ferguson M, et al. Efficacy of anal fistula plug in closure of cryptoglandular fistulas: long-term follow-up. *Dis Colon Rectum* 2006;49:1817–21.

Christoforidis D, Etzioni DA, Goldberg SM, et al. Treatment of complex anal fistulas with the collagen fistula plug. *Dis Colon Rectum* 2008;51:1482–7.

Corman M, Abcarian H, Bailey HR, et al. The surgisis AFP anal fistula plug: report of a consensus conference. *Colorectal Dis* 2008;10:17–22.

Ellis CN, Rostas JW, Greiner FG. Long-term outcomes with the use of bioprosthetic plugs for the management of complex anal fistulas. *Dis Colon Rectum* 2010;53:798–802.

Ky AJ, Sylla P, Steinhagen R, et al. Collagen fistula plug for the treatment of anal fistulas. *Dis Colon Rectum* 2008;51:838–43.

Lawes DA, Efron JE, Abbas M, et al. Early experience with the bioabsorbable anal fistula plug. *World J Surg* 2008;32:1157–9.

McGee MF, Champagne BJ, Stulberg JJ, et al. Tract length predicts successful closure with anal fistula in cryptoglandular fistulas. *Dis Colon Rectum* 2010;53:1116–20.

O'Connor LM, Champagne BJ, Ferguson M, et al. Efficacy of anal fistula plug in closure of Crohn's anorectal fistulas. *Dis Colon Rectum* 2006;49:1569–73.

Robb BW, Vogler SA, Nussbaum MN, et al. Early experience using porcine small intestinal submucosa to repair fistula-in-ano. *Dis Colon Rectum* 2004;47:609.

Safar B, Jobanputra S, Sands D, et al. Anal fistula plug: initial experience and outcomes. *Dis Colon Rectum* 2009;52:248–52.

Schultz DJ, Brasel KJ, Spinelli KS, et al. Porcine small intestine submucosa as a treatment for enterocutaneous fistulas. *J Am Coll Surg* 2002;194(4):541–3.

Schwandner T, Roblick MH, Kierer W, et al. Surgical treatment of complex anal fistulas with the anal fistula plug: a prospective, multicenter study. *Dis Colon Rectum* 2009;52:1578–83.

van Koperen PJ, Bemelman WA, Gerhards MF, et al. The anal fistula plug treatment compared with the mucosal advancement flap for cryptoglandular high transsphincteric perianal fistula: a double-blinded multicenter randomized trial. *Dis Colon Rectum* 2011;54: 387–93.

van Koperen PJ, D'Hoore A, Wolthuis AM, et al. Anal fistula plug for closure of difficult anorectal fistula: a prospective study. *Dis Colon Rectum* 2007;50:2168–72.

Wang JY, Garcia-Aguilar J, Sternberg JA, et al. Treatment of transsphincteric anal fistulas: are fistula plugs an acceptable alternative? *Dis Colon Rectum* 2009;52:692–97.

Part II: Anal Fistula

8 Ligation of the Intersphincteric Fistula Tract (LIFT)

Husein Moloo, Joshua I. S. Bleier, and Stanley M. Goldberg

Introduction

The treatment of fistula-in-ano is difficult and there are a variety of treatment options. To approach fistula repair in a systematic manner, the anatomy must be accurately understood; Parks provides a useful anatomic classification (1). In addition, in a separate paper, he described patients who have fistulas whose treatment place them at higher risk of developing impairment of continence (2)—the term "complex" fistula is based on a modification of Parks classification (3).

Complex fistulas are defined as those that traverse >30% of the external sphincter (high transsphincteric, suprasphincteric, and extrasphincteric fistulas according to Parks (2)), are anterior in a female, have multiple tracks, are recurrent, in patients with pre-existing continence issues, irradiation, or Crohn's (3).

Historically, approaches to these fistulas were quite varied. Lay-open fistulotomy, while successful, results in incontinence due to destruction of significant portions of the sphincter complex. Sphincter-sparing approaches such as advancement flaps and core-out fistulectomies were morbid and have varying success. Current methods to treat these fistulas include the fistula plug, fibrin glue, cutting seton, and advancement flaps with varying rates of success and impact on continence (4–9). There is no consensus on the best approach to this difficult problem (3).

INDICATIONS/CONTRAINDICATIONS

The ligation of the intersphincteric fistula tract (LIFT) is a promising new sphincter-sparing procedure first described by Rojanasakul et al. in 2007 (10). The main concept in the LIFT procedure is identification of the intersphincteric fistula tract (in the intersphincteric groove) with its subsequent ligation. There is no division of the sphincter muscle, and theoretically, continence should be preserved. This technique has been used on low and high trans-sphincteric fistulas as well as suprasphincteric and extrasphincteric fistulas (10).

Our current indications for the surgery are

- low transsphincteric fistulas
- high transsphincteric fistulas
- potentially suprasphincteric/extrasphincteric fistulas where the tract traverses the intersphincteric space
- recurrent fistulas
- pre-existing continence issues
- multiple tracks

In our opinion, contraindications to this approach are few, but may include

- active perineal sepsis
- active inflammatory bowel disease
- malignancy

It is an evolving technique with literature that continues to mature; as such, these indications and contraindications will likely change. The experience thus far is that a LIFT can be used in almost any type of fistula as long as a portion of the tract traverses the intersphincteric space.

Certainly, there are fistulas that may be more difficult to treat with a higher failure rate including fistulas secondary to Crohn's or radiation and rectovaginal fistulas. As more studies are done, these questions will hopefully be answered.

 # PREOPERATIVE PLANNING

There is no need to preoperatively admit the patient to the hospital. An outpatient preparation with two disposable phosphate enemas per rectum or a full bowel preparation can be done at the surgeon's discretion. No preoperative antibiotic therapy is required. The authors opinion is that insertion of a seton for 8–12 weeks prior to performing the LIFT is useful for (1) eliminating the sepsis in the area and (2) for maturation of the fistula tract.

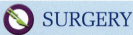 # SURGERY

Positioning

The patient is placed in the prone jackknife position; tape is used to retract the buttocks. The perianal area is then prepped and draped in order that the local anesthetic is infiltrated in as clean a field as possible. Local anesthetic with epinephrine is used to help decrease the amount of bleeding, which also helps with visualization.

Technique

1. Identification of the intersphincteric fistula tract:
   - Lockhart–Mummery probes can be used to traverse the fistula tract and identify the internal opening.
   - If a seton is not in place and there is difficulty finding the internal opening, we have found hydrogen peroxide to be helpful in aiding identification.
   - If the tract is long and curving doing a partial fistulotomy and following the granulation tissue to identify the tract up to the external sphincter can be done and

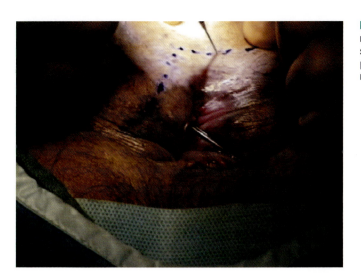

Figure 8.1 The skin incision is marked out overlying the intersphincteric groove. The fistula probe is exiting through the internal opening.

then it is usually easier to identify the internal opening once a shorter and more direct tract for the probe has been created.

2. A curvilinear skin incision is marked over the intersphincteric groove (Fig. 8.1):
   - The intersphincteric groove can be demonstrated by placing the sphincter on gentle stretch with operating anoscope and using the back of a dissecting forceps to demonstrate the groove.
   - A 3–4 cm incision is usually sufficient for exposure.
   - To facilitate visualization through the incision the Lone Star retractor™ (CooperSurgical, Inc., Trumbull, CT, USA) can be utilized.
3. Dissection of the fistula tract (Fig. 8.2):
   - A combination of blunt and sharp dissection can be used in the intersphincteric groove to identify the tract.
   - The semirigid fistula probe is used to guide the dissection.
   - If a seton has been used, the fistula tract is much easier to define.
   - A fine-tipped right angle dissector can also be used to get around the tract and delineate it more clearly.
4. Ligation and division of the fistula tract (Fig. 8.3):
   - To maintain identification of the tract once it is divided, ties may be placed on either side of the tract and a portion of the tract can be removed or the tract can simply be divided.
   - Ligation of the tract is then done on both sides, that is, at its entrance into the external and internal sphincter in the intersphincteric space.
   - The authors have found that suture ligation of the tract appears to be an effective method to achieve this. We have been using 2-0 Vicryl sutures to do this although other absorbable sutures are likely to be as effective.
   - Hydrogen peroxide can also be introduced through the external opening to ensure there has been a secure ligation on the external sphincter portion of the intersphincteric tract.
   - Hydrogen peroxide can be introduced into the interasphinteric space to ensure closure of the tract traversing the internal sphincter.
5. Addressing the fistula openings:
   - Presently, we do nothing to the internal except for some gentle curetting to make sure no infectious source is left.
   - The external opening is left open and usually widened; the tract is curetted to remove the granulation and epithelialized tissue
6. Closure:
   - The dissection cavity is irrigated.
   - The sphincters and cavity can be reapproximated with interrupted absorbable suture.

Figure 8.2 The fistula tract, with the probe through it for ease of identification, is dissected free in the intersphincteric space.

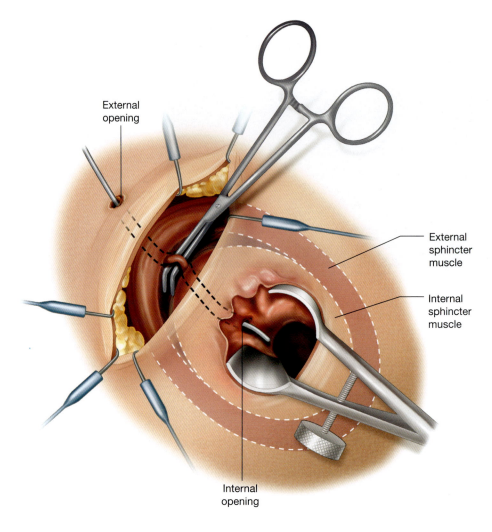

External opening

External sphincter muscle

Internal sphincter muscle

Internal opening

Figure 8.3 The probe is removed, and fistula tract is ligated and divided.

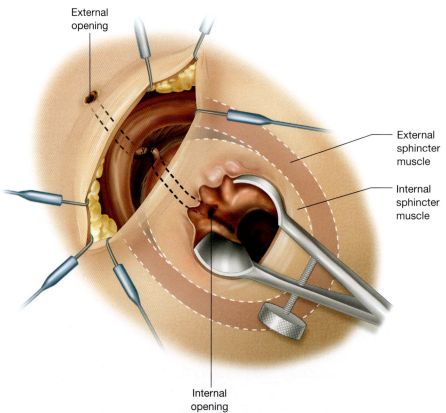

External opening

External sphincter muscle

Internal sphincter muscle

Internal opening

- The skin is then approximated with simple interrupted absorbable sutures. We prefer chromic.

 ## POSTOPERATIVE MANAGEMENT

The LIFT is performed as outpatient surgery and all patients in the authors' series have been sent home on the day of surgery. Appropriate analgesia for pain from the incision is needed usually consisting of oral acetaminophen, paracetamol, or opioid-based analgesics. An anti-inflammatory is also useful for attaining adequate pain control (over-the-counter ibuprofen™ is usually sufficient although cyclo-oxygenase inhibitors or other NSAIDs may be used).

Patients are usually seen approximately 1 month after the surgery and depending on the progress made, a second follow-up visit is scheduled at approximately the 3-month mark. The progress of the patient and surgeon preference will usually dictate when these visits take place.

 ## COMPLICATIONS

The experience with the LIFT continues to evolve. Thus far, we have not seen any major complications with a very low minor complication rate. In our first 39 patients, there were only two minor complications: a postoperative fissure in one individual and ongoing anal pain in another individual. In the latter patient, an examination under anesthesia was done and failed to identify any pathology to explain the ongoing pain.

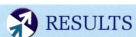 ## RESULTS

There are three groups that have now reported on this procedure. In the first paper by Rojanasakul et al., there was a 94% success rate reported on 18 patients with predominantly trans-sphincteric fistulas; there was one suprasphincteric and one extrasphincteric fistula at an unknown period of follow-up. Their experience continues to grow and in a personal communication with Dr. Rojanasakul, approximately 100 patients have now had a LIFT; the success rate has dropped to 85%.

A group from Malaysia (Shanwani et al.) recently presented their data at the annual meeting of the American Society of Colon and Rectal Surgeons in Hollywood, FL, 2009 (11). With a median follow-up of 9 months, they report a 82% success rate in 45 patients and a median operative time of 67.5 minutes.

In our series of 39 patients, we have a 60% success rate with a median follow-up of approximately 5 months. Although our success rate is lower, it is one with which we are quite encouraged since our patient population not only contains high trans-sphincteric, rectovaginal, horseshoe, and suprasphincteric fistulas but represents a population of patients who have had a median of two attempted repairs. Methods of previous repair include fibrin plugs, advancement flaps, fibrin glue, defunctioning stomas, and cutting setons.

None of the above series report any issues with continence nor did they utilize any standardized pre- or postoperative questionnaires to quantify fecal incontinence (12). All seem to uniformly agree, however, that this procedure is a simple technique that is easy to learn and theoretically is sphincter sparing. In our series and the Malaysian one, the LIFT procedure has been used successfully for recurrent fistulas after failed LIFT procedures (13).

One issue for consideration in the investigation of this new sphincter-sparing technique, and indeed, for all anorectal surgery in general is that perhaps we as surgeons should be presenting our patients with questionnaires to obtain an objective result of how issues have progressed (or regressed) with an intervention. For example, if an incontinence score was routinely used pre- and postoperatively, we would have a better understanding of how the surgery affects the patient's quality of life and continence.

Part II: Anal Fistula

Currently, there is growing individual and anecdotal experience with the LIFT technique. We are currently conducting a multicentered, randomized, controlled trial comparing the LIFT procedure to the fistula plug, another established sphincter-sparing approach to complex fistula. By using appropriate study design, uniform surgical technique, and standardized assessment methods for continence, quality of life, and follow-up, we hope to objectively describe the true efficacy of this procedure and establish it in the armamentarium of all surgeons who encounter fistula disease.

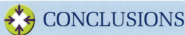 CONCLUSIONS

The LIFT procedure is a new technique that can be used to manage the difficult problem of fistula-in-ano. It is simple, inexpensive, quick, and has a success rate at least as good or better as all current sphincter-preserving options (based on early results). This success rate may change with longer follow-up and more studies; if the rate of closure remains anywhere near 40–60%, then this procedure would be a useful addition to the approach to complex anal fistulae. Importantly, the LIFT procedure does not burn any bridges with respect to using other types of approaches (including another LIFT) in patients who recur.

Acknowledgments

The authors wish to acknowledge Dr. Arun Rojanasakul and his team for their innovation, collegiality, and academic fellowship in the development and teaching of this new procedure.

Recommended References and Readings

1. Parks AG, Gordon PH, Hardcastle JD. A classification of fistula-in-ano. *Br J Surg* 1976;63(1):1–12.
2. Parks AG, Stitz RW. The treatment of high fistula-in-ano. *Dis Colon Rectum* 1976;19(6):487–99.
3. Whiteford MH, Kilkenny J III, Hyman N, et al. Practice parameters for the treatment of perianal abscess and fistula-in-ano (revised). *Dis Colon Rectum* 2005;48(7):1337–42.
4. Buchanan GN, Bartram CI, Phillips RK, et al. Efficacy of fibrin sealant in the management of complex anal fistula: a prospective trial. *Dis Colon Rectum* 2003;46(9):1167–74.
5. Christoforidis D, Etzioni DA, Goldberg SM, et al. Treatment of complex anal fistulas with the collagen fistula plug. *Dis Colon Rectum* 2008;51(10):1482–7.
6. van der Hagen SJ, Baeten CG, Soeters PB, van Gemert WG. Long-term outcome following mucosal advancement flap for high perianal fistulas and fistulotomy for low perianal fistulas: recurrent perianal fistulas: failure of treatment or recurrent patient disease? *Int J Colorectal Dis* 2006;21(8):784–90.
7. Lawes DA, Efron JE, Abbas M, Heppell J, Young-Fadok TM. Early experience with the bioabsorbable anal fistula plug. *World J Surg* 2008;32(6):1157–9.
8. Ortiz H, Marzo J. Endorectal flap advancement repair and fistulectomy for high trans-sphincteric and suprasphincteric fistulas. *Br J Surg* 2000;87(12):1680–3.
9. Sentovich SM. Fibrin glue for anal fistulas: long-term results. *Dis Colon Rectum* 2003;46(4):498–502.
10. Rojanasakul A, Pattanaarun J, Sahakitrungruang C, Tantiphlachiva K. Total anal sphincter saving technique for fistula-in-ano; the ligation of Intersphincteric fistula tract. *J Med Assoc Thai* 2007;90(3):581–6.
11. Shanwani A, Nor AM, Amri N. The Ligation of Intersphincteric Fistula Tract (LIFT) for Fistula-in-ano: Sphincter Saving Technique. ASCRS Meeting 2009, Hollywood, FL. Podium #S13, Abstract #580775, DCR (Diseases of Colon and Rectum) 2010;53(1):39–42.
12. Jorge JMN, Wexner S. Etiology and management of fecal incontinence. *Dis Colon Rectum* 1993;36:77–97.
13. Bleir JIS, Moloo H, Goldberg SM. Ligation of the Intersphincteric Fistula Tract (LIFT): An Effective New Technique for Complex Fistulas. DCR (Diseases of Colon and Rectum), 2010;53(1):43–46.

9 Transperineal Approach

C. Neal Ellis

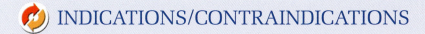

INDICATIONS/CONTRAINDICATIONS

Indications

Inflammatory, infectious, traumatic, or radiation injuries can result in a fistula between the rectum and the vagina. These fistulas allow the passage of intestinal contents and gas through the vagina with associated inflammation and irritation and usually result in significant psychosocial and sexual dysfunction. Given the morbidity of these fistulas, surgical management is indicated for any patient who is medically able to undergo a surgical procedure.

Selection of the Procedure

There is no one technique that is considered the "gold standard" for the management of rectovaginal fistulas. Instead, the surgical technique chosen depends on the training and experience of the surgeon, the etiology and anatomy or the fistula, and the presence or absence of a sphincter defect and incontinence. Options include fistulotomy with repair of the perineal body and sphincters, some type of local tissue flap, and transperineal ligation of the intersphincteric fistula tract (LIFT).

Fistulotomy with perineoproctotomy recreates a fourth-degree perineal laceration and provides excellent exposure allowing complete identification and excision of the fistula and all of its extensions followed by a precise, layer by layer closure of the vaginal and rectal walls and the perineal body. This approach is usually reserved for women with a rectovaginal fistula and a sphincter defect with incontinence. This approach can address both problems by combining closure of the fistula with overlapping sphincter repair (1).

A local tissue flap is another option for the management of rectovaginal fistulas. They can be constructed from the rectal mucosa, submucosa and circular muscle (mucosal flap), the anoderm (island pedicle flap), or the labial fat pad (Martius flap). These flaps can be created and used to cover the rectal side of the fistula (2,3). Possible complications of these flaps include creation of a mucosal ectropion with resultant mucus leakage and rectal bleeding (mucosal flap), and dyspareunia (Martius flap) (4,5).

The most recent addition for the management of rectovaginal fistulas is the transperineal LIFT. While LIFT alone has been successfully used for other anal fistulas, the one publication using LIFT for rectovaginal fistulas added a bioprosthetic graft to cover the closure of the fistula tract (2). This is the technique which will be described in this chapter.

Contraindications

The only absolute contraindication to the LIFT procedure for rectovaginal fistula is the medical inability to tolerate a surgical procedure. Relative contraindications include an acute fistula resulting from obstetric trauma or fistulas associated with acute inflammation.

The treatment of rectovaginal fistulas in patients with Crohn's disease is a special problem. Given the recurrent nature of the disease, patient satisfaction and the reduction in the number of septic events should be considered in addition to fistula recurrence rates. Also the chronic diarrhea associated with Crohn's disease will make any associated sphincter defect even more problematic. Many would consider active anorectal Crohn's a contraindication to the surgical repair of a rectovaginal fistula (6). For these patients, the use of a noncutting seton to reduce the number of perianal septic events may be a better choice.

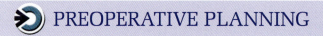

PREOPERATIVE PLANNING

History and Physical Examination

The initial step in the evaluation of a patient with a suspected rectovaginal fistula is a problem-specific history and physical examination. The patient should be questioned for any history of inflammatory bowel disease, diverticular disease, or cancers of colon, rectal, anal, or gynecologic origin. It is important to determine whether the patient has had any vaginal deliveries complicated by a significant perineal injury, gynecologic or colorectal surgical procedures, or radiation therapy. The degree of continence should be assessed. In general, the success of a rectovaginal fistula repair is related more to the underlying etiology and associated patient factors than to the technique of management.

Physical examination should include inspection of the anus and perineum. The thickness of the perineal body is determined by bidigital examination. The resting tone of the anus and the amount of voluntary squeeze are assessed by digital rectal examination. Anoscopic, proctoscopic, and vaginal speculum examination will frequently provide useful information regarding the etiology and anatomy of the fistula. Rectovaginal fistulas are usually easily identified with the above evaluation. If not, a vaginal tampon can be placed and an enema of dilute methylene blue can be administered. After 10 minutes, the tampon is removed and inspected for any blue staining.

Radiologic Evaluation

If the fistula is not apparent after the above evaluation, computerized tomography with oral and transanal contrast or magnetic resonance imaging of the abdomen and pelvis may be helpful for identifying the presence of a fistula and providing information on the etiology and anatomy of the fistula.

Transanal ultrasonography can also provide important information in the evaluation of patients with a rectovaginal fistula. Ultrasonography can be used to identify defects of the internal and external anal sphincter. This is particularly important for patients with associated incontinence or whose history suggests that the fistula is related to obstetric trauma (7).

Timing of Surgery

Rectovaginal fistulas associated with obstetric trauma may present either immediately post partum from an unrecognized injury or 7 to 10 days later, after failure of the primary repair of an obstetric injury. For patients with these acute obstetric fistulas, a period of observation is indicated as a small number of these fistulas will subsequently close spontaneously (8).

For patients with rectovaginal fistulas from other causes, it is important to have a period of nonoperative management to allow any acute inflammation of the fistula to resolve and to optimize the condition of the local tissues which will be used in the repair. A loose seton may be placed as a drain to prevent recurrent abscess formation and allow the fistula tract to mature. Severely symptomatic patients may require fecal diversion to relieve patient symptoms and allow the inflammation to resolve.

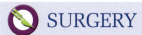 SURGERY

Positioning

Transperineal LIFT for rectovaginal fistulas is usually performed with the patient in the prone jackknife position (Fig. 9.1). For rare patients who cannot be placed in the prone jackknife position because of morbid obesity or other reasons, the procedure can be performed in lithotomy position.

Anesthesia

Transperineal LIFT has been performed with local, regional, and general anesthesia. The anesthetic technique selected is at the discretion of the patient, surgeon, and anesthesiologist. Perioperative antibiotics may be given if indicated in the judgment of the surgeon.

Dissection

A transverse incision is made over the mid-portion of the perineal body with dissection performed through the subcutaneous tissue to identify the intersphincteric groove. Dissection is continued in the intersphincteric plane mobilizing the internal sphincter and rectal mucosa posteriorly through approximately one-third of the circumference of the

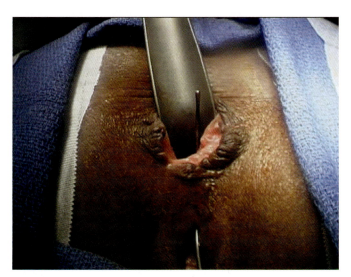

Figure 9.1 The procedure is usually performed with the patient in the prone jackknife position with the buttocks taped apart.

Part III: Rectovaginal Fistula

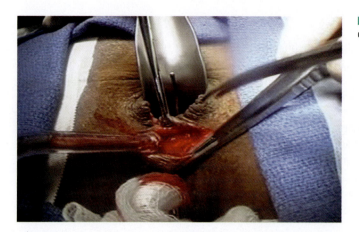

Figure 9.2 Dissection is carried out in the intersphincteric plane.

anus and rectum (Fig. 9.2). When the fistula tract is encountered, it is transected in this plane (Fig. 9.3). The dissection in the rectovaginal septum is continued at least 2 cm proximal to the transected fistula tract and laterally to identify the levator ani muscles.

Management of the Fistula Tract

After the dissection is complete, the fistula openings in the rectal and vaginal mucosa are closed with 3/0 interrupted, absorbable sutures. If there is an associated muscle injury, an end-to-end sphincteroplasty and/or levatorplasty can be performed. The bioprosthetic graft is trimmed to the appropriate width and placed into the intersphincteric space. It is important to ensure that there is at least 1–2 cm of overlap of the bioprosthetic on all sides of the rectal and vaginal closures. The bioprosthetic is sutured to the levator ani muscles laterally and the external sphincter distally with multiple, interrupted 3/0 absorbable sutures to prevent migration of the bioprosthetic (Fig. 9.4).

Wound Closure

The skin is very loosely approximated with interrupted 3/0 absorbable sutures to allow drainage of any fluid that may collect in the rectovaginal septum (Fig. 9.5). No drains are used.

 POSTOPERATIVE MANAGEMENT

Postoperatively, patients are usually discharged home on the day of surgery with narcotic analgesics, fiber supplements, and laxatives. No postoperative antibiotics are

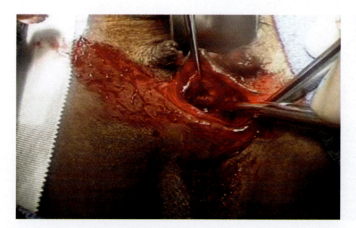

Figure 9.3 The fistula tract is transected in the intersphincteric plane. (Note the fistula opening in the internal sphincter).

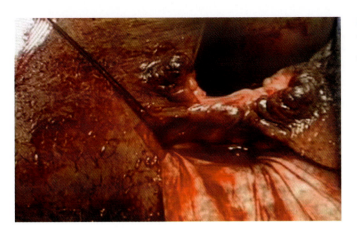

Figure 9.4 The bioprosthetic is sutured to completely cover the closure of each end of the fistula tract with at least 1 cm of overlap.

prescribed. Patients are encouraged to follow a diet high in fiber with adequate water intake. They are encouraged to engage in modest physical activity such as walking and light household duties but to refrain from sexual activity for 3 weeks. Sitz baths, three to four times daily as needed for comfort and after bowel movements, are recommended. Clinic visits are scheduled in 7–10 days and every 2–3 weeks thereafter until the perineal wound is healed.

 ## COMPLICATIONS

The most common complications associated with this procedure are those associated with any anorectal surgical procedure; urinary retention, and local sepsis. The incidence of abscess in the rectovaginal septum can be diminished by ensuring that there is adequate drainage of the surgical site.

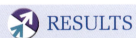 ## RESULTS

There is one published case series utilizing a transperineal LIFT with a bioprosthetic graft (Surgisis ES, Cook Surgical Inc., Bloomington, IN, USA) to repair the rectovaginal fistula in 27 patients with a mean followup of 12 months (range 6–22 months). Overall, there were five (19%) fistula recurrences. In this series, LIFT with a bioprosthetic graft was initially offered to 14 women who had failed at least two attempts at flap repair of their rectovaginal fistula. In this group the fistula recurred in four (29%) patients. An additional 13 patients underwent a transperineal LIFT as the initial attempt at repair of their rectovaginal fistula with the fistula recurring in one (8%) of these patients (2).

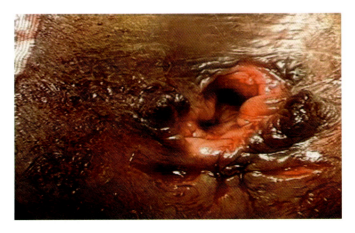

Figure 9.5 The incision is loosely closed to allow drainage from the wound.

Part III: Rectovaginal Fistula

✳ CONCLUSIONS

The use of transperineal LIFT with a bioprosthetic graft for the management of rectovaginal fistulas is a new technique that in the early experience seems to yield results equal to if not superior to other methods of management.

Recommended References and Readings

1. Chew SS, Rieger NA. Transperineal repair of obsteric-related anovaginal fistula. *Aust N Z Obstet Gynaecol* 2004;44:68–71.
2. Ellis CN. Outcomes after repair of rectovaginal fistulas using bioprosthetics. *Dis Colon Rectum* 2008;51:1084–8.
3. Zimmerman DD, Gosselink MP, Briel JW, Schouten WR. The outcome of transanal advancement flap repair is not improved by an additional labial fat flap transposition. *Tech Coloprocto* 2002;6: 37–42.
4. Devesa JM, Devesa M, Velasco GR, et al. Benign rectovaginal fistulas: management and results of a personal series. *Tech Coloproctol* 2007;11:128–34.
5. Petrou SP, Jones J, Parra RO. Martius flap harvest site: patient self-perception. *J Urol* 2002;167:2098–9.
6. Michelassi F, Melis M, Rubin M, Hurst RD. Surgical treatment of anorectal complications in Crohn's disease. *Surgery* 2000; 128: 597–603.
7. Yee LF, Birnbaum EH, Read TE, et al. Use of endoanal ultrasound in patients with rectovaginal fistulas. *Dis Colon Rectum* 1999;42:1057–64.
8. Goldaber KG, Wendel PJ, McIntire DD, et al. Postpartum perineal morbidity after fourth-degree perineal repair. *Am J Obstet Gynecol* 1993;168:489–93.

10 Transanal Repair

Ann C. Lowry

 ## INDICATIONS/CONTRAINDICATIONS

Rectovaginal fistulas, communications between the rectum and the vagina, may occur at any level of the vagina. Most commonly, the fistula originates low in the rectum and ends in the lower portion of the vagina. Obstetrical trauma, infection, and inflammatory bowel disease are the most common etiologies but some fistulas are congenital while others result from malignancy, radiation, or operative trauma.

Although rectovaginal fistulas caused by obstetrical trauma may close within the first few months postpartum, the majority of these fistulas require operative repair. Low, relatively small fistulas caused by infection or trauma are amenable to local repairs without diversion. They may be approached through the rectum, vagina, or perineum. More complex fistulas often require the interposition of muscles under the protection of temporary diversion. Such fistulas include ones located high in the rectum, caused by inflammatory bowel disease, radiation or malignancy, or large in size.

The choice of the local repair depends upon the status of the anal sphincter and the surrounding tissues. Given the nature of the injury, many women with a rectovaginal fistula caused by an obstetrical injury will also have an anterior sphincter defect. Without appropriate evaluation, sphincter dysfunction may be difficult to detect clinically as the passage of flatus and stool through the vagina may mask the symptoms of fecal incontinence. If a sphincter defect is identified then a transperineal repair is more appropriate than a transanal approach.

If there is no associated sphincter defect, the choice between a transvaginal and transanal approach for the initial repair is largely the surgeon's preference. Proponents of the transanal approach argue that the rectum is the high pressure side, so a secure repair of that side is critical to success.

The condition of the rectum and surrounding tissue must also be considered. Repair should be avoided if active infection or inflammation is present within the rectum or the perianal tissue. Perianal sepsis should be adequately drained; in many instances, a noncutting seton is helpful in controlling sepsis and allowing a surrounding cavity to close. An alternative approach should be chosen if an anal or rectal stricture or significant scarring is identified in the rectal wall. In patients with Crohn's disease, a transanal approach is contraindicated in the presence of active proctitis. Even without active proctitis, surgical repair of a rectovaginal fistula in a woman with Crohn's disease should be carefully considered. Successful control of symptoms is reported with medical management using azathioprine, metronidazole, and more recently with biologic medication. Given the high rate of recurrence and the possibility of worsening of the patient's symptoms after surgery, repair should only be undertaken in women who have failed other options and still have significant symptoms without active proctitis.

PREOPERATIVE PLANNING

While the passage of flatus or stool through the vagina is pathognomonic of a rectovaginal fistula, the presence and anatomy of the fistula must be confirmed before surgery. In addition, evaluation of the anal sphincter and bowel symptoms must be complete. The underlying etiology largely determines the specific investigations required.

A careful history is necessary to determine the preoperative evaluation needed. Any history of anorectal or gynecologic malignancy should prompt a thorough investigation for recurrence, both in the rectovaginal septum and pelvis. Prior treatment with radiation should be specifically elicited. Issues related to continence should also be documented. Patients with a history of a difficult delivery or previous anorectal surgery are at significant risk of a sphincter defect. One study found that 100% of women presenting with an obstetric rectovaginal fistula had evidence of an anterior sphincter defect (1). Bowel function as well as signs/symptoms of inflammatory bowel disease should also be targeted as possible areas for workup.

The site of a rectovaginal fistula can usually be readily identified during digital examination as a palpable dimple in the anterior midline. The rectal opening is frequently visible on anoscopy, but in some women the diagnosis may be elusive. A methylene blue test may confirm the presence of a communication and aid in locating the site. During this test, the patient is placed in prone position and a vaginal tampon is inserted; a 20–30 ml enema colored with methylene blue is then administered. Staining on the tampon is diagnostic of a rectovaginal fistula, assuming no spillage of dye. If this test does not confirm a fistula, an examination under anesthesia or radiologic evaluation is necessary.

The examiner should also look for findings suggestive of Crohn's disease and/or any evidence of local sepsis. Findings of fluctuance, cellulitis, or any other signs of active infection should prompt an examination under anesthesia and drainage with or without placement of seton(s) or drain(s). Any mass discovered on examination should be biopsied to exclude malignancy. In patients with a prior history of anorectal or gynecologic malignancy, the threshold for a biopsy should be especially low. In patients with a history of radiation treatment for malignancy, an examination under anesthesia with biopsies is often necessary. Assessment of a patient's sphincter function including resting tone, presence of circumferential motion, and change in tone when asked to squeeze should be included in the examination.

Radiographic tests may help identify an elusive fistula. Vaginography may detect a fistula and demonstrate the anatomy. The test is performed by instilling contrast into the vagina through a catheter with the balloon inflated to occlude the vaginal opening. The technique has a sensitivity of 79–100% for the detection of the fistula tract. Vaginography is most helpful for colovaginal and enterovaginal fistulae; it is less useful for low rectovaginal fistulae (2,3).

Computed tomography scans may identify the fistula tract and characterize the surrounding tissue. Contrast material in the vagina after oral or rectal administration is diagnostic of a fistula. Suggestive evidence includes air or fluid in the vagina if there is no history of recent instrumentation. Magnetic resonance imaging (MRI) and endorectal ultrasound are also useful in identifying fistulae; the injection of hydrogen peroxide into fistulae has been shown to increase the yield of ultrasonography (4). Vaginal gel inserted prior to a pelvic MRI may be beneficial. At present, there is no clear gold standard test to detect elusive fistulae.

Endoanal ultrasound and MRI also have a role in assessing the structural integrity of the anal sphincter (Fig. 10.1). Comparison of endoanal ultrasound and MRI reveals

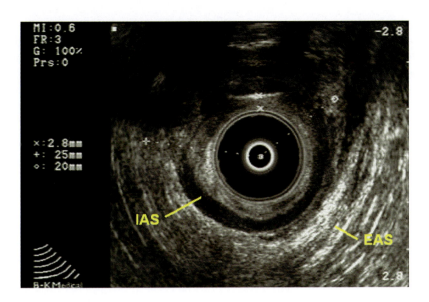

Figure 10.1 An ultrasound demonstrating a thin perineal body, anterior defect in the internal anal sphincter and external anal sphincter muscles.

them to be essentially equivalent in detection of a sphincter defect (5). If a limited sphincter injury is identified, anorectal physiology may be helpful in determining whether sphincter repair should be part of the chosen procedure.

Evaluation of the intestinal tract by colonoscopy and contrast studies is indicated in patients with known or suspected inflammatory bowel disease.

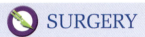 # SURGERY

Options for Transanal Repairs

Transanal approaches are appropriate choices for the repair of rectovaginal fistulas without associated anal sphincter injuries. While multiple transanal techniques for repair of rectovaginal fistulas exist in the literature, three of those techniques will be discussed in this chapter. Endorectal advancement flaps have the longest history, with the most data available. However, there are reports of postoperative incontinence with that approach (6–8). In attempt to avoid that complication, two recently described techniques, insertion of a fistula plug and the LIFT (ligation of intersphincteric fistula tract) are gaining popularity.

The preoperative preparation and positioning are similar for all three procedures.

Preoperative Preparation

Smoking is associated with a higher failure rate for repairs of complex anal fistulas (9,10). Although there is no definite evidence proving benefit, theoretically cessation of smoking would be beneficial. Patients undergo a mechanical bowel preparation prior to surgery to try to reduce the risk of sepsis and postoperative constipation; that recommendation is based upon clinical experience rather than high-level evidence. Intravenous antibiotics are administered immediately prior to the surgery. Oral antibiotics are not utilized. A urinary catheter is not routinely utilized.

Anesthesia and Positioning

General, regional, and local anesthesia with sedation may be used effectively for these procedures. Many surgeons prefer general anesthesia for improved patient comfort in the prone position. The patient is placed in the prone jackknife position with her hips over a padded roll. The arms are typically on padded arm boards with the patient's arms extended. The buttocks are taped apart for exposure. The prone position allows optimal exposure of the surgical field and comfortable access for the surgeon and assistant; a headlight aids visualization significantly.

Technique

Endorectal Advancement Flap

Advancement flaps aim to eradicate rectovaginal fistula by occluding the internal opening of the tract with healthy tissue. Using a bivalve anoscope for exposure, a probe is passed from the vagina to identify the internal opening (Fig. 10.2). Starting just distal to the internal opening of the fistula, a U-shaped flap is outlined with electrocautery. The base of the flap should be 2–3 times as wide as the apex to ensure adequate blood supply of the flap (Fig. 10.3). The dissection commences distally and includes mucosa, submucosa, and circular muscle (Fig. 10.4). If the flap is too thin, the blood supply may be jeopardized. Continuing in this plane, the flap is raised for a distance sufficient to allow a tension-free repair, usually 4–5 cm (Fig. 10.5). Care should be taken to avoid creating a hole in the flap. With adequate mobilization, the distal end of the flap should easily lay at the anal verge. The fistula tract is then debrided, not excised. The internal sphincter muscle lateral to the incision is bilaterally freed from the overlying anoderm and the underlying external sphincter muscle for a short distance. The edges of the internal sphincter muscle are approximated over the fistula opening with long-acting absorbable suture in one or two layers (Fig. 10.6). Hemostasis is carefully achieved to avoid a hematoma. The distal end of the flap including the fistula site is trimmed and the flap sutured in place with interrupted 3-0 absorbable sutures (Fig. 10.7). The vaginal side is left open for drainage.

Insertion of Fistula Plug

In 2007, the results of a consensus conference regarding the anal fistula plug were published. The following technique describes the determined best practices (11). Using an anoscope for exposure, a probe is passed from the vagina to identify the internal opening (Fig. 10.2). Irrigation of the tract with either saline or diluted hydrogen peroxide is recommended. Debridement, curettage, or excision of the tract is discouraged other than if the

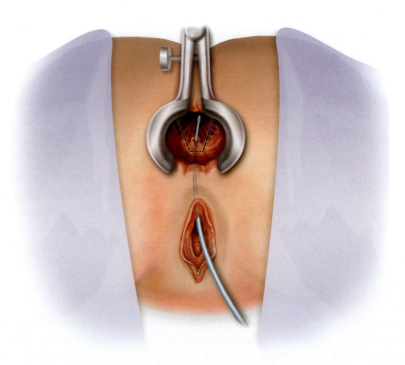

Figure 10.2 A probe demonstrates the fistula tract.

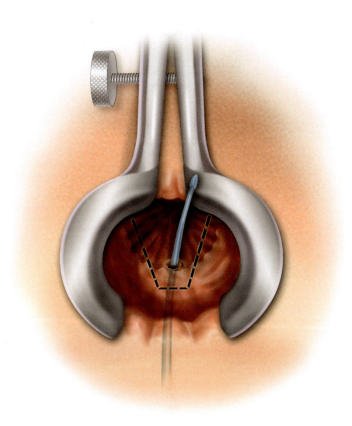

Figure 10.3 Outline of endorectal advancement flap with adequate width.

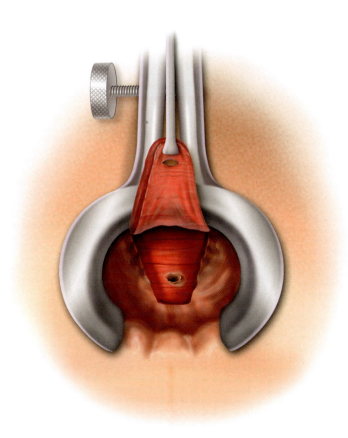

Figure 10.4 Depth of flap containing mucosa, submucosa, and circular muscle.

Part III: Rectovaginal Fistula

Figure 10.5 Adequate mobilization to avoid tension.

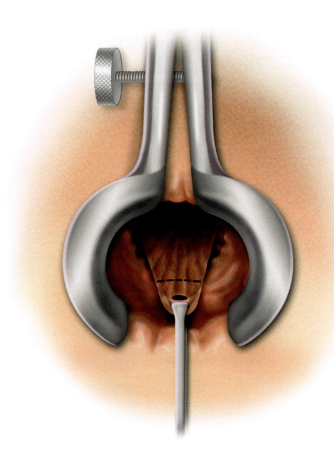

Figure 10.6 Closure of internal sphincter.

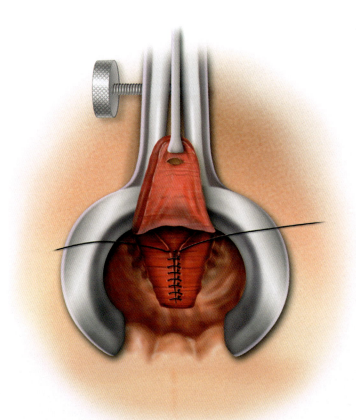

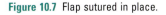
Figure 10.7 Flap sutured in place.

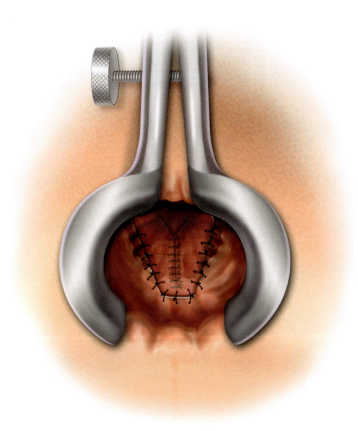

internal opening is epithelialized. In that situation, limited mobilization and debridement of the mucosal edges may be considered before suture placement. The plug should be prepared according to the manufacturer's instructions. One end of the suture is tied to the probe and the other to the narrow end of the plug. Using the suture as a guide, the plug is then gently passed from the internal opening to the external opening until the plug is snug in the tract (Fig. 10.8). Any excess plug should be trimmed at the internal opening. The plug is sutured in place with 2-0 long-term absorbable-braided suture (Fig. 10.9). The figure of eight anchoring suture should incorporate the internal sphincter muscle bilaterally and pass through the center of the plug. There is a controversy over the need for imbrication of the mucosa over the plug; many surgeons recommend a figure of eight suture to bury the end of the plug. Any excess plug on the vaginal side is then trimmed at the level of the vaginal wall but not sutured to the vaginal wall.

Recently, a fistula plug was developed specifically for rectovaginal fistulas because of higher failure rates reported from plug dislodgement from short fistula tracks. The modification involves the addition of a "button" to the plug; that end of the plug is inserted on the rectal side of the fistula track. The initial portion of the technique is the same as described above. The plug is inserted through the rectal opening using a suture as a guide until the button portion is snug against the mucosa. The plug is then sutured in place with four 2-0 absorbable sutures passed the mucosa, internal sphincter, and specially designed holes on the button (Fig. 10.10). Some surgeons also anchor the plug near the opening in the vaginal wall after which the excess fistula plug is trimmed.

LIFT Procedure

The LIFT procedure was originally described by Rojanasakul as a sphincter-sparing operation for transsphincteric fistulas (12). The concept is the identification of the fistula tract in the intersphincteric space with subsequent ligation and division of the tract. Recently, a modification with the insertion of bioprosthetic material between the ligated

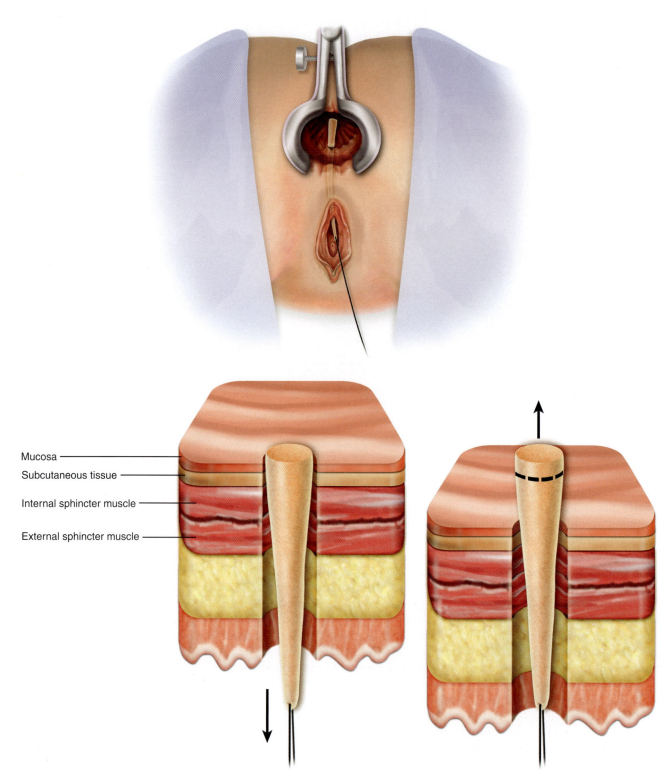

Mucosa

Subcutaneous tissue

Internal sphincter muscle

External sphincter muscle

Figure 10.8 Fistula plug pulled through tract.

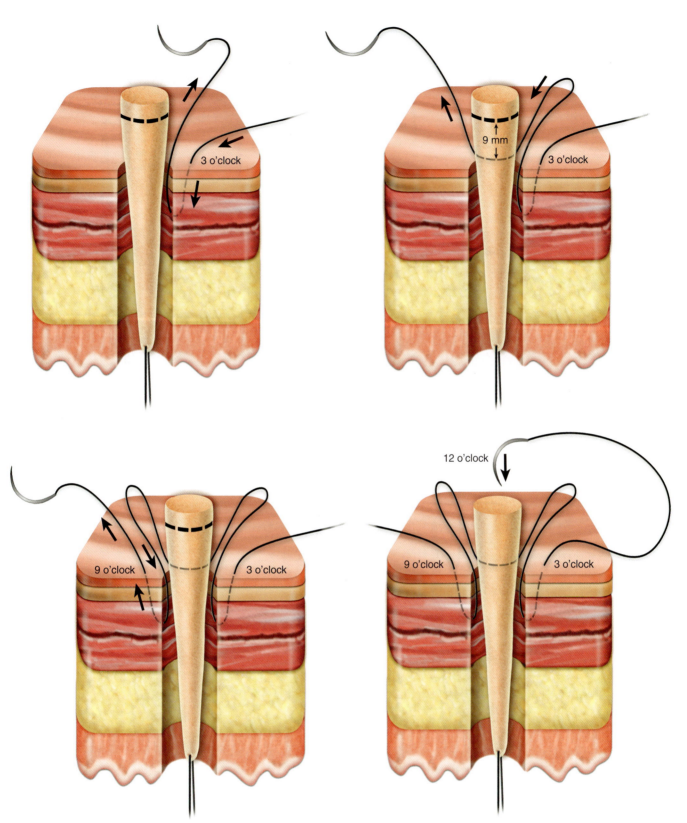

Figure 10.8 (*Continued*)

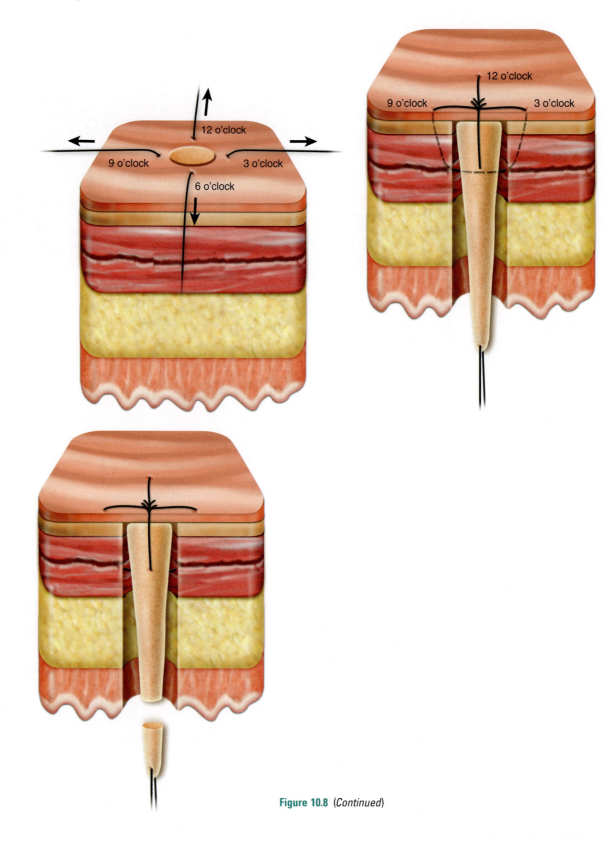

Figure 10.8 (*Continued*)

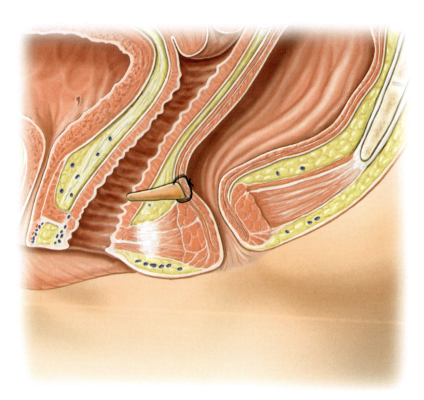

Figure 10.9 Fistula plug sutured in place.

ends was described. For low rectovaginal fistulas passing through an intact sphincter complex, this technique might be considered. A probe is passed through the fistula tract. A curvilinear skin incision just lateral to the intersphincteric groove is outlined; the incision involves about 25% of the circumference of the anal canal centered on the probe (Fig. 10.11). The intersphincteric groove is identified and the incision is deepened between the internal and external sphincters. Leaving the probe in place facilitates

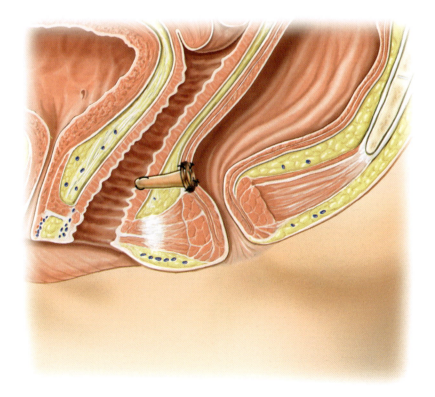

Figure 10.10 Rectovaginal fistula plug sutured in place.

Figure 10.11 Incision for LIFT procedure.

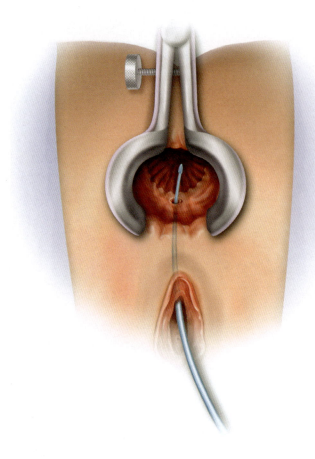

the identification of the fistula tract (Fig. 10.12). The tract is dissected from the surrounding tissue and encircled. The tract is ligated and divided; often the ligation is reinforced with a suture ligature (Fig. 10.13). The internal opening is then closed with an absorbable suture. For fistula in anorectal region, some surgeons core out the external opening and remnant fistula tract; excision of the vaginal opening and residual tract anteriorly is not recommended for rectovaginal fistulas. When insertion of a

Figure 10.12 Identification of fistula tract in intersphincteric space.

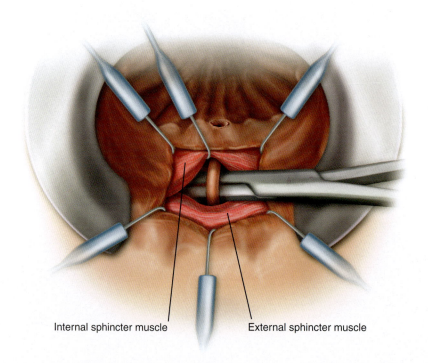

Internal sphincter muscle   External sphincter muscle

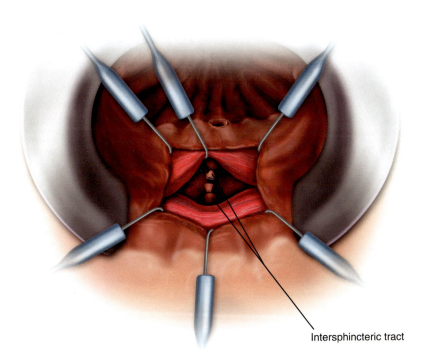

Figure 10.13 Ligation and division of fistula tract.

Intersphincteric tract

bioprosthetic material is planned, the dissection is continued several centimeters proximal to the fistula tract. After closure of the internal opening, the bioprosthetic graft is placed into the intersphincteric space and anchored with absorbable suture to the sphincter muscles. The deep sutures are placed first and then passed through the graft; the graft can then be parachuted into the proper location (Fig. 10.14). The bioprosthetic material should overlap the fistula tract closure by 1–2 cm on all sides. The wound is then irrigated and loosely closed with absorbable suture material.

Figure 10.14 Insertion of bioprosthetic material to separate ends of the divided tract.

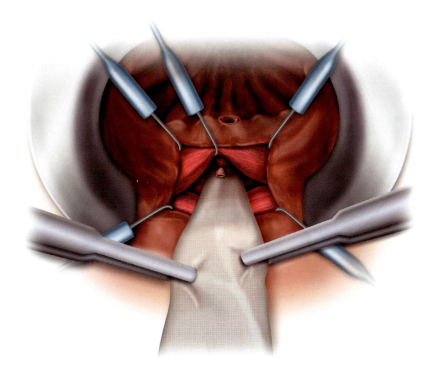

Part III: Rectovaginal Fistula

POSTOPERATIVE MANAGEMENT

Patients typically resume a normal diet with fiber supplements to prevent constipation. Stimulant laxatives are avoided as diarrhea will affect healing as much as constipation. If frequent loose stools occur, they should be controlled with antidiarrheal medication after evaluation for infection. Postdischarge instructions include avoidance of intercourse and the use of tampons for 6 weeks. Avoidance of any strenuous activity, exercise, or lifting is recommended for at least 2 weeks, particularly after the insertion of a fistula plug.

 COMPLICATIONS

All three procedures have low complication rates. However, bleeding, hematoma formation, perianal sepsis, and thrombosed hemorrhoids have been reported. Dislodgement of the fistula plug occurs with some frequency. Incontinence has also been reported after endorectal advancement flap. Studies reporting results of advancement flaps in patients with fistula-in-ano document altered continence in 21–40% of patients (6–8). The lack of standardized measures of continence in these reports makes objective comparison challenging. In some cases, the incontinence is unmasked sphincter dysfunction after the rectovaginal fistula is repaired. In that case, incontinence of stool and flatus may occur. If the external sphincter muscle is intact, the typical symptoms are incontinence of flatus or soiling. Incontinence has not been reported after insertion of the fistula plug or the LIFT procedure, although detailed studies with standardized questionnaires are rare.

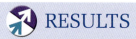 RESULTS

Endorectal Advancement Flaps

The literature contains widely varying success rates for endorectal advancement flaps for rectovaginal fistulas (Table 10.1) (6–8,13–19). Size of the series, mixed etiologies, frequent inclusion of additional procedures, and length of the follow-up are likely to contribute to the variation. It is important to note that success rates are measured in terms of fistula closure, and measures of continence are rarely included. In some series, inflammatory bowel disease and number of previous repairs inversely relates to successful outcome. Smoking has been linked to failure of endorectal advancement flaps, possibly the result of impairments in mucosal blood flow (9,10). It is not known whether smoking cessation prior to surgery can increase the rates of success.

TABLE 10.1		Recent Results of Endorectal Advancement Flaps for Rectovaginal Fistulas		
Author	Year	Number of patients	Success rate (%)	Comments
Tsang	1998	27	41	All obstetric
Hyman	1999	12	91	Etiology not reported
Joo	1998	20	75	Ultimate success, all Crohn's
Baig	2000	19	74	7 concomitant sphincteroplasty
Mizrahi	2002	32	56	Mixture of etiologies
Sonoda	2002	37	43	Mixture of etiologies
Zimmerman	2002	21	48	6 concomitant sphincteroplasty 12 labial flap transposition
Casadesus	2006	12	75	Vaginal advancement flap
Uribe	2007	56	93	Endorectal advancement flaps; 4 failures successfully rerepaired
Abbas	2008	8	50	All were recurrent prior to repair

Fistula Plug

The reported results of insertion of fistula plugs for trans-sphincteric fistulas are highly variable (20–24). Only small series exist specifically regarding the use of the fistula plug for rectovaginal fistulas. Ellis reported a series of 34 patients treated for rectovaginal fistulas with bioprosthetic material; seven patients had a fistula plug inserted. Successful closure occurred in 86% of those patients (25). In comparison, Thekkinkatill and co-authors documented a successful repair with a fistula plug in two out of nine patients with fistulas involving the vagina (26). The effectiveness of the plug designed for rectovaginal fistulas was recently examined in one series of 12 patients (27). Successful healing was achieved in three out of five rectovaginal fistulas and four out of seven pouch-vaginal fistulas. A total of 20 plug placements were performed, yielding a procedural success rate of 35% and an overall success rate of 58%. Larger series are necessary before the true efficacy of either of the fistula plugs in these patients is known.

LIFT Procedure

The few published studies of the results of the LIFT procedure report success rates ranging from 57–94% (12,28–30). Only one study included patients with rectovaginal fistulas and the results were not analyzed separately. Ellis reported the only series evaluating the use of bioprosthetic material added to the LIFT procedure in patients with rectovaginal fistulas (25). An unspecified number of patients underwent concomitant sphincter reconstruction. Overall, healing was achieved in 81% of 27 patients. In 13 patients, for whom this technique was the initial repair, closure occurred in 12 patients (92%). As with the fistula plug, more extensive experience from different centers is needed to determine the role of this procedure in the management of women with rectovaginal fistulas.

Choice of Procedure

There are no comparative studies of these three alternative approaches in patients with rectovaginal fistulas. The appeal of the fistula plug is its minimally invasive nature and avoidance of disturbance of sphincter function. In addition, the planes for an advancement flap or transperineal repair are not violated if failure occurs. However, the true efficacy is far from clear and the plug is expensive. It is too early to determine the role of the LIFT procedure with or without bioprosthetic material. Larger studies and data on postoperative continence are needed. In addition, theoretically, the technique is only applicable to those women with a rectovaginal fistula and intact sphincter muscle. Considerable, though varied, data exist for endorectal advancement flaps for rectovaginal fistulas, with few comparative studies. Two studies comparing different techniques in patients with fistula in anorectal region were published recently. Both studies were retrospective; one reported healing in 63% of 43 patients after endorectal advancement flap and in 32% of 37 patients after insertion of a fistula plug (22). The other reported very similar results: 62% of 26 patients healed after endorectal advancement flap repair and 34% of 29 patients healed after plug insertion (23). Three randomized controlled trials are currently recruiting patients (www.clinicaltrials.gov) (31). While the results may not be completely transferrable to patients with rectovaginal fistulas, the data should be useful.

✴ CONCLUSIONS

Rectovaginal fistulas remain vexing problems for the patients as well as the surgeons. Transanal approaches are appropriate for women with rectovaginal fistulas and intact sphincter muscles as long as there is no active inflammatory or malignant process present. No procedure is clearly preferable among the alternatives. Endorectal advancement flaps have the highest reported success rates but carry a risk of postoperative incontinence. Insufficient experience exists with the alternative procedures to understand their roles. Comparative studies, particularly randomized controlled trials, are necessary to determine the optimal procedure.

Recommended References and Readings

1. Yee LF, Birnbaum EF. Use of endoanal ultrasound in patients with rectovaginal fistulas. *Dis Colon Rectum* 1999;42:1057–64.
2. Bird D, Taylor D, Lee P. Vaginography: the investigation of choice for vaginal fistulae? *Aust N Z J Surg* 1993;63:894–6.
3. Giordano P, Drew PJ, Taylor D, Duthie G, Lee PW, Monson JR. Vaginography: investigation of choice for clinically suspected vaginal fistulas. *Dis Colon Rectum* 1996;39:568–72.
4. Sudol-Szopinska I, Jakubowski W, Szcepkowski M. Contrast enhanced endosonography for the diagnosis of anal and anovaginal fistulas. *J Clin Ultrasound* 2002;30:145–50.
5. Stoker J, Rociu E, Schouten WR, Lameris JS. Anovaginal and rectovaginal fistulas: endoluminal sonography versus endoluminal MR imaging. *Am J Roentgenol* 2002;178:737–41.
6. Mizrahi N, Wexner SD, Zmora O, et al. Endorectal advancement flap: are there predictors of failure? *Dis Colon Rectum* 2002;45:1616–21.
7. Sonoda T, Hull T, Piedmonte MR, Fazio VW. Outcomes of primary repair of anorectal and rectovaginal fistulas using endorectal advancement flap. *Dis Colon Rectum* 2002;45:1622–8.
8. Uribe N, Millian M, Minguez M, et al. Clinical and manometric results of endorectal advancement flap for complex anal fistula. *Int J Colorectal Dis* 2007;22:259–64.
9. Zimmerman DD, Gosselink MP. Smoking impairs rectal mucosal blood flow-a pilot study. *Dis Colon Rectum* 2005;48:1228–32.
10. Ellis CN, Rostas JW, Greiner FG. Long-term outcomes with the use of bioprosthetics plugs for the management of complex anal fistulas. *Dis Colon Rectum* 2010;53:798–802.
11. The surgisis AFP anal fistula plug: report of a consensus conference. *Colorectal Disease* 2007; 10:17–20.
12. Rojanasakul A, Pattanaarun J, Sahakitrungruang C, Tantiphlachiva K. Total anal sphincter saving technique for fistula-in ano; the ligation of the intersphincteric fistula tract. *J Med Assoc Thai* 2007;90:581–5.
13. Tsang C, Madoff RD, Wong WD, et al. Anal sphincter integrity and function influences outcome in rectovaginal fistula repair. *Dis Colon Rectum* 1998;41:1141–6.
14. Hyman N. Endoanal advancement flap repair for complex anal fistula. *Am J Surg* 1998;178:337–40.
15. Joo JS, Weiss EG, Nogueras JJ, Wexner SD. Endorectal advancement flap in perianal Crohn's disease. *Am Surg* 1998;64:147–50.
16. Baig MK, Zhao RH, et al. Simple rectovaginal fistulas. *Int J Colorectal D* 2000;15:323–7.
17. Zimmerman DD, Gosselink MP, Briel JW, Schouten WR. The outcome of transanal advancement flap repair of rectovaginal fistulas is not improved by additional labia fat flap transposition. *Tech Coloproctol* 2002;6:37–42.
18. Casadeus D, Villasana L, Sanchez IM, Diaz H, Chavez M, Diaz A. Treatment of rectovaginal fistula: a 5 year review. *Aust N Z J Obstet Gynaecol* 2006;46:49–51.
19. Abbas MA, Lemus-Rangel R, Hamadani A. Long term outcome of endorectal advancement flap for complex anorectal fistulae. *Am Surg* 2008;74:921–4.
20. Owen G, Keshava A, Stewart P, et al. Plugs unplugged. Anal fistula plug: the concord experience. *Aust N Z J Surg* 2010;80:341–3.
21. McGee MF, Champagne BJ, Stulbberg JJ Reynolds H, Marderstein E, Delaney CP. Tract length predicts successful closure with anal fistula plug in cryptoglandular fistulas. *Dis Colon Rectum* 2010;53:1116–20.
22. Christoforidis D, Pieh MC, Madoff RD, Mellgren AF. Treatment of transsphincteric anal fistulas by endorectal advancement flap or collagen fistula plug: a comparative study. *Dis Colon Rectum* 2009;52:18–22.
23. Wang JY, Garcia-Aguilar J, Sternberg JA, Abel ME, Varma MG. Treatment of transsphincteric anal fistulas: are fistula plugs an acceptable alternative? *Dis Colon Rectum* 2009;52:692–7.
24. Champagne BJ, O'Connor LM, Ferguson M, Orangio GR, Schertzer ME, Armstrong DN. Efficacyof anal fistula plug in closure of cryptoglandular fistulas: long term follow-up. *Dis Colon Rectum* 2006;49:1817–21.
25. Ellis CN. Outcomes of repair of rectovaginal fistulas using bioprosthetics. *Dis Colon Rectum* 2008;51:1084–8.
26. Thekkinkattil DK, Botterill I, et al. Efficacy of the anal fistula plug in complex anal fistulae. *Colorectal Disease* 2009;11:584–7.
27. Gonsalves S, Sagar P, Lengyel J, Morrison C, Dunham R. Assessment of the efficacy of the rectovaginal button fistula plug for the treatment of ileal pouch-vaginal and rectovaginal fistulas. *Dis Colon Rectum* 2009;52:1877–81.
28. Alfred K, Roslani K, Chittawatanarat K, et al. Short-term outcomes of the ligation of intersphincteric fistula tract (LIFT) procedure for treatment of fistula-in-ano: a single institution experience in Singapore. *Dis Colon Rectum* 2008;51:696–7.
29. Shanwani A, Nor AM, Amri N. Ligation of the intersphincteric fistula tract (LIFT): a sphincter-saving technique for fistula-in ano. *Dis Colon Rectum* 2010;53:39–42.
30. Bleier JI, Moloo H, Goldberg SM. Ligation of the intersphincteric fistula tract: an effective new technique for complex fistulas. *Dis Colon Rectum* 2010;53:43–6.
31. van Koperen PJ, Bemelman WA, et al. The anal fistula plug versus the mucosal advancement flap for treatment of anorectal fistula (PLUG trial). *BMC Surg* 2008;8:11.

11 Overlapping Repair

Brooke Gurland and Tracy Hull

 ## INDICATIONS/CONTRAINDICATIONS

In otherwise healthy younger women, direct sphincter trauma or neuropathic injuries from vaginal deliveries are the principal causative factors in the development of fecal incontinence (1). Prospective studies using anal physiologic testing have shown that anal sphincter injuries can occur after vaginal deliveries without any visible signs of perineal trauma in 11.5–35% of patients (2). A delayed presentation of fecal incontinence can also occur as the effects of menopause summate with those of pelvic muscular and neurologic injuries to produce overt symptoms of urinary incontinence, pelvic organ prolapse, and fecal incontinence (3,4).

In the United States, sphincteroplasty is the most commonly performed procedure for fecal incontinence. Overlapping anal sphincter repair is the operation of choice for the incontinent female with an anatomically disrupted external anal sphincter (EAS) muscle. It can be performed for any type of injury to the EAS muscle, such as those due to anorectal surgery or trauma, but is most commonly performed for obstetric injury.

Transanal ultrasound, manometry, and pudendal nerve latencies are important diagnostic studies in the evaluation of patients with fecal incontinence. These tests help to delineate other etiologies of fecal incontinence. These tests provide us with objective evaluation of anal neuromuscular function that would not be otherwise detected on clinical examination. Anal sphincter injuries are detected by a break in the muscular ring visualized on 2-D or 3-D anal ultrasonography. Defects may be reported as EAS, internal anal sphincter (IAS), or combined injuries.

Bilateral, not unilateral, pudendal neuropathy is associated with diminished sphincter function and higher incontinence scores. In some studies, bilateral prolonged pudendal nerve latencies have been shown to be a poor prognostic indicator in patients undergoing anal sphincter repair and are a relative contraindication to sphincter repair (5). However, the significance of pudendal nerve terminal latencies has been debated by others.

PREOPERATIVE PLANNING

A detailed bowel history is performed to assess stool consistency and frequency of bowel movements (BMs). Loose watery BMs may be difficult to control even in the setting of normal sphincter function and evaluation of diarrhea should be initiated before considering sphincter repair. Bulking agents and constipating medications are recommended as first-line therapy to minimize BMs, thus decreasing incontinent episodes.

The following information should be collected regarding fecal accidents: urgent versus passive incontinence, type of incontinence (gas, liquid, solid, mucus), frequency, and quantity of fecal incontinnce (FI). A validated incontinence scoring system should be used (6). Women with more predictable bowel habits but with FI of solid stool tend to improve postoperatively compared to women with bothersome gas incontinence that is frequently not corrected with sphincter repair. It is very important to set realistic expectations with the patients about their anticipated postsphincteroplasty bowel control.

Physical examination of the perineum should reveal visible contraction of the sphincter muscle, and no evidence of rectal prolapse. Absence of sphincter contractions during perineal examinations can be a poor prognostic indicator.

Overlapping sphincter repair is generally performed without a diverting stoma unless there is a complex injury with a cloacal defect, redo sphincter repair, or complex rectal-vaginal fistula.

Preoperative management includes the following:

- Appropriate patient selection
- Setting realistic postoperative continence expectations
- Mechanical bowel preparation 24 hours before the onset of surgery
- A single dose of intravenous antibiotics administered prior to the surgery

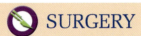 **SURGERY**

Operative Positioning

- The patient is positioned in the prone jackknife position on a Kraske Roll.
- The procedure is performed under general or spinal anesthesia.
- Large tapes are used to separate the buttocks for exposure of the anus.
- Although we prefer prone jackknife position, this procedure can also be performed in lithotomy, which may be preferable if the patient is undergoing a concomitant urinary or prolapse procedure.

Operative Technique

A number of different techniques have been described for sphincteroplasty and the choice of technique is operator-dependant. Some authors advocate an en bloc overlapping sphincteroplasty, avoiding separating the internal and external sphincters (7) (see sphincteroplasty video), while others deliberately try to restore normal anatomy (8).

- Sterile preparation of the perianal area, vagina, and perineum is performed.
- A foley catheter is placed in the bladder.
- Injection of the perineal body with 0.25% bupivacaine with 1:100,000 epinephrine.
- An anterior 120-degree curvilinear incision is made along the perineum with a 15-blade scalpel to allow dissection and mobilization of the sphincter muscle and scar.
- Sharp dissection is used until we adequately identify the anatomy.
- The skin edges are grasped with Allis clamps for exposure and flaps are developed toward the anal verge and the vagina. Care is taken not to "button hole" the skin.
- Lateral dissection, where the muscle anatomy is intact, can help to identify the proper plane of dissection. The EAS is the medial border of the ischiorectal fossa and identification of the ischiorectal fat is useful landmark to identify the lateral border of dissection.

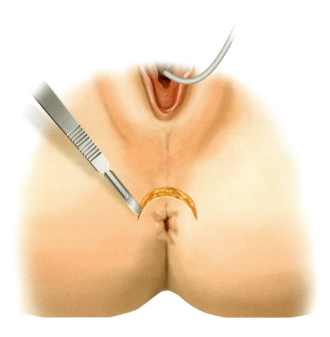

Figure 11.1 A curvilinear incision is made along the perineal body.

■ The scar tissue is divided through the midline if the sphincters halves are joined by scar. It is important to preserve all scar tissue in order to anchor the sutures. In other cases, the muscles edges are retracted laterally and grasped with Allis clamps.
■ After adequate mobilization, an en bloc overlapping of the EAS/IAS complex is performed.

   Other authors advocate anterior levatorplasty, IAS imbrication, and overlapping EAS repair (8,9).

■ Incision and dissection are performed as noted during EAS/ IAS overlap (Fig. 11.1).
■ The intersphincteric space is then mobilized from lateral to medial to the area of the midline scar and external and internal anal sphincters are separated (Fig. 11.2).
■ The repair starts with apposition of the levator muscles with interrupted 3, 2.0 polydioxanone monofilament delayed absorption suture.

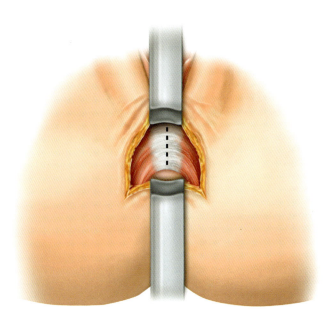

Figure 11.2 The sphincter scar is divided but not excised.

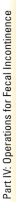

Part IV: Operations for Fecal Incontinence

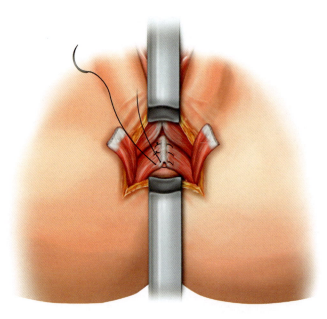

Figure 11.3 The internal anal sphincter is imbricated when a layered repair is performed.

- The internal muscle fibers are identified and imbricated with 3, 3.0 sutures (Fig. 11.3).
- The EAS is overlapped and four mattress sutures are used to approximate the ends 2.0 sutures (Fig. 11.4).
- Careful hemostasis is maintained with electrocautery throughout the procedure.
- The wound is irrigated with tetracycline infused antibiotic solution.
- The tapes are loosened prior to skin closure.
- The edges of the wound are approximated in a V-shape or longitudinally with interrupted 3.0 absorbable mattress sutures (Fig. 11.5). The center of the wound can be left open, a small drain inserted, or the wound can be closed (Fig. 11.6).
- The perineal body is bulkier than it was preoperatively.

→ POSTOPERATIVE MANAGEMENT

Postoperative management requires keeping the stools soft, the area clean, and pain tolerable; patients are kept overnight 1–2 days. There is no consensus on the routine

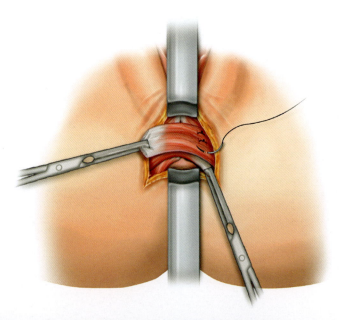

Figure 11.4 The external anal sphincter is overlapped.

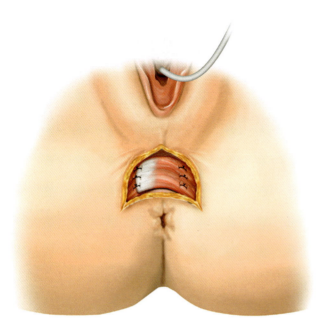

Figure 11.5 The edges of the wound are approximated in a V-shape or longitudinally with interrupted 3.0 absorbable mattress sutures.

administration of postoperative oral antibiotics at discharge. The patient is discharged on stool softeners. Maintaining the patient nothing by mouth and constipated does not have any proven benefit (10).

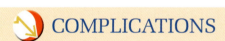 COMPLICATIONS

Complications that may occur in the early postoperative period include formation of a hematoma or seroma. This complication can be treated by opening the wound and evacuating the hematoma or seroma. Fecal impaction can cause disruption of the repair. Late complications include abscess formation and wound breakdown. Abscesses require drainage, wound breakdown usually heals secondarily, and rarely does this require secondary suturing. The patient's main complaint after surgery is pain from the perineal wound.

- Hematoma
- Seroma

Figure 11.6 The center of the wound is left open for drainage.

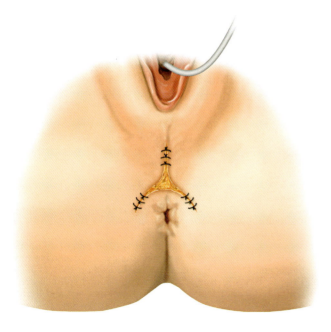

TABLE 11.1	Sphincteroplasty Series				
Author	**Year**	**N**	**Age (years)**	**FU (months) mean (range)**	**Outcomes (Good/ Excellent) N(%)**
Gibbs and Hooks (15)	1993	36	47 (20–74)	43 (4 m–9.5 years)	24 (73)
Malouf et al. (16)	2000	55	43 (26–67)	77 (60–96)	23 (50)
Halverson and Hull (17)	2002	44	38.5 (22–80)*	62.5 (47–141)	30 (68)
Bravo-Gutierrez et al. (18)	2004	182	37 (not reported)	10 (7–16 years)	24 (23)
Barisic et al. (19)	2006	65	35.9 (18–64)	80.1 (not reported)	31 (48)
Mevik et al. (20)	2009	29	45 (6–77)	84 (74–185)	9 (53)
Oom et al. (21)	2009	172	58 (30–85)*	111 (12–207)	44 (37)
Johnson et al. (22)	20108	33	36 (22–75)*	103 (62–162)	21 (64)

*Reported as median.

- Fecal impaction
- Abscess
- Wound dehiscence

RESULTS

Early symptom improvement is noted after sphincteroplasty (11,12). However, 5- and 10-year follow-up reveals a decline in continence and increasing fecal accidents (13,14). It is difficult to compare between series because many are retrospective, surgical technique varies, and the patient population is heterogeneous.

- Early symptom improvement up to 90% in some series (12).
- Deterioration of FI over time with return to base line in 10 years.
- Improvement after sphincteroplasty is noted but it is not to the level that it was before the sphincter injury.

CONCLUSIONS

Overlapping sphincter repair remains the treatment of choice for patients with EAS defects. However, continence declines on a long-term follow-up. This may occur because of the weakening of the muscle due to normal aging or repair breakdown. New techniques exist that involve sphincter augmentation with biologic graft material but long-term results are not available. When patients have recurrent symptoms of fecal incontinence after an initial successful repair, re-evaluation is beneficial and other options such as redo sphincteroplasty, sacral nerve stimulation, or artificial bowel sphincter may be offered.

Recommended References and Readings

1. Sultan AH, Kamm MA, Hudson CN, Thomas JM, Bartram CI. Anal-sphincter disruption during vaginal delivery. *N Engl J Med* 1993;329:64–70.
2. Willis S, Faridi A, Schelzig S, et al. Childbirth and incontinence: a prospective study on anal sphincter morphology and function before and early after vaginal delivery. *Arch Surg* 2002;387:101–7.
3. Nichols C, Ramakrishnan V, Gill E, Hurt W. Anal incontinence in women with and those without pelvic floor disorders. *Obstet Gynecol* 2005;106(6):1266–71.
4. Donnelly VS, Fynes M, O'Connell PR, O'Herlihy C. The influence of oestrogen replacement on faecal incontinence in post menopausal women. *Br J Obstet Gynaecol* 1997;104:311–5.

5. Gilliland R, Altomare D, Moreira H, Oliveira L, Gilliland JE, Wexner SD. Pudendal neuropathy is predictive of failure following anterior overlapping sphincteroplasty. *Dis Colon Rectum* 1998;41:1516–22.
6. Jorge JMN, Wexner S. Etiology and management of fecal incontinence. *Dis Colon Rectum* 1993;36:77–97.
7. Galandiuk S, Roth LA, Greene QJ. Anal incontinence-sphincter ani repair: indications, techniques, outcome. *Langenbecks Arch Surg* 2009;394:425–33.
8. Wexner S, Marchetti F, Jagelman DG. The role of sphincteroplasty for fecal incontinence reevaluated: a prospective physiologic and functional review. *Dis Colon Rectum* 1991;34:22–30.
9. Evan C, Davis K, Kumar D. Overlapping anal sphincter repair and anterior levatorplasty: effect of patient's age and duration of follow-up. *Int J Colorectal Dis* 2006;21:795–801.

10. Nessim A, Wexner S, Agachan F, et al. Is bowel confinement necessary after anorectal reconstructive surgery? A prospective, randomized, surgeon-blinded trial. *Dis Colon Rectum* 1999;42:16–23.
11. Karoui S, Leroi M, Koning E, Menard JF, Michot F, Denis P. Results of sphincteroplasty in 86 patients with anal incontinence. *Dis Colon Rectum* 2000;43:813–20.
12. Grey BR, Sheldon RR, Telford KJ, Kiff ES. Anterior anal sphincter repair can be long term benefit: a 12-year case cohort from a single surgeon. *BMC Surg* 2007;7:1.
13. Zutshi M, Hull T, Bast J, Halverson A, Na J. Ten-year outcome after anal sphincter repair for fecal incontinence. *Dis Colon Rectum* 2009;52:1089–94.
14. Gutierrez AB, Madoff RD, Lowry AC Parker SC, Buie WD, Baxter NN. Long term results of anterior sphincteroplasty. *Dis Colon Rectum* 2004;47:727–32.
15. Gibbs DH, Hooks VH, 3rd. Overlapping sphincteroplasty for acquired anal incontinence. *South Med J* 1993;86:1376–80.
16. Malouf AJ, Norton CS, Engel AF, et al. Long-term results of overlapping anterior anal-sphincter repair for obstetric trauma. *Lancet* 2000;355:260–5.
17. Halverson AL, Hull TL. Long-term outcome of overlapping anal sphincter repair. *Dis Colon Rectum* 2002;45:345–8.
18. Bravo Gutierrez A, Madoff RD, Lowry AC, et al. Long-term results of anterior sphincteroplasty. *Dis Colon Rectum* 2004;47:727–31; discussion 731–2.
19. Barisic GI, Krivokapic ZV, Markovic VA, et al. Outcome of overlapping anal sphincter repair after 3 months and after a mean of 80 months. *Int J Colorectal Dis* 2006;21:52–6.
20. Mevik K, Norderval S, Kileng H, et al. Long-term results after anterior sphincteroplasty for anal incontinence. *Scand J Surg* 2009;98:234–8.
21. Oom DM, Gosselink MP, Schouten WR. Anterior sphincteroplasty for fecal incontinence: a single center experience in the era of sacral neuromodulation. *Dis Colon Rectum* 2009;52:1681–7.
22. Johnson E, Carlsen E, Steen TB, et al. Short- and long-term results of secondary anterior sphincteroplasty in 33 patients with obstetric injury. *Acta Obstet Gynecol Scand* 2010;89: 1466–2.

Part IV: Operations for Fecal Incontinence

12 Dynamic Graciloplasty

Cornelius Baeten and S. Breukink

Introduction

Continence is a subtle coordinated action of several factors including peristalsis, stool consistency, rectal capacity, anorectal sensibility, pelvic floor muscles, central neural intactness, and an intact sphincter. After the sphincter is damaged the quality of the other factors will determine patients' continence. In the presence of fecal incontinence, it is mandatory to investigate all these variables. The best methods to evaluate the sphincter function are endosonography and anal manometry in order to obtain insight into the anatomy and contractility of the internal and external sphincter. One of the last resorts for incontinent patients is the dynamic graciloplasty. Gracileplasty is the transposition of the gracilis muscle from the upper leg to encircle the anus (1). This muscle transposition seems an ideal solution as the anus is reinforced with a fresh muscle. This muscle seems to have no other function in the human body but auxiliary to endorotation and adduction of the leg, and can be harvested without affecting performance in the lower limb.

The procedure is termed dynamic graciloplasty as the muscle is stimulated and therefore able to contract longer without any fatigue. A normal skeletal muscle is not capable for long-term contraction; the muscle will fatigue and within a few minutes it is not capable to recontract. This means that a normal transposition can never give a functional replacement of the original anal sphincters.

ANATOMY AND PHYSIOLOGY

The gracilis muscle is the most superficial muscle in the medial aspect of the upper leg (Fig. 12.1). Its vascular supply consists of several arteries. The main artery, the vein, and the gracilis nerve enter the muscle at 8 cm from the origin of the gracilis very reliably. The main artery derives from the arteria femoris profunda. The number of peripheral arteries vary among people ranging from zero to five, and even shows variability in the same patient between sides. To harvest and rotate the muscles all of

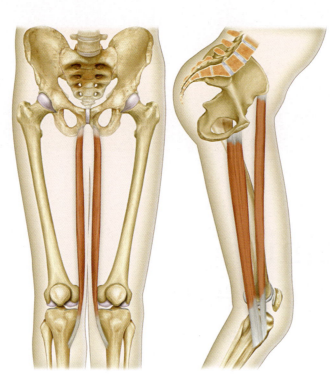

Figure 12.1 Gracilis muscle origo at os pubis and insertion at pes anserinus.

the peripheral arteries must be divided. In over 95% of patients the vascular bed inside the muscle will supply even the most distal part of the gracilis muscle (2).

The veins always accompany the arteries. The obturator nerve supplies the gracilis nerve. The origin of the muscle is the wide attachment at the pubic bone. The distal tendon of the gracilis muscle joins with the tendons of the sartorius and semi-tendinosus to form the "pes anserinus" (goose's foot). The part of the gracilis distally from the neurovascular bundle is available for transposition around the anus. At the top the gracilis is wider, and while running downward it tapers to the distal tendon. The form and location of the gracilis provide the most ideal muscle to construct a sphincter.

Microscopically the fiber pattern of most skeletal muscles is very similar to the muscle fibers of the gracilis. The majority of the fibers consist of type II fibers which are forceful, but fatigue-prone, capable of a short-term contraction hence unsuitable for sphincter function.

The first dynamic graciloplasty was described in 1988 (3). The muscle was stimulated with electrical pulses, inducing a change in fiber pattern of the muscle. Type 1 fibers were gradually replaced by type 2 fibers, which are less force-full but not loosely fatigable. The dynamic graciloplasty was capable of long-term contraction of the gracilis muscle (4,5), and it resembled the fiber pattern of the original anal sphincter (6). Contracting the gracilis muscle voluntarily was no longer necessary as the implanted stimulator forced the muscle to a continuous contraction. By switching off the stimulator, we allow muscle relaxation followed by evacuation.

 ## INDICATIONS

The dynamic graciloplasty should only be utilized after most other therapies have proven to be unsuitable or have failed. It can be the last step before a consideration of permanent colostomy.

The patient has to be informed about all pros and cons of the operation. The choice for a left or a right graciloplasty depends on the condition of the muscles, innervations, vascularization, or surgeon's preference. Patient hand dominance has no influence on choice of side.

The patient is positioned with the legs in stirrups to have good access to the upper leg, the perineum, and the lower abdomen. The skin is prepared and the patient receives systemic antibiotics.

Dynamic graciloplasty is always performed under general anesthesia. Spinal or epidural anesthesia is possible but can be psychologically demanding on the awake patient.

 # SURGERY

The operation starts with an incision in the median aspect of the upper leg. The sub-cutis is divided and the first muscle visible is the gracilis muscle. The gracilis is not encapsulated by the Fascia Lata. The dorsal side provides a safe entrance to free the gracilis muscle. With index finger the gracilis can now be encircled and drawn from its bed. In doing this, several peripheral arteries are stretched (Fig. 12.2).

The small arteries are divided by ligation of both ends or by coagulation. The gracilis should be freed first about halfway the upper leg. The sartorius muscle partially covers the gracilis and should not be mistaken for the gracilis muscle. The gracilis is now freed up to its distal tendon. The gracilis tendon can be divided some centimeters proximal from its insertion. The gracilis now lies free in the upper leg and can be drawn to medial with a clamp on the distal tendon. The proximal part of the muscle can now be freed up to the neurovascular bundle that invariably can be found at the lateral side, 8 cm from the origo. The neurovascular bundle must be preserved. Damaging the nerve, the artery and the vein will necrotize the muscle. The medial aspect of the proximal part of the gracilis can be freed from the subcutaneous tissue. The only structure that can be found here are the small arteries to the dermis, which can be coagulated. The gracilis muscle is now distally free (only attached to its origin and its neurovascular bundle); while preparing for the next part of the operation, it can be protected by tucking it in the perianal subcutaneous pocket.

The author prefers two small incisions; one over the proximal neurovascular pedicle and one over the distal tendon. The perforating vessels can then be controlled through those small incisions using an energy source such as an Ultracision™ scissors or a bipolar cutting scissors.

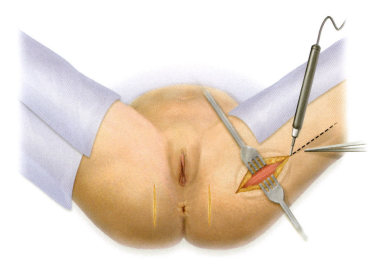

Figure 12.2 Incision upper leg and lateral of the anus.

Figure 12.3 Creation of tunnels around the anus.

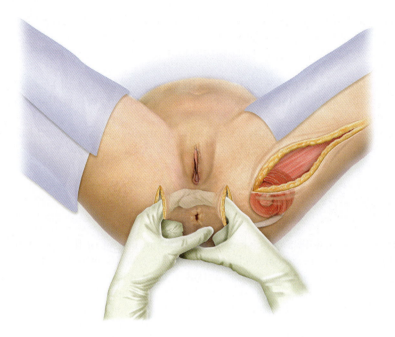

The operation continues with the creation of the tunnels around the anus. Two incisions are made lateral to the anus (Fig. 12.3). Using fingers, a tunnel can be bluntly created through these incisions, the dorsal side first. The tip of the coccygeal bone is the guiding point for the tunnel. Then both index fingers are directed frontally in the direction of the labia (or scrotum in males) and never directly to the midline, as there is almost always significant scar tissue between anus and vagina. A blunt dissection at this location would give too much traction on the tissue increasing a risk of perforation. The correct way to proceed is to sharply dissect the tissue between the rectum and the vagina and to keep the bowel and vaginal layer intact. If this maneuver is not possible an auxiliary incision in the posterior vagina may be safer. A vaginal incision will always heal, but a rectal enterotomy never heals spontaneously, with great risk of infection should it occur. In that case it is advisable to complete the gracilis operation without the implantation of the neurostimulator. After creating the perianal tunnels, a connection has to be made toward the wound in the upper thigh (Fig. 12.4). As the very strong fascia lata cannot be passed bluntly, I personally prefer to puncture it with a strong

Figure 12.4 Creation of connection between perianal tunnels and wound in upper leg.

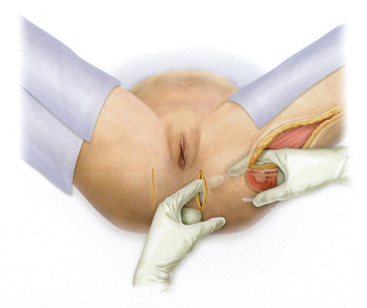

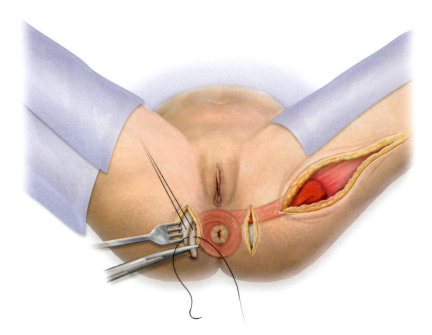

Figure 12.5 Gracilis is brought in gamma figuration around the anus.

clamp. By spreading the clamp the subcutaneous tunnel can be widened to ensure a patent conduit leading the gracilis muscle toward the anus. Muscle entrapment in the tunnel could cause necrosis of the distal part of the gracilis. The gracilis can be wrapped around the anus in various forms (Fig. 12.5).

1. In case of a long muscle and a short tendon, an alpha loop is the best configuration in which the first turn is anterior to the anus and then posterior, and the attachment of the tendon is made behind the bulk of the muscle at the descending part of the ipsilateral pubic bone, preventing an entrapment of the bulk of the gracilis.
2. In case of a long muscular and a long tendinous part of the gracilis, a gamma loop can be made. The first turn is at the anterior side, the second at the posterior side, and the tendon passes the anterior tunnel a second time and is attached at the contralateral descending ramus of the pubic bone (Fig. 12.6).

Figure 12.6 Two electrodes are tunneled from transposed gracilis to the stimulator in the pocket.

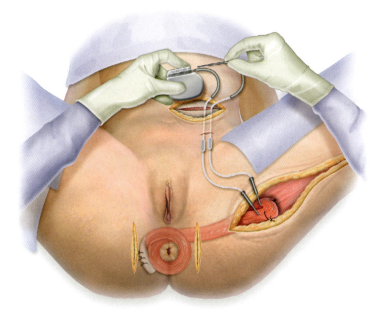

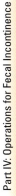

Part IV: Operations for Fecal Incontinence

3. When there is a weak spot in the posterior side of the anus, an omega loop can be made. The gracilis is first positioned through the posterior tunnel, then through the anterior one, and finally through the posterior one again and sutured to the ramus inferior of the ipsi- or contralateral pubic bone.

All sutures are made with nonresorbable monofilament material.

There are two strategies possible to make this graciloplasty dynamic: (1) One can stop the operation at this point and continue some weeks later or (2) one can finish the procedure now.

1. When the wrap around the anus is completed and the configuration to be used is known, it is wise to retract the gracilis back into the upper leg. This method allows sufficient space to place a suture through the periosteum of the inferior ramus of the pubic bone. This step cannot be done when the view is obstructed by the bulk of the gracilis. Once the suture is placed the gracilis muscle can be brought around the anus again and the distal tendon is now fixed to the periosteal suture. All wounds can be closed in two layers; stimulation can be done in a second phase a few weeks later.

Before training, the patient is seen at the outpatient clinic to examine the wounds and to ensure that they are free of infections. Normally the gracilis can be contracted voluntarily for only a short time. An active contraction means that the muscle is vital and the innervation is intact. The force of the voluntary contraction is the maximum force the muscle can generate. The electrically stimulated force is never higher than the voluntary force.

When there is no sign of infection and the muscle works properly the indication for the second operation is confirmed. For this second intervention, the leg and the lower abdomen are prepped and draped after legs are positioned in stirrups. The proximal part of the gracilis can be found by making an incision more proximal to the leg incision. Here the turning point of the gracilis is found. An intramuscular electrode can be brought through the muscle and fixed to the epimysium.

This electrode will serve as the positive pole or the anode. The second electrode is brought through the gracilis close by the entrance point of the nerve. This location can be found by stimulating the introduction needle. A forceful contraction with a low voltage means that the needle is in the right location, close to the nerve.

This electrode is the negative pole or the cathode. The contractions can be seen through the perineum or felt by rectal examination. The threshold is determined by the lowest voltage causing a detectable contraction. Both electrodes can now be tunneled toward a pocket (Fig. 12.6). In the lower abdomen the electrodes are connected with a stimulator which is placed in the pocket.

2. The stimulation of the gracilis muscle can also be executed during the first operation. In this case the procedure of the graciloplasty is similar until the placement of the non-absorbable sutures through the periosteum. The gracilis muscle retracted in the upper leg can be straightened into the wound. It is very easy to place the electrodes in the stretched muscle and to anchor them to the epimysium. At the moment the cathode is connected and enough current is delivered and the muscle starts to contract. The contraction can be so forceful that it is difficult to hold the muscle. The threshold can be found by lowering the voltage to the level which gives minimal visible contraction. The muscle can now be pulled toward the perineal tunnels and positioned in gamma, alpha, or omega position as decided before and anchored to the periost. The two electrodes are tunneled toward the pocket that is made in the lower abdomen. The pocket is made underneath the fascia of the rectus muscle. The leads can now be connected to the stimulator. The stimulator is placed in the pocket and the surplus of the electrodes is tucked behind the stimulator. It is necessary to position the non-insulated part of the stimulator, where the manufactuer's name is visible, in such a way to be accessible for programming at a later time. After this, wounds are closed.

The comparison between the direct and the indirect method of stimulation revealed that the direct implant is easier, and the patient needs anesthesia only once. Moreover, the two-phase operation is better when there is a higher chance of infection.

ELECTRICAL TRAINING

The muscle cannot be immediately trained but should be allowed to rest for at least one month. After a few weeks the stimulator is programmed in a cyclic mode or in a very low frequency. This setting is maintained for 2 weeks, after which the frequency is increased and maintained for another 2 weeks. The frequency is subsequently doubled again every 2 weeks. In these 6 to 8 weeks, the gracilis muscle has changed from a voluntary, high-twitch, fatigable muscle into an automatic, stimulator-driven, infatigable, slow-twitch muscle. During training the current is set to the extent that the stimulation is felt, but not higher, because this may be painful. When stimulation has resulted in continuous contraction (no undulating effect can be seen or felt), the training is completed and the ideal stimulation has been reached.

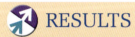 RESULTS

Usually the wounds heal without problems but in some cases infections develop. When this happens in the upper thigh or in the incisions lateral of the anus the wounds can be opened for drainage. Normally these wounds have a good secondary healing. The transposed gracilis will survive such infections without any problem. Should the infection come into contact with the foreign material like the electrodes and the stimulator, a more significant complication may ensue which if not resolved by antibiotics may require explantation. The preoperative administration of local antibiotics is not always enough to prevent infections. In our hospital Gentamycin is used as a local antibiotic. For some time Garamycin sponges were used, but soon abandoned due to high association with seroma formation.

Anorectal perforation during tunnel creation is responsible for most infections, most commonly it occurs anteriorly where there is a high degree of scarring.

Positive reported results for dynamic graciloplasty vary from 40 to 80%. Long-term results show a decrease of success (8–12). A review of my personal series after 10 years showed a success rate of only 40%. Presently we have other alternative therapies for severe fecal incontinence like artificial bowel sphincter (ABS) or sacral nerve stimulation. Indications for dynamic graciloplasty include severe birth lesions with a cloaca-like defect of the sphincters , and fecal incontinence in patients who are not candidates for newer alternatives.

CONCLUSION

Dynamic graciloplasty is an operation for very severe fecal incontinence when all other methods have been tried and proven unsuccessful. It is especially indicated when there is a serious loss of tissue between rectum and vagina.

In the opinion of the author, it is unfortunate that this procedure is unavailable in the United States. Despite the availability of the newer procedures such as sacral nerve stimulation or ABS, significant tissue loss makes stimulation impossible and coverage of the ABS unatainable. Even though the long-term success rate is only 40%, the only alternative in these patients is a permanent stoma. This procedure should be available in the armamentarium of the surgeon wishing to provide care for the incontinent patient.

Recommended References and Readings

1. Pickrell KL, Broadbent TR, Masters FW, Metzger JT. Construction of a rectal sphincter and restoration of anal continence by transplanting the gracilis muscle; a report of four cases in children. *Ann Surg* 1952;135(6):853–62.
2. Geerdes BP, Kurvers HA, Konsten J, et al. Assessment of ischaemia of the distal part of the gracilis muscle during transposition for anal dynamic graciloplasty. *Br J Surg* 1997;84(8):1127–9.
3. Baeten C, Spaans F, Fluks A. An implanted neuromuscular stimulator for fecal continence following previously implanted gracilis muscle. Report of a case. *Dis Colon Rectum* 1988;31(2):134–7.
4. Pette D, Vrbová G. Adaptation of mammalian skeletal muscle fibers to chronic electrical stimulation. *Rev Physiol Biochem Pharmacol* 1992;120:115–202. Review. No abstract available.
5. Baeten CG, Konsten J, Spaans F, et al. Dynamic graciloplasty for treatment of faecal incontinence. *Lancet* 1991;338(8776):1163–5.
6. Konsten J, Baeten CG, Havenith MG, Soeters PB. Morphology of dynamic graciloplasty compared with the anal sphincter. *Dis Colon Rectum* 1993;36(6):559–63.
7. Baeten CG, Geerdes BP, Adang EM, et al. Anal dynamic graciloplasty in the treatment of intractable fecal incontinence. *N Engl J Med* 1995;332(24):1600–5.
8. Rongen MJ, Uludag O, El Naggar K, et al. Long-term follow-up of dynamic graciloplasty for fecal incontinence. *Dis Colon Rectum* 2003;46(6):716–21.
9. Madoff RD, Rosen HR, Baeten CG, et al. Safety and efficacy of dynamic muscle plasty for anal incontinence: lessons from a prospective, multicenter trial. *Gastroenterology* 1999;116:549–56.
10. Konsten J, Rongen MJ, Ogunbiyi OA, et al. Comparison of epineural or intramuscular nerve electrodes for stimulated graciloplasty. *Dis Colon Rectum* 2001;44(4):581–6.
11. Saunders JR, Williams NS, Eccersley AJ. The combination of electrically stimulated gracilis neoanal sphincter and continent colonic conduit: a step forward for total anorectal reconstruction? *Dis Colon Rectum* 2004;47(3):354-63; discussion 363–6.
12. Grandjean P, Acker M, Madoff R, et al. Dynamic myoplasty: surgical transfer and stimulation of skeletal muscle for functional substitution or enhancement. *J Rehabil Res Dev* 1996;33(2):133–44. Review.

13 Artificial Bowel Sphincter

Paul-Antoine Lehur and Steven Wexner

 ## INDICATIONS/CONTRAINDICATIONS

Many factors, both anal and extra-anal, contribute to fecal continence. The artificial bowel sphincter (ABS) was designed to restore/create a high-pressure zone in the anal canal in a static manner, without the need for voluntary input to increase pressure.

The ABS corrects the loss of resting anal pressure. It would thus be fallacious to assume that normal continence can be restored by this means, even though the functional results obtained can be highly satisfactory.

- The best indications for the ABS are lesions of the anal sphincters unresponsive to or ineligible for local repair and unresponsive or ineligible for sacral nerve stimulation (SNS). Optimal results are also contingent upon preservation of extra-anal sphincter mechanisms of continence including normal transit time, rectal volume and compliance, and anorectal sensitivity. Thus, the ABS may be recommended, in young subjects, when the chances for successful local (direct) sphincter repair are poor (Fig. 13.1).
- In cases of incontinence resulting from sequelae of anal agenesis, there is a lower chance of success. The lack of anal sensitivity and/or a rectal reservoir and the existence of associated colonic motor disorders make all techniques of sphincteric substitution more uncertain. There are no available data to help predict ABS success in this indication, although some patients seem to be better served with techniques of antegrade colonic enemas (Malone procedure).
- In cases of neurogenic or neurologic fecal incontinence, it is essential to take into account possible associated dyschezia and excessive perineal descent. The ABS creates an obstacle to rectal evacuation, which can sometimes cause considerable evacuationary difficulties. Continence will not be restored if evacuation is compromised as a result. However, an objective assessment of the state of preoperative transit is not always easy because patients have often modified their diet to avoid incontinence or have had recourse to antidiarrheic treatments. A history of rectal prolapse or treatment for prolapse should be sought before considering implantation of an ABS, insofar as these conditions are indicative of disturbances in the defecation process.

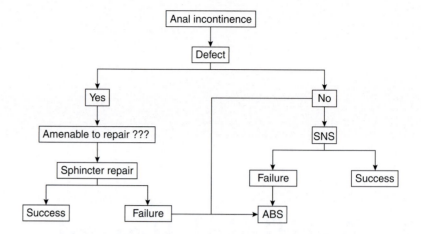

- Although the role of the ABS in anoperineal reconstructions after rectal amputation has not yet been fully defined, radiation therapy is probably a relative although not absolute contradiction.
- Implantation of an ABS is possible after failure of gracicloplasty and in some cases is a planned second stage after a gracicloplasty.
- Likewise, reimplantation of the device can take place immediately after explantation when all or part of the device has to be replaced because of a mechanical failure, or later (6-month interval) in the event of an infection after all inflammatory processes have disappeared.
- Globally, the ABS is suitable for well-motivated, selected patients with fecal incontinence
  - of more than a year's duration
  - whose condition is regarded as an important personal, familial, and/or social handicap
  - as an alternative to definitive colostomy
  - who are able to manipulate the control pump as required
  - with sufficient intellectual capacity to understand the functioning of the device and to ensure regular rectal evacuation.

The success of the ABS technique depends on serious consideration of the selection criteria and potential contraindications listed in Table 13.1.

PLACE OF THE ABS IN THE ERA OF THE SACRAL NERVE STIMULATION

Recently in a systematic review from Australia (9), the role and place of the ABS was challenged. On the basis of a full review of the literature, the authors concluded that "there was insufficient evidence on the safety and effectiveness of ABS implantation

TABLE 13.1	**Indications and Contraindications for Artificial Bowel Sphincter**
Type of indication	**Clinical settings**
Good	Traumatic sphincter disruption; neurologic incontinence; neurogenic (idiopathic) incontinence; failure or contraindications to sacral nerve stimulation
Relative	Imperforate anus/anal agenesis; severely scarred perineum; thin rectovaginal septum; advanced age, diabetes, severe digital arthritis; anorectal reconstruction after abdominoperineal excision
Contraindications	Excessive perineal descent; severe constipation; irradiated perineum; perineal sepsis (past or present); Crohn's disease; anal intercourse

. . . and for most patients, the procedure was of uncertain benefit." Such a statement is clearly not reflective of the practices of either of the authors.

Clearly, SNS has strong and unique advantages as a minimally invasive procedure, and in terms of testing phase, allows a screening process that provides unique patient selection and efficiency. Therefore, both authors have successfully utilized the adaptation of SNS. The SNS procedure however is not a panacea and may not be viable in patients with severe muscle loss. Therefore, there is still a place for a sphincteric replacement, with an ABS in cases of unresponsiveness to or ineligibility for SNS.

Any referral center for the surgical treatment of fecal incontinence must offer a range of options including ABS implantation, SNS, and antegrade irrigation through the colon.

The authors (Paul-Antoine Lehur) experience with both ABS and SNS offered a unique opportunity to compare their respective results. "We compared 15 SNS patients in a case-control study to 15 patients treated with an ABS. Both groups were similar regarding age, gender, incontinence severity, and conservative treatment failure. Preoperative manometric studies were similar in both groups. Results of the study showed that quality of life evaluation was similar in both groups, whereas incontinence and constipation scores were significantly different. As expected, greater improvement in continence is obtained after ABS implantation at the significant price in term of exacerbated obstructed defecation" (6).

DEVICE DESCRIPTION AND FUNCTIONING

The Acticon Neosphincter ABS Device—Description

The Acticon Neosphincter ABS (American Medical Systems [AMS], Minnetonka, MN, USA) is a totally implantable device made of solid silicone rubber. It comprises three parts: a perianal occlusive cuff, a control pump with a septum, and a pressure-regulating balloon. These three components are linked together by subcutaneous kink-resistant tubing (Fig. 13.2).

- The occlusive cuff is implanted in the upper part of the anal canal, and the closing system incorporated into the cuff uses the initial part of the tubing. The cuff comes in different models with respect to length (9–14 cm) and height (2.0 cm or 2.9 cm).

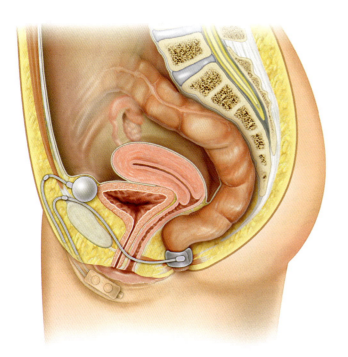

Figure 13.2 The Acticon Neosphincter™ artificial bowel sphincter implanted in a female patient.

The choice of the cuff, an important intraoperative consideration, is determined by measurements made during the implantation procedure.

▓ The pressure-regulating balloon, which is implanted in a pocket created in the subperitoneal space, controls the level of pressure applied on the anal canal by cuff closure. Available pressures range from 80–110 cm H2O in 10-cm gradations. Thus, the occlusive effect of the cuff depends on its size (length and height) that determines whether it fits more or less tightly around the anal canal and the pressure level chosen for the balloon.

▓ The control pump is implanted in subcutaneous tissues of the scrotum in men and of the labia majora in women. The hard upper part of the pump contains a resistance regulating the rate of fluid circulation throughout the system and a deactivation button allowing fluid cycling to be stopped by external action. The soft lower part of the pump is squeezed repeatedly to transfer fluid within the device. A septum placed at the bottom of this soft part is intended for postoperative use in case a small amount of liquid needs to be injected. The principle of this septum is similar to that of an implantable portacath.

The Acticon Neosphincter ABS Device—Functioning

The ABS functions semiautomatically:

▓ The cuff automatically ensures continuous anal closure at low pressures, close to normal physiological resting pressure. The regulating balloon transmits pressure to the occlusive cuff through the tubing, and the pressure is applied uniformly and nearly circularly to the upper part of the anal canal, restoring a barrier and isolating the rectum from outside.

▓ Defecation is initiated by the patient. Anal opening is achieved by transferring the pressurized fluid from the cuff toward the balloon by means of the control pump. The fluid is transferred by 5–20 squeezes on the pump, each evacuating approximately around 0.5 cc from the cuff, thereby lowering anal pressure and opening the anal canal to expel stool. Suitable compliance allows the volume of the pressure-regulating balloon to transiently increase to receive the several cubic centimeters of fluid contained in the cuff.

▓ Anal closure automatically occurs in 5–8 minutes by passive fluid transfer and a progressive return to baseline pressure in the cuff. The balloon recovers its initial volume during this period, thereby restoring equal pressure throughout the system (Fig. 13.3).

The system can be temporarily deactivated to allow the cuff to be empty and the anal canal to be continuously open. This arrangement can be used during the postoperative period to avoid manipulation of the cuff and pump during the healing period. Deactivation for 6–8 weeks is desirable after implantation to ensure tissue integration of the device. The system can then be activated simply by firmly squeezing the control pump, a procedure not requiring anesthesia performed during an office visit. Deactivation of the cuff in its open position is also necessary for transanal endoscopic procedures in order to avoid any tear or damage to the cuff during the passage of the endoscope. Deactivation during bowel preparation for radiologic or surgical procedures may also be desirable.

PREOPERATIVE CARE

Preoperative care includes careful cutaneous and bowel preparation over a 48-hour period.

▓ Skin prep: Two douches of the patient are performed daily with an iodinated solution

▓ Bowel prep: A complete colonic preparation is done, including X-prep and enemas until fluid becomes clear. There is no need for a colostomy, except in the case of

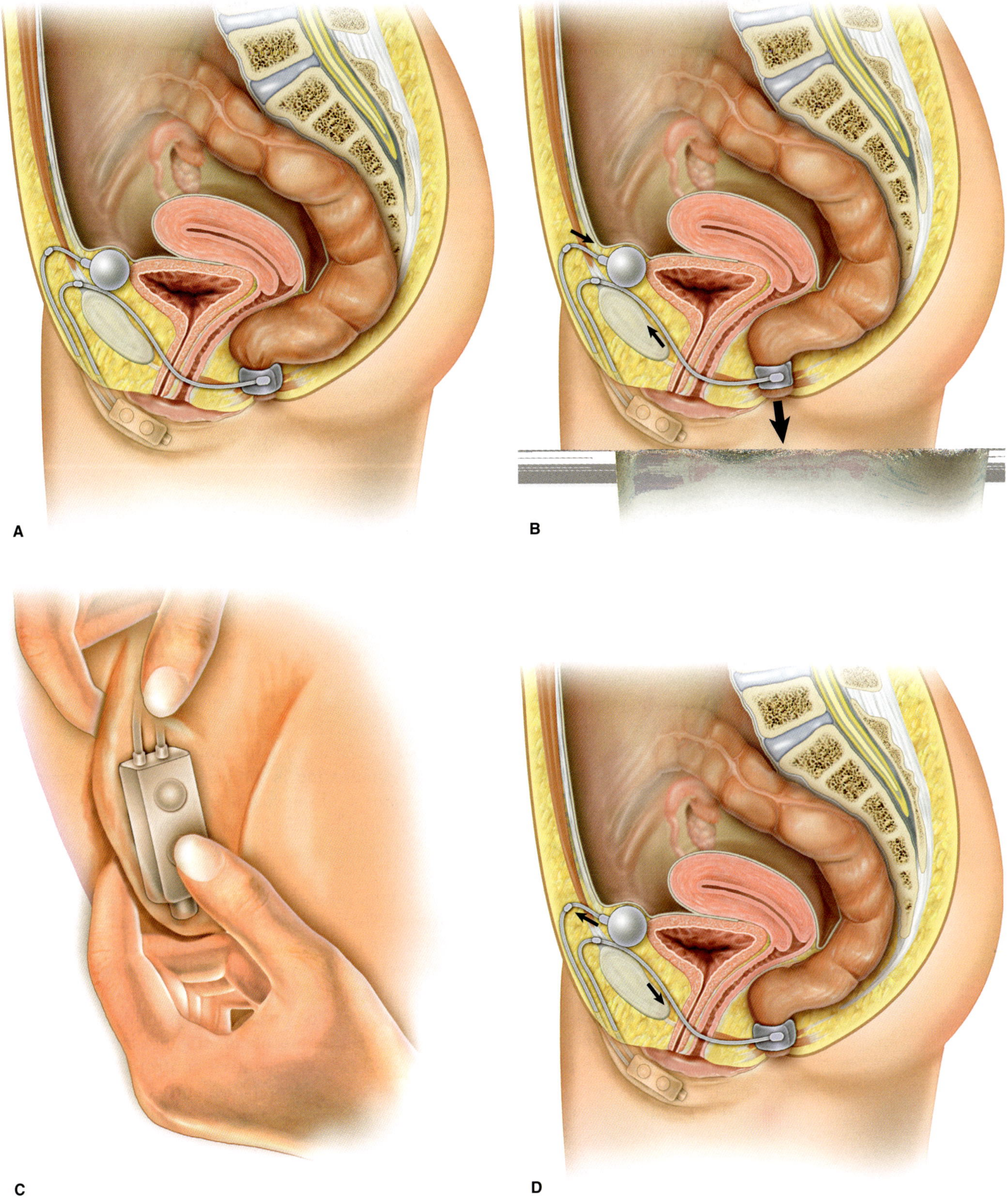

Figure 13.3 Functioning of the artificial bowel sphincter. **A.** Anal cuff closure. **B.** Opening of the cuff by pumping on the control pump. **C.** ABS control pump manipulation. **D.** Automatic closure of the cuff after evacuation.

diarrheic patients in whom contamination of the perineal wound may occur from too rapid a resumption of bowel movements.

▪ Antibiotic prophylaxis based on a third-generation cephalosporin and an aminoglycoside is administered in a single dose at the induction of anesthesia.

The author (Steven Wexner) recently performed in a multivariate analysis of 51 ABS implantations (in 47 patients and identified two independent risk factors for early-stage infectious complication after ABS implantation (defined as occurring before ABS activation): an early return of stool passage (before day 2) and an history of perianal infection (17).

This finding reinforces the need for a perfect bowel preparation (what has been called a chemical transient colostomy). Avoiding stool contamination of the perineal wound (or even the operative field at time of operation) is imperative.

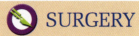 ## SURGERY

Operative Position

▪ Lithotomy position: The operative position of the patient should allow a combined perineal and abdominal access.

Operative Technique

▪ Perineal incision and perianal tunnel creation

The first phase of the operation involves placement of the perianal occlusive cuff. A single perianal incision can be used, allowing rectovaginal or rectourethral separation (5–6 cm) from which a perianal tunnel can be created around the anal canal by blunt dissection. Alternatively, bilateral incisions can be made laterally on both sides of the anus, following the example of graciloplasty procedure. A transvaginal approach has also been proposed (P Lee, MD. Portland, OR, USA). The length of the occlusive cuff is then determined using a specially designed sizer. The cuff should not narrow the anal canal, which would hinder evacuation. Rectal examination is the best means of determining the caliber obtained. In the event of perforation of the vagina or rectum at this point in the dissection, implantation of the ABS should be deferred or possibly abandoned.

▪ Device preparation

Once the perianal tunnel has been made, preparation of the ABS device can begin on a sterile table intended for this purpose. Tissue, blood, and any potentially aggressive surgical material are excluded from this area in order to avoid possible alteration of the device. All three components of the system are carefully bled of any air bubbles, which might prevent cycling of the pressurization fluid. This rather delicate preparation should be entrusted to a nurse trained in the technique. The pressurization fluid is an isotonic solution as the artificial sphincter walls are semipermeable membranes and radiopaque (except in the case of iodine allergy) to allow postoperative control of fluid movements in the system. The fluid is extemporaneously prepared and composed of Telebrix 12 sodium (53%) and sterile water (47%) although other possible solutions are described by AMS company.

▪ Cuff implantation – Connection to the abdominal site – Pressurization

The perianal cuff is the first component put into place. Tubing from the cuff is then tunneled subcutaneously to the abdominal incision with a special atraumatic, long needle. The rectus abdominis is split to provide access to the subperitoneal space lateral to the bladder. A pocket is created in this space to lodge the pressure-regulating balloon. The cuff is first pressurized by connection with the balloon, which is filled with 55 cc of radiopaque fluid. The amount of fluid kept in the cuff after pressurization is carefully measured when emptying the balloon; it is usually between 4 cc and 8 cc. It indicates the volume of fluid that the patient will have to transfer by pumping to open the cuff and evacuate.

- Balloon implantation – Control pump placement – Connections – Wound closures

The balloon is then implanted empty and filled with 40 cc of radiopaque fluid, a volume at which the pressure delivered to the cuff corresponds to values determined by the manufacturer (usually between 80 cm and 110 cm of water). One of the authors (Steven Wexner) routinely overfills the balloon with an additional 5 cc. The aponeurosis is carefully closed during this step. The control pump is then positioned. As this is the only component that the patient will feel and manipulate, it needs to be perfectly accessible. The occlusive cuff and the pressure-regulating balloon are connected to the pump. The kink-resistant tubes are identified by a color code (black from the balloon and clear from the cuff). Connections are made with special "quick connectors," preventing any air bubbles from entering the system. After assessing that cycling is correct, the incisions are closed without drainage.

- Device deactivation

The device is deactivated at the end of the procedure by pressing firmly on the deactivation button.

- Operative duration

In our experience, the entire procedure lasts between 90–120 minutes.

POSTOPERATIVE MANAGEMENT

- Postoperative care

The patient is maintained on a liquid diet for three days to avoid an early bowel movement. The anal wound is regularly cleaned. The mean length of hospital stay is 3–10 days in the absence of complications. The patient is discharged once evacuation has become normal and the incisions are healed.

- Activation of the ABS

The patient is readmitted 6 to 10 weeks later for 1 day during which the artificial sphincter is activated. A firm pressure on the control pump unblocks the deactivation button, allowing the empty cuff to fill and play its occlusive role. The patient is given the necessary instructions for opening the sphincter (cuff), allowing regular defecation, possibly initiated with small enemas in case of difficulty.

FOLLOW-UP OF PATIENTS WITH ABS IMPLANTS—RECOMMENDATIONS

Is it necessary to follow up patients who have received implants? This point is debatable, as the device is easy to operate and its use rapidly becomes natural for the patient. The patient could be instructed to return in the event of incontinence recurrence, which would be a good arrangement for persons living far from the implantation center.

However, we require regular follow-up for our patients, not only for research purposes, but also to verify the proper use of the device, its efficacy in restoring satisfactory anorectal function, and the possible occurrence of complications. Postoperative evaluation is based on simple annual examinations (clinical, plain X-rays, and anorectal manometry).

- Clinical evaluation relative to fecal continence and rectal evacuation is performed best by questionnaires. Efficacy of the device in restoring satisfactory quality of life can also be assessed by specific questionnaires. Such evaluations are currently in progress and appear to justify the financial investment involved in the use of artificial sphincters.

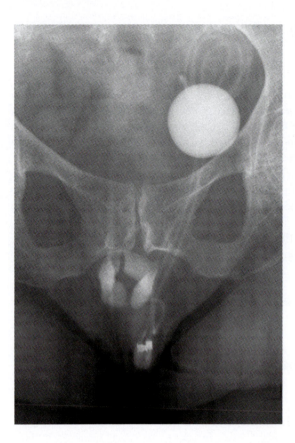

Figure 13.4 Radiological aspect of the artificial bowel sphincter inflated with a radiopaque fluid.

The clinical examination checks the proper positioning of the control pump and its accessibility, the efficacy of anal closure by digital rectal examination, and the quality of anal opening after manipulation of the pump by the patient. Local tolerance of the artificial sphincter is also assessed. It is important during the first postoperative months to detect any migration of the cuff. If it is too close to the anal margin, there is risk of skin damage and erosion, leading to contamination of the material and explantation. If detected early enough, this complication can be corrected by reoperation and repositioning the cuff higher in the pelvic floor. This repositioning can be achieved by redoing the perineal incision and simply unbuttoning the deactivated cuff.

- Pressurization of the ABS with a radiopaque fluid allows very simple radiological monitoring (Fig. 13.4).
  - In the immediate postoperative period, device deactivation can easily be checked by plain pelvic X-rays.
  - During activation, a series of X-rays can be used to analyze fluid transfer through the device and thus visualize the ABS function. These images can also be used for reference purposes in the event of subsequent device dysfunction.
  - Endoanal ultrasonography can also be performed during the monitoring procedure. This examination, though not routinely undertaken, is considered a valid means of assessing the thickness of tissues encircled by the cuff and detecting any possible atrophy, which would be suggestive of ulceration of the device in the anal canal.
- Anal manometry, an important aspect of postimplantation monitoring, precisely and objectively estimates the efficiency of the ABS (Fig. 13.5). We consider it important to determine three manometric parameters systematically:
  - Basal pressure with the ABS closed indicates the capacity of the device to create a high-pressure zone in the anal canal. A significant increase compared with preoperative values contributes to restoring fecal continence.
  - Basal pressure with the ABS opened by the patient represents residual anal pressure. When low, it is indicative of a wide anal opening and easy defecation, whereas high residual pressure could account for postoperative dyschezia.

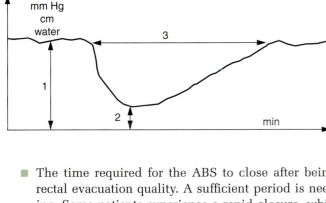

Figure 13.5 Anal manometry of a normally functioning artificial bowel sphincter.

- resting anal pressure with the cuff closed (pressurized)
- resting anal pressure with the cuff open (empty)
- time of anal closure

- The time required for the ABS to close after being opened is also indicative of rectal evacuation quality. A sufficient period is needed to obtain complete emptying. Some patients experience a rapid closure, which may also be responsible for dyschezia. Closure time can range from 2–10 minutes (15).
- Anal manometry can also be used to assess whether the patient is correctly manipulating the device. Pumping quality, which needs to be slow to be efficient, and that of the resulting anal opening can be evaluated on a screen image for the patient's benefit, during biofeedback sessions.

COMPLICATIONS

The main outcome endpoints regarding complications include infection, revision surgery, and explantation of the device are given in Table 13.2. The overall incidence of permanent explantation of the ABS in the published series varied between 17 and 31% with follow-up periods of between 10 and 58 months. Revision surgery with replacement of part of or the entire device occurred in 7–25% of patients. Complications leading to explantation included perioperative infection, failure of wound healing, erosion of part of the device through the skin or the anal canal, late infection, and mechanical malfunction of the device due to cuff (frequent) or balloon (rare) rupture.

RESULTS AND RECOMMENDATIONS

Recently Published Results of the ABS and Personal Series

Several centers in Europe (1–3,5,12), the United States (13,17,18), and Australia (11) have adopted the ABS to treat severe fecal incontinence not amenable to local repair. Reports with larger numbers of cases and longer follow-up have recently appeared, providing a better assessment of this technique.

- Continence: successful results have been respectively obtained in groups from Spain; Italy; Minneapolis, MN, USA; Weston, Fl, USA; Rouen, France; and Nantes, France,

TABLE 13.2	Results with the Artificial Bowel Sphincter				
	Number	Infection rate (%)	Revision surgery (%)	Explant rate (%)	Mean follow-up (months)
Wong et al. (18)	112	25	46	37	18
Ortiz et al. (12)	22	9	50	32	26
Altomare et al. (1)	28	18	32	25	19
Parker et al. (13)	37	34	37	40	39
Michot et al. (8)	25	7	28	20	34
Lehur unpublished series	32	0	53	31	26
Wexner et al. (17)	51				

in 15 out of 24 (62.5%), 21 out of 28 (75%), 17 out of 35 (49%), 22 out of 30 (73%), and 23 out of 32 (72%) cases. As did others, we found improvement in quality of life after ABS implantation.

- Quality of life: In a series of 16 patients consecutively receiving implants and a follow-up of 25 months, there was significant improvement in the four separate quality-of-life domains explored in the Fecal Incontinence Quality of Life. Scores were recorded, with a linear correlation between improvement over time in the quality-of-life index and evaluation of continence measured by a clinical score (4).

- ABS reimplantation after failure: In many series, patients have undergone successful reimplantation after failure of a previous implantation related to infection, ulceration, or mechanical breakdown. In the Nantes series of 32 patients receiving implants (unpublished), 10 were explanted, but five of them underwent reimplantation with success. All, or portion, of the device can be replaced when revision surgery is needed. The series of Parker et al, reported the risk of infection following revision to be 19%, lower than after primary implantation (34%). Their success rate in this setting was 65% (13/21 cases) (13). Patients choosing ABS therapy must be aware of the risk of revision surgery. They usually accept redo surgery in case of complications, as they greatly appreciate the benefit obtained with the device.

- Results of the ABS in anorectal reconstruction following abdominoperineal excision: Romano et al reported using the ABS in this setting in a series of eight patients of whom four are reported to have good neoanal function (14). Our personal experience is based on five patients in whom an ABS was implanted around a perineal colostomy built after curative rectal excision for T1–2 node-negative (N0) cancer. Four of them have had preoperative radiotherapy. Device implantation was feasible and uneventful. In four patients, leaks and urgency significantly decreased, but colonic retrograde enemas were maintained. Dietary restriction was loosened. Quality of life improved, and these four patients considered the device a useful adjunct. In this limited experience, implantation of an artificial sphincter around a perineal colostomy following APR for cancer appeared feasible and safe, even following previous radiotherapy. Tolerance at midterm was satisfactory. Continence and quality of life significantly improved (5).

Recently Published Recommendations for the Management of Fecal Incontinence

Over the past 2 years, the Standards Practice Task Force of The American Society of Colon and Rectal Surgeons (US) and the National Institute for Clinical Excellence (UK) have published recommendations for the management of fecal incontinence (16,10).

- Practice Parameters for the Treatment of Fecal Incontinence of the American Society of Colon and Rectal Surgeons (2007): "The ABS has a role in the treatment of severe fecal incontinence, especially in patients with significant sphincter disruption. Level of Evidence: III; Grade of Recommendation: B".

- NICE (2008):". . .If a trial of SNS is unsuccessful, an individual can be considered for a neosphincter, for which the two options are a stimulated graciloplasty or an ABS. People should be informed of the potential benefits and limitations of both procedures. Those offered these procedures should be informed that they may experience evacuatory disorders and/or serious infection, either of which may necessitate removal of the device. People being considered for either procedure should be assessed and managed at a specialist center with experience of performing these procedures. If an ABS is to be used, there are special arrangements that should be followed, as indicated in NICE interventional procedures guidance 66."

CONCLUSIONS

The role of the ABS must be put in perspective along with the other new minimally invasive approaches to anal incontinence, namely, SNS.

■ Although morbidity and the need for revisional surgery is high following implantation of the ABS, the outcome in terms of continence and improvement in quality of life is significantly satisfactory.

■ Patient selection is mandatory to achieve the best results.

■ Late mechanical failure is a concern and suggests that modification of the device from the manufacturing company (AMS) is needed as is continuous evaluation from surgeons.

■ In case of nonresponse to conservative treatment, local repair, or SNS, the ABS is an effective solution for motivated patients and experienced surgeons.

Recommended References and Readings

1. Altomare DF, Dodi G, La Torre F, Romano G, Melega E, Rinaldi M. Multicentre retrospective analysis of the outcome of artificial anal sphincter implantation for severe faecal incontinence. *Br J Surg* 2001;88:1481–6.
2. Casal E, San Ildefonso A, Carracedo R, Facal C, Sánchez JA. Artificial bowel sphincter in severe anal incontinence. *Colorectal Dis* 2004;6:180–4.
3. Christiansen J, Rasmussen OO, Lindorff-Larsen K. Long-term results of artificial anal sphincter implantation for severe anal incontinence. *Ann Surg* 1999;230:45–8.
4. Lehur PA, Zerbib F, Glemain P, Neunlist M, Bruley des Varannes S. Comparison of quality of life and anorectal function after artificial sphincter implantation. *Dis Colon Rectum* 2002;45:508–13.
5. Marchal F, Doucet C, Lechaux D, Lasser P, Lehur PA. Secondary implantation of an artificial sphincter after abdominoperineal resection and pseudocontinent perineal colostomy for rectal cancer. *Gastroenterol Clin Biol* 2005;29:425–8.
6. Meurette G, La Torre M, Regenet N, Robert-Yap J, Lehur PA. Value of sacral nerve stimulation in the treatment of severe faecal incontinence: A comparison to the artificial bowel sphincter. *Colorectal Dis* 2008;11:631–5.
7. Michot F, Costaglioli B, Leroi AM, Denis P. Artificial anal sphincter in severe fecal incontinence: outcome of prospective experience with 37 patients in one institution. *Ann Surg* 2003;237:52–6.
8. Michot F, Tuech JJ, Lefebure B, Bridoux V, Denis P. A new implantation procedure of artificial sphincter for anal incontinence: the trans-vaginal approach. *Dis Colon Rectum* 2007;50:1401–4.
9. Mundy L, Merlin TL, Maddern GJ, Hiller JE. Systematic review of safety and effectiveness of an artificial bowel sphincter for faecal incontinence. *Br J Surg* 2004;91:665–72.
10. NICE clinical guideline 49: Faecal incontinence: the management of faecal incontinence in adults. http://www.nice.org.uk/CG049.
11. O'Brien PE, Dixon JB, Skinner S, Laurie C, Khera A, Fonda D. A prospective randomised controlled clinical trial of placement of the artificial bowel sphincter (Acticon Neosphincter) for the control of fecal incontinence. *Dis Colon Rectum* 2004;47:1852–60.
12. Ortiz H, Armendariz P, DeMiguel M, Ruiz MD, Alós R, Roig JV. Complications and functional outcome following artificial anal sphincter implantation. *Br J Surg* 2002;89:877–81.
13. Parker SC, Spencer MP, Madoff RD. Artificial bowel sphincter: long-term experience at a single institution. *Dis Colon Rectum* 2003;46:722–9.
14. Romano G, La Torre F, Cutini G, Bianco F, Esposito P, Montori A. Total anorectal reconstruction with the artificial bowel sphincter: report of eight cases. *Dis Colon Rectum* 2003;46:730–4.
15. Savoye G, Leroi AM, Denis P, Michot F. Manometric assessment of an artificial bowel sphincter. *Br J Surg* 2000;87:586–9.
16. Tjandra JJ, Dykes SL, Kumar RR, et al. and Standards Practice Task Force of The American Society of Colon and Rectal Surgeons. Practice parameters for the treatment of fecal incontinence. *Dis Colon Rectum* 2007;50:1497–1507.
17. Wexner SD, Jin HY, Weiss EG, Nogueras JJ, Li VK. Factors associated with failure of the artificial bowel sphincter—A study of over 50 cases from Cleveland Clinic Florida. *Dis Colon Rectum*, 2009;52:1550–7.
18. Wong WD, Congilosi S, Spencer M, et al. The safety and efficacy of the artificial bowel sphincter for faecal incontinence: results from a multicenter cohort study. *Dis Colon Rectum* 2002;45:1139–53.

14 Sacral Nerve Stimulation

Klaus E. Matzel

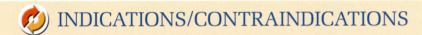

INDICATIONS/CONTRAINDICATIONS

Operative intervention for fecal incontinence should only be considered when conservative treatments have failed to result in adequate symptom relief.

The spectrum of indications for sacral nerve stimulation (SNS) is continually evolving. Since its first use for the treatment of fecal incontinence in 1994, its application has broadened. Initial indications were a very distinct population: patients presenting with fecal incontinence and residual function of a weak, but structurally intact, striated muscular anal sphincter and pelvic floor. However, the following findings widened the spectrum of indications:

- The effect of SNS is not confined to the muscle relevant to continence.
- Temporary test stimulation is low risk.
- The result of a positive test stimulation is highly predictive of the clinical outcome of chronic therapeutic stimulation.

Today, test stimulation is liberally used, not only in established indications, but also to explore potential new indications, both for specific etiologies leading to incontinence and for other pathological conditions of the colorectum resulting in functional disorder. Permanent stimulation is directed by the clinical effectiveness of test stimulation.

Test stimulation is used on a pragmatic trial-and-error basis as it is clinically efficient and minimally invasive and because no other reliable clinical or physiologic predictor for a positive outcome of chronic SNS with a permanent neurostimulation device exists.

- Patients are appropriate for test stimulation if they have existing, even if residual, voluntary anal sphincteric function or existing reflex sphincteric activity, indicating a nerve–muscle connection (confirmed by intact anocutaneous reflex activity, reflex contraction during sneezing or coughing, or a muscle response to pudendal stimulation with the St. Mark's electrode).

Permanent stimulation with a fully implanted device is usually indicated if the trial stimulation results in >50% improvement symptom.

In addition to general contraindications (unfit for surgery or prone placement, bleeding diathesis), contraindications for test stimulation and implantation of the permanent device include the following:

- Pathologic conditions of the sacrum preventing adequate electrode placement (such as congenital malformations)
- Skin disease (especially septic) at the area of implantation
- Micturition disorders that are considered contraindications for SNS
- Pregnancy
- Psychological instability, mental instability, or retardation that would impede understanding and handling the device programmer
- The presence of devices incompatible with the implanted neurostimulator (cardiac pacemaker or implantable defibrillator)
- The need for magnetic resonance imaging (MRI) in diagnosing or treating any other medical condition (the current generation of stimulation systems is not MRI-safe).

 ## PREOPERATIVE PLANNING

Preoperative planning is pragmatic and algorithmic. The decision making relies solely on documentation of the pretreatment bowel pattern and its change during temporary stimulation. It is helpful to know whether the patients retain voluntary sphincter/pelvic floor contractions or if reflex contraction can be provoked by a pin-prick test or coughing or sneezing. If both are missing, SNS is less promising.

Success of treatment (and of test stimulation) depends on appropriate electrode placement; preoperative sacral imaging in two planes will identify individual variances in bone anatomy and sacral foramina configuration. Preoperative bowel cleansing is not necessary.

For implantation of the permanent device, the position of the implantable pulse generator (INS) should be discussed with the patient and marked preoperatively. The patient must be able to reach it with the handheld programmer to activate and deactivate it or to change stimulation amplitude in a preset range. Interference with personal habits or clothing should be avoided.

 ## SURGERY

Concept

Permanent SNS is indicated if trial stimulation results in symptom relief. Usually, a 50% reduction in the number of incontinent episodes or days with incontinence is considered adequate. The trial must be long enough to confirm these changes.

The SNS procedure consists of three steps:

- In the first diagnostic stage, acute percutaneous nerve evaluation (PNE), the accessibility of the nerve/s through the sacral foramen and the feasibility of electrode placement are determined.
- PNE assesses the relevance of each sacral spinal nerve to anal sphincteric contraction and anal canal closure/pelvic floor contraction. This information can help perform the following:
  - Distinguish between the true functional capability of the striated anal sphincteric muscles and the patient's ability to make full voluntary use of them
  - Identify the individual pattern of peripheral innervation and demonstrate individual differences of the somatomotor/somatosensory innervation
  - Detect and determine the site of a possible lesion of the peripheral anal sphincteric nerve supply
  - Identify the optimal site for future stimulation

■ In the second diagnostic step, the therapeutic potential of stimulation is assessed by temporarily stimulating the sacral nerve identified during acute testing. As a therapeutic trial, it serves to select patients who may benefit from permanent neurostimulation.

■ In the third step, the aims is to improve symptoms permanently with continuous low-frequency stimulation.

PNE and permanent implantation can be performed under local or general anesthesia.

■ If general anesthesia is used, muscle relaxants must be avoided. They will suppress the motor reaction when the sacral nerves are stimulated and complicate identification of the optimal position for the electrode.

■ If local anesthesia is used, accidental blockade of the relevant sacral spinal nerves must be avoided, as the technique of electrode placement depends on a conducting nerve.

Anatomy

Technically, the most important part of the procedure at all stages—acute testing, subchronic test stimulation, and permanent implantation—is the appropriate placement of the electrode. It should be positioned close to the exit of the sacral spinal nerves through the ventral opening of the sacral foramen, at the site where the nerves enter the pelvic cavity and proximal to the formation of the sacral plexus.

Distinct, palpable, bony anatomic landmarks help identify the sacral foramina. Most commonly, S3 is used for stimulation; during the procedure, it is also used as a reference site for orientation to place electrodes on S4 or S2.

The following landmarks help identify the foramina (Fig. 14.1):

■ The spinal processes mark the midline. Variations can occur, mostly distally.

■ The S3 foramen level is located medial to the upper edge of the greater sciatic notch.

■ The S3 foramen level (upper edge) corresponds to half the distance between the upper edge of the sacrum (lumbar–sacral junction) and the tip of the coccyx.

■ The S4 level corresponds with the sacral crest. Soft tissue coverage is least at S4 level.

■ The foramina are located 1–2 cm from the midline, which is marked by the palpable spinal processes. (The arrangement of the foramina relative to the midline may vary from parallel to a more V-shaped pattern.)

■ The distance between the levels of the sacral foramina is approximately 1.5 cm.

Neurostimulation Devices for SNS: Main Components

■ Test Stimulation Lead, Medtronic Model 3057: Unipolar lead designed to be implanted adjacent to the sacral nerve for temporary stimulation.

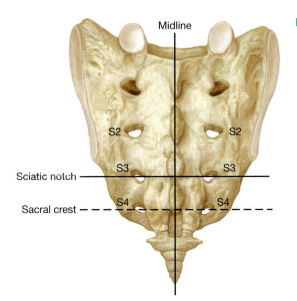

Figure 14.1 Sacrum with landmarks for palpation.

- InterStim® Tined Lead, Medtronic Model 3889: A quadripolar in-line lead containing four cylindrical electrodes equal in length and spaced equidistantly. The lead has tines and marker bands. The tines anchor the lead, and the marker bands indicate lead depth and tine deployment during percutaneous implantation with a lead introducer.
- InterStim® Tined Lead, Medtronic Model 3093: A quadripolar like Model 3889, but with a different electrode arrangement. The lead contains three cylindrical electrodes equal in length and spaced equidistantly and one extended (coiled) electrode approximately three times longer than the other three cylindrical electrodes.
- InterStim® Implantable Neurostimulator, Medtronic Model 3023: A neurostimulator producing electrical pulses for stimulation with a variety of parameters, modes, and polarities. The implantable neurostimulator connects with an extension Model 3095, and the extension lead connects with a lead through which a stimulation program is delivered.
- InterStim® II Implantable Neurostimulator, Medtronic Model 3058: Like Model 3023 above, a neurostimulator producing electrical pulses for stimulation with a variety of parameters, modes, and polarities. However, this is smaller, carries a smaller battery, and does not require a connecting cable to the electrode lead.
- N'Vision Clinician Programmer, Medtronic Model 8840: Used by physicians with an 8870 Application Card (software) to program and communicate via telemetry with an InterStim or InterStim II neurostimulator.
- iCon Patient Programmer, Medtronic Model 3037: To use with the InterStim (3023) or InterStim II (3058) neurostimulator. This handheld unit allows the patient to turn the neurostimulator on or off, change preset programs, adjust the amplitude within preset limits, and check the status of the neurostimulator and programmer batteries.

Patient Positioning

The patient is positioned prone (if fluoroscopy with lateral imaging of the sacrum is used on an X-ray-capable operating table).

- The pelvis is elevated and supported. The legs and feet are fixed, but should be movable, as concomitant movements of the ipsilateral leg and foot during stimulation may aid electrode placement (Fig. 14.2).
- The buttocks are taped to allow visual access to the anus and perineum. Taping should not be so tight as to counteract stimulation-induced contraction of the anus and the pelvic floor, which can be delicate.
- The operative field (sacrum and buttock) is draped and sterile.
- Visualization of a motor response of the anus and perianal area, as well as the feet, must be ensured.
- Perioperative antibiotic prophylaxis is advised for implantation of permanent devices.

Acute Percutaneous Nerve Evaluation

For acute PNE, needle electrodes (Medtronic Model 041828 or 041829 Foramen Needles), not isolated at the tip and top, are inserted into the dorsal sacral foramina of the

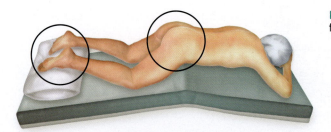

Figure 14.2 Patient positioning: pelvic floor, anus, and feet must be visible.

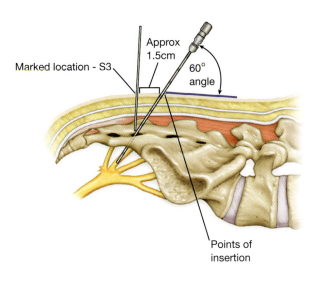

Figure 14.3 Acute needle electrode insertion: 1.5 cm cephalad to the foramen.

potentially relevant nerve—most commonly S3, but also S2 and S4. Placement is mainly guided by sacral bony landmarks and can be supported and confirmed by fluoroscopy.

- Identification of the sacral foramina: A distinct sensation of entering the dorsal opening of the foramen, perforating rigid ligamentous structures (as compared with hitting the periosteum of the sacrum), will be experienced.
- Needle electrode positioning: The angle of insertion should be acute to minimize the risk of nerve or vascular damage, which is 60 degrees at the level of the skin (Fig. 14.3). As the needle has to cross soft tissue before entering the foramen, its entrance point should be cephalad to the position of the foramen.
- Optimizing positioning: Once the foramen is entered, the needle electrode should be moved in a ventral direction (or back) with intermittent stimulation of graduated amplitude (beginning with low amplitudes). Gentle movements in millimeter steps with intermittent stimulation will help optimize positioning. Markers on the needle electrode indicate the depth of placement.
- Response to stimulation: A motor response of the pelvic floor and the anus (if general anesthesia) or a sensory response (if local anesthesia) will optimize the positioning of the needle electrode.

Although the effect of stimulation on the pelvic floor and the lower extremity activity may vary among individuals, the following motor responses are generally typical:

- S2 stimulation results in a clamp-like contraction of the perineal muscles and an outward rotation of the ipsilateral leg.
- S3 stimulation leads to contraction of the levator ani and external anal sphincter, resulting in a bellows-like movement and circular contraction of the anus, along with plantar flexion of the first and second toes.
- S4 stimulation produces a bellows-like contraction of the levator ani and circular contraction of the anus without movement of leg, foot, or toe.

Concomitant reactions of the leg/foot/toe can be observed, but are not essential. Their presence does not indicate a superior position of the electrode or a better clinical outcome.

If a sensory response is used to guide the placement of the electrode, it can range from a tingling "pins-and-needles" sensation to the perception of a contracting muscle in the perianal, anal, perineal, or vaginal area.

The electrode position is optimal when the motor/sensory response is most pronounced and the applied current is lowest.

If acute PNE successfully elicits the required reaction, an electrode is inserted for subchronic PNE. Therefore, the inner stylet of the needle electrode is removed, while keeping the needle sheath in the position.

Part IV: Operations for Fecal Incontinence

Subchronic PNE

Two technical options are available for assessing the clinical effect of temporary stimulation before permanent implantation:

1. A temporary, percutaneously placed, test stimulation lead (or multiple leads) (Medtronic 041830, Temporary Screening Lead), which will be removed at the end of the trial period.
2. The so-called tined lead, a quadripolar electrode placed operatively (Seldinger technique) with the aid of fluoroscopy. If testing is clinically successful, this electrode will remain in place for permanent stimulation. This procedure is stage 1 of the "two-stage implant."

After acute PNE, the needle stylet is removed, but the needle sheath stays in place.

■ For a temporary electrode, it will be inserted through the sheath of the placed needle electrode and maneuvered to the appropriate sacral nerve. Intermittent stimulation is used to confirm positioning. The sheath is then withdrawn and the electrode is secured by adhesive dressing and its position again confirmed by stimulation and radiography, either intraoperatively with fluoroscopy or postoperatively with a two-plane sacral radiograph or fluoroscopy.
■ If the "two-stage" option is used, an introducer guide is placed after placing a stylet through the sheath of the needle electrode and removing the sheath, to direct the placement of the quadripolar tined lead electrode (details are given below).

For screening, both types of electrodes are connected with an extension cable to an external pulse generator (Medtronic Screener 3625) (Fig. 14.4). The "two-stage" option has an extension cable connected to the electrode at the location of the future placement of the INS and tunneled percutaneously, usually to a site remote from the future position of the INS (most commonly the contralateral side) (Fig. 14.5). A sterile dressing is used to decrease the risk of infection at the skin or perforation of the extension cable during the course of the test stimulation.

Stimulation Setting

With temporary electrodes, only unipolar test stimulation with the external stimulator is possible. The parameters used are the same as for permanent stimulation (see below).

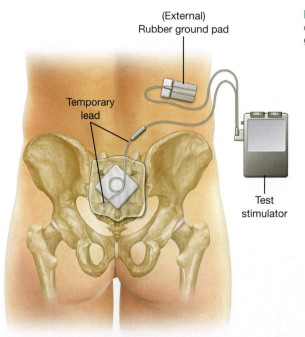

(External)
Rubber ground pad

Temporary lead

Test stimulator

Figure 14.4 Test stimulation with temporary electrode connected to an external pulse generator with ground pad.

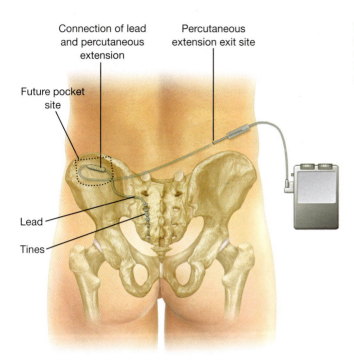

Connection of lead
and percutaneous
extension

Percutaneous
extension exit site

Future pocket
site

Lead

Tines

Figure 14.5 Test stimulation with tined lead electrode connected with an extension cable to an external pulse generator. No ground pad needed.

If multiple temporary electrodes have been placed, the one with the best sensory/motor response and the lowest threshold is chosen. At the end of the screening phase, the percutaneously placed temporary test stimulation lead is removed and a permanent system consisting of an electrode and INS is implanted. This step is usually performed several weeks after screening to ensure intact skin conditions.

If a tined lead has been placed as the first stage in the two-stage procedure, uni- or bipolar stimulation can be applied by setting the external pulse generator accordingly; bipolar stimulation is preferred. If the test is successful, the percutaneous extension is removed and only the INS is added (the second stage of the two-stage implant). If the test fails, the tined lead is removed by operative intervention: the electrode is extracted after skin incision and exposure of its entrance into the soft tissue covering the sacrum dorsally fluoroscopy is advised to ensure complete removal of the electrode.

During the test stimulation, patients are instructed to interrupt stimulation only for defecation and micturition. Bowel habits are documented with standardized bowel diaries and compared with similarly documented pretreatment levels.

Permanent Implant

When test stimulation demonstrates a 50% improvement in symptoms, permanent SNS is usually considered.

- The electrode is inserted with a minimally invasive Seldinger technique. Intraoperative neurostimulation and fluoroscopy are used to direct placement.
- After positioning the needle electrode close to the site where the target nerve enters the pelvic cavity the needle is removed, leaving the sheath in place; through this a stylet is placed to guide an introducer. To enter the skin with the introducer usually a skin incision is placed. This should be sufficiently long to adequately cover and bury the electrode, which will be bent in this position. The depth of introducer placement is guided with a radiopaque marker close to its tip. The position of the introducer is monitored by fluoroscopy (Fig. 14.6).
- Once the introducer is in the required position (radiopaque marker in the lower third of the sacral canal), the stylet is removed and the tined lead quadripolar electrode lead is pushed in (Fig. 14.6).

■ The electrode lead carries four electrode contacts, each of which can be individually stimulated. Intermittent stimulation and imaging optimize positioning. Ideally, the electrode should be parallel to the nerve (Fig. 14.7) in a caudolateral position with all four contacts resulting in an adequate motor/sensory response at low-amplitude stimulation. The introducer permits only ventral or dorsal movement. If a different direction is required, the procedure must be restarted with the needle electrodes placed at a different angle.

■ When positioning is optimal, the electrode is anchored: the introducer is gently withdrawn and the tines of the lead unfold to fix the electrode in the surrounding tissues (Fig. 14.8).

■ The pulse generator (INS) is then placed in a subcutaneous pocket, most commonly in the buttock, medial to the dorsal axillary line, distant from prominent bone structures, such as the iliac crest. The position should be preoperatively discussed with

Figure 14.6 Placement of the tined lead electrode with fluoroscopy.

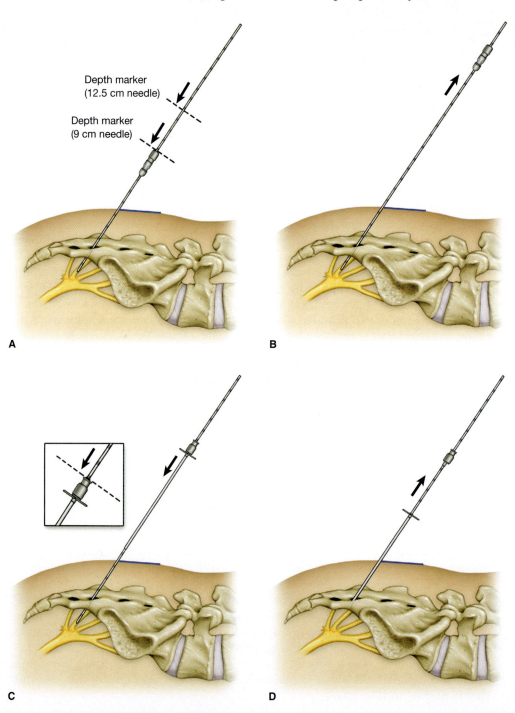

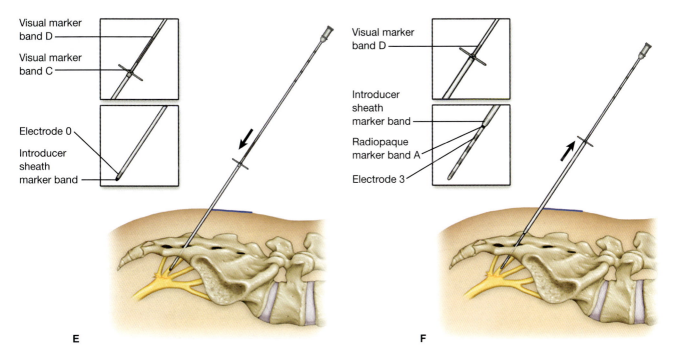

Figure 14.6 (*Continued*)

the patient and marked. The skin incision and subcutaneous dissection for the pocket should be large enough to cover the INS, but not so wide as to permit device rotation. In patients unable to reach around the buttocks to place the handheld programmer above the INS, the pocket can be placed in the abdominal wall.

■ Two INS models are currently available (as mentioned earlier): a smaller one with a direct connector to the electrode; and a larger one, requiring the use of an additional connecting cable. Either way, the electrode or the connecting cable is tunneled with a tunneling device subcutaneously to the position of the INS. Care should be taken to avoid proximity of the electrode/connecting cable track to bony structures. If a tined electrode has been used for test stimulation it will remain in place and be connected after removal of the percutaneous extension that connected it to the external pulse generator.

■ After connection with the electrode/connecting cable, the INS is buried in the pocket but should not be sutured to the muscle. Care must be taken to place the INS with the nonisolated surface facing upward to ensure programming. Redundant connecting cable/electrode should be placed around or behind the INS, but not in front of it to avoid interference with programming. The INS pocket is closed with a subcutaneous and skin layer of sutures.

During the operative placement of the electrode and the INS the electrode's position can accidently be changed by any manipulation. Repeated stimulation is recommended to ensure that this has not occurred and to confirm the function of the various implanted hardware components.

Bilateral implantation of foramen electrodes is uncommon, as it has not been systematically proven to be more effective than unilateral stimulation. However, it may be chosen if it improved the outcome of the screening phase. Bilateral electrodes can be connected to two single INS devices or to a dual-channel INS that allows separate programming.

POSTOPERATIVE MANAGEMENT

■ The INS should be postoperatively imaged to serve as a reference if complications occur and dislodgement is a concern.

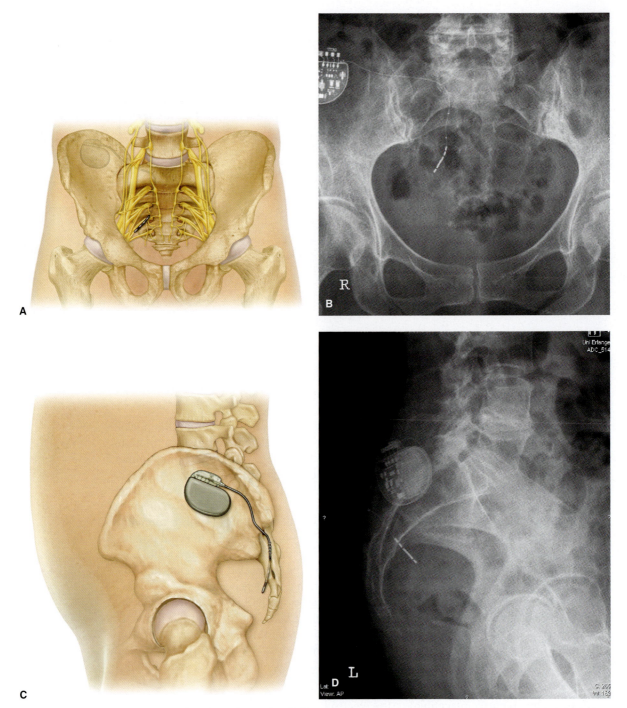

Figure 14.7 A. Position of the electrode: schematic drawing. **B.** X-ray, anteroposterior and lateral view. **C.** Position of the electrode: schematic drawing. **D.** X-ray, lateral view.

- The pulse generator is activated early in the postoperative course, usually on the day of surgery. Patients must be able to cooperate because the programming is largely based on their perception of the stimulation effect.

- For the screening phase, unipolar stimulation is applied (as mentioned earlier) if temporary electrodes are used: usually frequency of 14 Hz, pulse width of 210 microseconds, continuous stimulation. The intensity is directed by patient perception: most commonly, a tingling, twitching sensation in the anal, perianal, perineal, or vaginal area (or a combination).

- For screening with a tined lead electrode, bipolar stimulation can be applied with the external pulse generator. The contact electrodes on the tined lead are programmed accordingly (as follows).

Figure 14.8 Tined lead fixed.

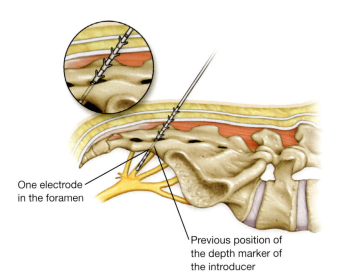

One electrode
in the foramen

Previous position of
the depth marker of
the introducer

For permanent therapeutic SNS, programming is based on the following principles.

- Each of the four electrode contacts of the tined lead can be programmed as anode, cathode, or neutral (switched off). In addition, the pulse generator can be programmed as anode or neutral.
- Bipolar stimulation is preferred to unipolar stimulation.
- Programming should be structured and documented, following an algorithm in the selection of the best parameters.
- The electrode combination most effective with regard to required intensity and the patient's perception of sensation or muscle contraction of the perineum and anal sphincter is chosen for permanent stimulation and has commonly been found to be: pulse width, 210 microseconds; frequency, 15 Hz; cylic (e.g., on:off, 5:1 seconds), or continuous stimulation. Parameter setting is done with the programmer by telemetry (Fig.14.9).

Figure 14.9 System components: tined lead electrode, InterStim II pulse generator. (Courtesy of Medtronic, Inc.)

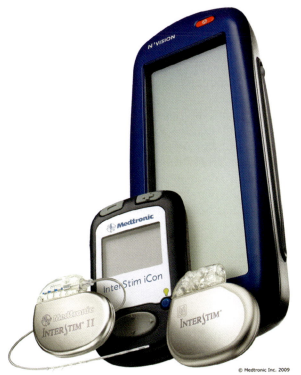

© Medtronic Inc. 2009

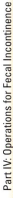

■ The intensity of stimulation is usually adapted to be above the individual patient's perception of muscular contraction or perianal sensation and is adjusted if necessary. Subsensory threshold stimulation has been shown to be effective also.

■ Patients are instructed to interrupt stimulation with the handheld programmer only for defecation and micturition. Urinary side effects such as retention and hydronephrosis have been reported with uninterrupted stimulation.

■ Patients can decrease or increase the intensity of stimulation in a preset range. This variation is usually done to ensure that the device is working (as adaptation to the perception of stimulation can be observed), and to adapt stimulation to variations in body positioning, such as decreased intensity during nighttime in a sleeping position, and to adjust to insufficient clinical effectiveness.

■ SNS therapy requires maintenance. A relevant portion of patients will require readjustment of the stimulation parameters to ensure constant optimal therapeutic effectiveness during follow-up.

COMPLICATIONS

■ Battery life of the INS is limited; battery size, current amplitude, and stimulation usage mainly determine lifespan, ranging from 4 to 7 years. A cycled program (alternating on and off for a set duration) or switching off the generator at regular intervals (such as during sleep) helps prolong it. As the current versions of the INS do not include rechargeable batteries, the INS needs to be exchanged in a minor surgical intervention once the battery is drained.

■ The INS and the electrodes are sensitive to magnetic fields and the manufacturer recommends removal if an MRI is needed. The device is also sensitive to unipolar cautery, and hence bipolar cautery is advised for surgical interventions.

■ The most frequent complications associated with chronic SNS are loss (or lack: inability to reproduce the therapeutic effect achieved during PNE) of efficacy in an estimated 12%, pain in 13%, infection in 4%, and adverse stimulation effects.

■ In general, one must establish whether the complication is a result of the treatment—either mechanical or functional. The latter can often be corrected by reprogramming. Even if a slight dislodgement of the electrode is involved, the arrangement of the contacts at the tip of the electrodes allows stimulation fields of various sizes and shapes, which may compensate for a minor dislodgement. The reprogramming should always be done in a structured manner. The algorithm of reprogramming is the same if adverse or uncomfortable stimulation effects occur.

■ If relevant electrode migration has occurred and reprogramming is ineffective, revisional surgery with repositioning is unavoidable. If potential loss of efficacy due to other (not mechanical) causes is suspected, reimplantation of a new electrode to a stimulation-naive sacral spinal nerve is advised.

■ Pain during therapy can also result simply from the presence of the device or from stimulation. To exclude pain owing to stimulation, the INS should be switched off for a period of time to clarify whether the pain is caused by the current.

■ Infections are rare and are usually apparent from clinical signs such as redness, warmth, and discharge. If not resolved with adequate antibiotic therapy (covering *Staphylococcus aureus*), removal of the device—most commonly the complete device—is unavoidable. Once the infection has been overcome, reimplantation of a new system can be considered.

■ In general, serious complications requiring device removal are rare (<5%), mostly prompted by infection or device malfunction.

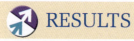 RESULTS

Since its first use in treating fecal incontinence, the clinical efficacy of SNS has been confirmed with reproducible results in multiple studies. These studies vary regarding

TABLE 14.1	Sacral Nerve Stimulation (SNS) for Fecal Incontinence						
				Incontinence episodes per week		Cleveland Clinic Incontinence Score	
Authors	Year	Number of patients	Follow-up (months)	Before SNS (baseline)	SNS (last FU)	Before SNS (baseline)	SNS (last FU)
Matzel et al.	2004	34	24*	16, 4	2, 0	nr	nr
Jarret et al.	2004	46	12*	7	1	14	6
Rasmussen et al.	2004	34	6	nr	nr	18	7
Leroi et al.	2005	34	7*	3, 5*	0, 5*	16*	10*
Holzer et al.	2007	29	35*	2, 3	0, 67	nr	nr
Hetzer et al.	2007	37	13	nr	nr	14	5
Tan et al.	2007	53	12	9, 5	3, 1	16	1, 2
Melenhorst et al.	2007	100	25.5	10, 4	1, 5	nr	nr
Vallet et al.	2008	32	37	nr	nr	16, 1	4, 9
Altomare et al.	2009	60	74	3, 5	0, 7	15	5
El-Gazzaz et al.	2009	24	28*	4.5	1.5	12	4.7
Wexner et al.	2010	120	28	9, 4	1, 4	nr	nr
Gallas et al.	2010	200	12*	4*	nr	14*	6, 5*
Michelsen et al.	2010	126	24	8, 3	0, 6	16	10

Note: Cleveland Clinic Fecal Incontinence Score: 0, fully continence; 20, worst incontinence.
*Denotes median, otherwise all data are presented as mean.
FU, follow-up; nr, not reported.
Source: Adapted from Matzel KE. *Colorect Dis* 2011 Mar;13(Suppl 2):10–14.

outcome criteria, but typically the frequency of involuntary loss of bowel content is the measure, although Cleveland Clinic Florida Incontinence Score and the ability to postpone the call for stool are also used. The majority of studies report a significant improvement in symptoms, short- and midterm, regardless of outcome measure (Table 14.1). With symptom improvement, quality of life is also increased. There is increasing evidence that the effect of SNS remains stable: a sustained clinical benefit has been demonstrated for up to 14 years.

Patient selection for permanent stimulation is uniform, directed by the outcome of the temporary test stimulation, which is highly predictive.

The range of indications for SNS in fecal incontinence has steadily evolved. Early application was confined to a distinct group of patients presenting with weak, but morphologically intact, anal sphincteric, and pelvic floor musculature. Based on the highly predictive value of a positive result to trial stimulation, which carries minimal risk, and the increasing knowledge that the effect of SNS is not limited to the muscle, but involves a variety of physiological functions contributing to continence, the use of PNE was expanded. This expansion resulted in a broader application of permanent SNS, even for patients with a structural defect of the internal and external anal sphincters. Today, SNS represents an essential part of the surgical armamentarium to treat fecal incontinence. It also carries potential for patients with concurrent fecal and urinary incontinence.

A systematic comparison with other surgical techniques—based on the existing level of evidence—has led to the current guidelines of the International Consultation of Incontinence (ICI). Surgical treatment of fecal incontinence is advised if conservative means do not result in adequate symptom relief. If fecal incontinence secondary to other underlying conditions is excluded, the choice of treatment is directed by the findings of endoanal ultrasound. In the treatment algorithm, SNS is central: it is recommended in patients presenting without a sphincteric lesion and as a therapeutic alternative to surgical repair in those with a sphincteric gap of up to 180 degrees. Although the results of the latter indication are more recent, limited to smaller series and midterm outcome, the findings are consistent.

✳ CONCLUSION

SNS has evolved to become an established treatment for fecal incontinence.

- The therapy is minimally invasive and relatively low risk.
- Patient selection is based on a therapeutic trial phase, which—if clinically efficient—is highly predictive of the outcome of permanent stimulation.
- The results of SNS are reproducible, and an increasing body of evidence indicates sustainability.
- The therapy requires maintenance.

Suggested Readings

Abrams P, Andersson KE, Birder L, et al. Fourth international consultation on incontinence recommendations of the international scientific committee: evaluation and treatment of urinary incontinence, pelvic organ prolapse, and faecal incontinence. *Neurourol Urodyn* 2010;29:213–40.

Colorect Dis 2011;13(Suppl 2).

Maeda Y, Lundby L, Buntzen S, et al. Suboptimal outcome following sacral nerve stimulation for faecal incontinence. *Br J Surg* 2011;98(1):140–7.

Maeda Y, Matzel K, Lundby L, et al. Postoperative issues of sacral nerve stimulation for faecal incontinence and constipation: a systematic literature review and treatment guideline. *Dis Colon Rectum* 2011 (accepted for publication).

Matzel KE, Stadelmaier U, Hohenfellner M, et al. Electrical stimulation of sacral spinal nerves for treatment of faecal incontinence. *Lancet* 1995;346(8983):1124–7.

Matzel KE, Kamm MA, Stösser M, et al. Sacral nerve stimulation for faecal incontinence: a multicenter study. *Lancet* 2004;363:1270–6.

Melenhorst J, Koch SM, Uludag O, et al. Sacral neuromodulation in patients with faecal incontinence: results of the first 100 permanent implantations. *Colorectal Dis* 2007;9:725–30.

Tan JJ, Chan M, Tjandra JJ. Evolving therapy for faecal incontinence. *Dis Colon Rectum* 2007;50:1950–6.

Wexner SD, Coller JA, Devroede G, et al. Sacral nerve stimulation for faecal incontinence: results of a 120-patient prospective multicenter study. *Ann Surg* 2010;251:441–9.

15 Delorme

Abdel Rahman A. Omer and Ian K.H. Scot

 ## INDICATIONS/CONTRAINDICATIONS

Rectal prolapse is a distressing condition that is usually associated with incontinence and bowel dysfunction. There are multiple operations that correct the anatomical disability with the possibility of improving the function. The Delorme procedure is one of the modalities of treating full thickness external rectal prolapse. In elderly patients and those who are not fit for major operations, the Delorme procedure has low morbidity and mortality rate compared to the other available procedures. It can also be offered to those patients who do not wish to go through a major procedure for reasons other than fitness.

The Delorme procedure should not be offered to patients with internal prolapse or intussusception or, as per the author's experience, those individuals in whom the distance between the distal part of the prolapse and the dentate line is fixed (due to previous surgery [e.g., procedure for prolapse and hemorrhoids], phenol injections, low rectal or anal pathology) or if the distance from the dentate line to the distal part of the prolapse is longer than 3 cm. It is also contraindicated for those patients who suffer from diarrheal bowel dysfunction and those individuals who cannot be properly positioned on the operating table. Attention should be paid to patients who suffer with inflammatory bowel diseases and those patients with a history of rectal irradiation, but each case should be individualized.

Patients should be made aware of the high recurrence rate, the possibility of redoing the procedure if needed and the fact that not much assurance can be given regarding the improvement of continence.

 ## PREOPERATIVE PLANNING

Patients who are offered the Delorme procedure for rectal prolapse should be fully investigated in order to exclude other colonic pathologies that can precipitate rectal prolapse such as low sigmoid or rectal tumors. Other than the full office (outpatient's clinic) assessment including digital examination, rigid sigmoidoscopy, and proctoscopy, patients should have an appropriate endoscopic examination (flexible sigmoidoscopy or colonoscopy) or a barium enema. Anal physiological studies and endoanal ultrasound tests are not a mandatory part of our routine preoperative assessment.

Patients should be given information leaflets, be well informed and consented about the procedure and told that the main objective of the procedure is treatment of the external rectal prolapse.

Two phosphate enemas administered 2 hours before the procedure are used for bowel preparations. Additional enemas can be given as necessary.

Prophylactic antibiotic are administered upon induction of general endotracheal anesthesia (the authors use gentamicin and metronidazole). Thromboembolic prophylaxis should be routinely employed in all patients. In general sequential compression stockings and if not medically contraindicated heparin or low molecular weight heparin may be employed.

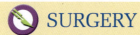 SURGERY

Anesthesia

The Delorme procedure is amendable to different modalities of anesthesia. Although general anesthesia is the most preferred modality, it is safe and acceptable to use spinal anesthesia. High-risk patients can have the procedure under caudal block or even local anesthesia with or without intravenous sedation.

Positioning

The author usually carries out the Delorme procedure with the patient in Lithotomy position. However the procedure can also be performed while the patient is in the prone jackknife or even the left lateral (SIMMs) position. The choice of position should be based upon the patient's ability to be in the surgical position for the duration of the operation, surgical access and patient's cardiac and respiratory needs.

Urinary bladder catheterization should be initiated under aseptic conditions.

Technique

1. Using the lone star circular retractor the anal verge is retracted in a circumferential pattern and the full prolapse is reproduced. The submucosal space is injected with 1:3,00,000 solution of normal saline with adrenaline in order to facilitate the separation of the mucosa from the rectal muscular tube. Using the diathermy blade the mucosa is circumferentially stripped holding its edge with a tissue forceps. This initial incision is made at a distance of approximately one centimeter cephalad to the dentate line. Diathermy scissors or dissecting scissors can be used. Any blood vessels encountered at this stage can be controlled using diathermy forceps (Fig. 15.1).

2. The mucosal and submucosal plane can be easily identified due to the solution injected in this space. The edges of the mucosa tube are held with gentle traction applied to facilitate further dissection. Avoidance of holes in the mucosal tube or injury to the muscle will facilitate the progression of the dissection. Further injections of the adrenaline solution may make the dissection easier. This process should continue till the apex of the intussusception is reached and the mucosal layer become adherent to the muscular layer. (Fig. 15.2)

3. At the apex of the prolapse a small incision is made in the mucosal tube at the anterior midline and the muscular plication commences. The authors prefer to use 2/0 Proline. Plication sutures are placed from the dentate line toward the apex of the prolapse including the dentate line mucosa and the proximal rectal mucosa at each end of the plication suture. The suture incorporates 1 cm of muscle with each pass and progresses another 1 cm to the point of next passage in a vertical line along the muscular tube. The suture is tagged with an artery forceps and hung on the circular

Figure 15.1

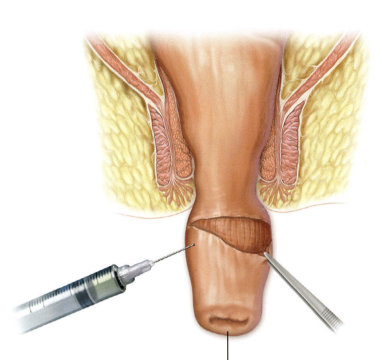

Rectal prolapse

retractor; this procedure is repeated at the posterior midline, left lateral and right lateral positions. The mucosa is then excised and sent for histology. The plication step is repeated between the quadrant sutures taking the number of vertical plication sutures to eight in total. These sutures then are tightened up and held on the artery forceps hanging on the retractor before being tied. (Fig. 15.3) The prolapse will be fully reduced and the plicated rectal tube will be sitting at the level of the sphincters.

Figure 15.2

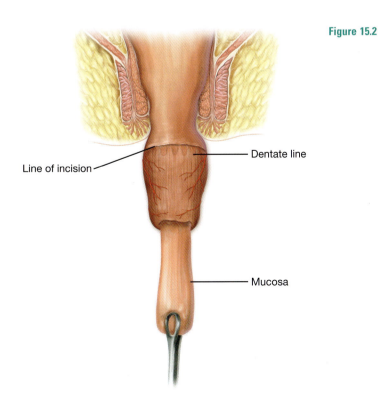

Line of incision

Dentate line

Mucosa

Figure 15.3

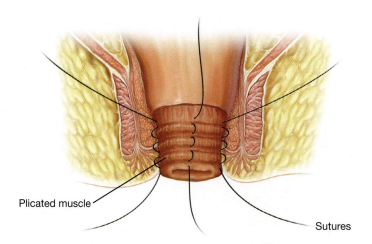

Plicated muscle

Sutures

4. The mucosal gaps at the rectoanal anastomosis are closed now using 2/0 Monocryl interrupted sutures. During the procedure, small muscular tears are included in the plication sutures and if a major defect inadvertently occurs, the surgeon may abandon the procedure and convert it to an Altemeier procedure.

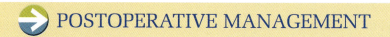

POSTOPERATIVE MANAGEMENT

Postoperative Plan

The postoperative plan is as follows:

- **Analgesia:** If the patient is under general anesthesia a pudendal block can be performed at the end of the operative procedure. Oral analgesia should be introduced early in the form of regular paracetamol and nonsteroidal analgesics. Patient controlled analgesia can be used but is rarely required.
- **Prophylactic antibiotics:** The patient is given extra two doses of oral Metronidazole.
- **Thromboembolic prophylaxes:** TEDS stockings and daily heparin or low molecular weight heparin should be offered to all patients until discharge unless there are contraindications.
- **Normal activities:** Patients should commence a regular diet as soon as possible, and early mobilization is encouraged. The urinary catheter should be removed at the end of the first postoperative day. If the patient is well, passing urine after removing the catheter, and opening their bowel normally, discharge from hospital should be considered.

 # COMPLICATIONS

Complications are uncommon, although self limiting bleeding and hematoma formation can take place. If significant bleeding continues, an examination under anesthesia is important for proper examination. Oversewing any bleeding points will provide satisfactory hemostasis. Although sepsis is rare, if it is suspected a CT scan or an MRI are indicated. Postoperative changes can make the radiological diagnosis of pelvic sepsis difficult. In that circumstance, empiric antibiotic therapy should be started and surgical intervention should be considered, if there is no improvement. An examination under anesthesia with transanal drainage of any septic focus may be indicated.

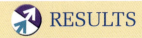

RESULTS

Prolapse repair using the Delorme procedure has a high recurrence rate (15%) in comparison to other prolapse operations but it delivers a high patient satisfaction rate. Both continence and quality of life may significantly improve.

CONCLUSIONS

The Delorme procedure is a simple safe operation which can be considered in patients of all ages. It can help some patients to regain continence due to improvement in anal sphincter physiological function. The problem of a high recurrence rate is balanced by the possibility to repeat the procedure as needed. It is a procedure that can be taught easily to trainees with anticipated good outcome.

Suggested Readings

Agachan F, Pfeifer J, Joo JS, Nogueras JJ, Weiss EG, Wexner SD. Results of perineal procedures for the treatment of rectal prolapse. *Am Surg* 1997;63(1):9–12.

Agachan F, Reissman P, Pfeifer J, Weiss EG, Nogueras JJ, Wexner SD. Comparison of three perineal procedures for the treatment of rectal prolapse. *South Med J* 1997;90(9):925–32.

Marchal F, Bresler L, Ayav A, et al. Long-term results of Delorme's procedure and Orr-Loygue rectopexy to treat complete rectal prolapse. *Dis Colon Rectum* 2005;48(9):1785–90.

Pescatori M, Interisano A, Stolfi VM, Zoffoli M. Delorme's operation and sphincteroplasty for rectal prolapse and fecal incontinence. *Int J Colorectal Dis* 1998;13(5–6):223–7.

Plusa SM, Charig JA, Balaji V, Watts A, Thompson MR. Physiological changes after Delorme's procedure for full-thickness rectal prolapse. *Br J Surg* 1995;82:1475–78.

Senapati A, Nicholls RJ, Thomson JP, Phillips RK. Results of Delorme's procedure for rectal prolapse. *Dis Colon Rectum* 1994;37(5):456–60.

Sielezneff I, Malouf A, Cesari J, Brunet C, Sarles JC, Sastre B. Selection criteria for internal rectal prolapse repair by Delorme's transrectal excision. *Dis Colon Rectum* 1999;42(3):367–73.

Tsunoda A, Yasuda N, Yokoyama N, Kamiyama G, Kusano M. Delorme's procedure for rectal prolapse: clinical and physiological analysis. *Dis Colon Rectum* 2003;46(9):1260–5.

Watkins BP, Landercasper J, Belzer GE, et al. Long-term follow-up of the modified Delorme procedure for rectal prolapse. *Arch Surg* 2003;138:498–503.

Watts AM, Thompson MR. Evaluation of Delorme's procedure as a treatment for full-thickness rectal prolapse. *Br J Surg* 2000;87(2):218–22.

16 Altemeier

Dana R. Sands

The optimal treatment of rectal prolapse has been debated for centuries. Numerous abdominal and perineal procedures have been described in the literature, which lead us to conclude that the "best" repair is one that is tailored to the individual patient. Many considerations are necessary to determine the correct approach, the most obvious being the patients' age and any coexistent comorbidities. Perineal approaches are invaluable for management of this problem in the elderly population.

Perineal approaches have traditionally been associated with higher recurrence rates, yet some of the more recently reported recurrence rates have been comparable to abdominal approaches (1–3), with the overall impression that this improvement is attributable to the addition of a levatoroplasty (4–7). Since the incidence of rectal prolapse is at its highest in the fifth, sixth, and seventh decades of life, the drawback of a higher recurrence rate is balanced by the reduction in perioperative morbidity. It is therefore necessary to appropriately counsel patients regarding a higher likelihood of recurrence, such as those undergoing a perineal procedure as a primary or repeat operation for the treatment of prolapse (4,8–12).

PERINEAL RECTOSIGMOIDECTOMY

First described by Mikulicz in 1889 (13), the perineal rectosigmoidectomy was subsequently advocated by Miles in 1933 (14). It was ultimately championed in the United States by Altemeier and Culbertson in the late 1960s, early 1970s and therefore now bears the eponymous name of Altemeier (15–17).

Traditionally, the Altemeier procedure involves a full thickness resection of the rectum, starting 1 cm proximal to the dentate line and can often include resection up to the sigmoid colon. The bowel is first everted and the prolapse is reproduced (Fig. 16.1). Following this maneuver, a full thickness incision is made 1–2 cm proximal to the dentate line (Fig. 16.2). Proximal dissection is undertaken until the peritoneal hernia sac is identified and opened (Fig. 16.3). This step is crucial in allowing the surgeon to assess the amount of sigmoid redundancy. The mesentery is sequentially divided until there is no further redundancy noted. This process is greatly expedited with the newer vessel sealing devices. Once all of the redundant bowel has been removed, the prolapse is amputated (Fig. 16.4). An anterior levatoroplasty can be performed at this point. The anastomosis is then performed (Fig. 16.5).

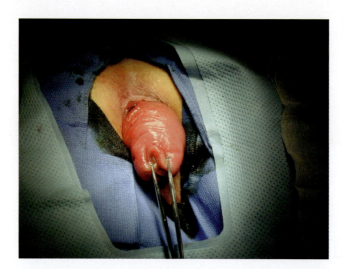

Figure 16.1

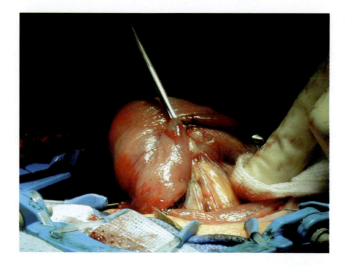

Figure 16.2

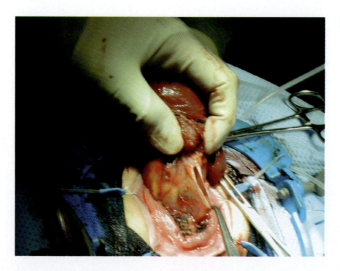

Figure 16.3

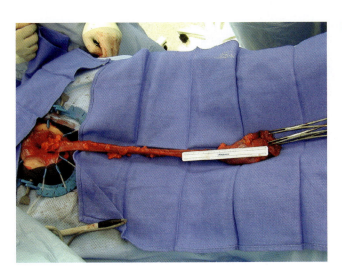

Figure 16.4

Perineal rectosigmoidectomy is the operation of choice for patients with an incarcerated, gangrenous rectal prolapse. In male patients, one of the most important complications has been sexual dysfunction secondary to extensive pelvic dissection and posterior rectopexy procedures, leading some surgeons to a recommend a perineal approach for young male patients (11,18).

Table 16.1 lists patients undergoing perineal rectosigmoidectomy with reported mortality rates of 0–5% and recurrence rates from 0 to 16%. One of the most important modifications to the perineal rectosigmoidectomy has been the addition of the levatoroplasty which will be addressed separately. Data listed include studies where an additional levatoroplasty was employed and those where it was not (1–4,6–8,11,17,19–24).

TABLE 16.1		Results of Perineal Rectosigmoidectomy for Rectal Prolapse						
Authors	N	Study	Levatorplasty	Mortality, # (%)	Continence, %	Constipation, %	Recurrence, # (%)	Follow-up, mo.
Altmeier et al., 1971[17]	106	Retrospective	No	0	Not stated	Not stated	3 (3)	228
Watts et al., 1985[23]	33	Retrospective	No	0	6 (+) 22 (−)	Not stated	0	23
Prasad et al., 1986[7]	25	Not stated	Yes	0	88 (+)	Not stated	0	Not stated
Williams et al., 1992[4]	56	Retrospective	No	0	46 (+)	Not stated	6 (11)	12
	11		Yes		91 (+)		0	
Johansen et al., 1993[34]	20	Not stated	No	1 (5)	21 (+)	Not stated	0	26
Ramanujam et al., 1994[22]	72	Not stated	No	0	67 (+)	Not stated	4 (6)	120
Deen et al., 1994[11]	10	Prospective	No	0	80 (+)	Not stated	1 (10)	18
Agachan et al., 1997[8]	32	Retrospective	No	0	(+)	Not stated	4 (13)	30
	21		Yes				1 (5)	30
Takesue et al., 1999[6]	10	Not stated	Yes (7)	0	(+)	Not stated	0	42
Kim et al., 1999[25]	183	Retrospective	No	Not stated	53 (+)	61 (+)	29 (16)	47
Kimmins et al., 2001[1]	63	Retrospective	Yes (29)	0	87 (+)	31.7	4 (6.3)	21
Zbar et al., 2002[2]	80	Retrospective	Yes	0	100 (+)	Not stated	3 (3.8)	22
Chun et al., 2004[27]	109	Retrospective	Yes	0	100 (+)	Not stated	18 (16.5)	29
Habr-Gama et al., 2006[3]	44	Retrospective	Yes	0	85.7 (+)	Not stated	3 (7.1)	49
Boccasanta et al., 2006[28]	40	RCT	Yes	Not stated	100(+)	Not stated	5 (12.5)	28
Altomare et al., 2008[29]	93	Retrospective	No Yes (73)	0	47 (+)	(+)	5 (25) 12 (16.4)	41

Abbreviations: (+), improvement; (−), worsening.
*Levatorplasty performed at surgeon's discretion.

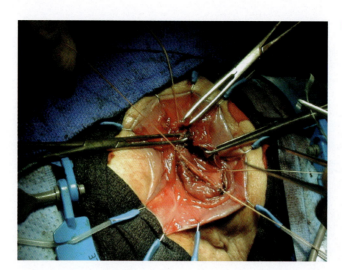

Figure 16.5

PERINEAL RECTOSIGMOIDECTOMY WITH LEVATOROPLASTY

The two main concerns that favor the addition of levatoroplasty include the high rate of fecal incontinence, typically reported preoperatively to be between 50 and 75% (10), and the prevention of recurrent prolapse (2). Because of both, the reduced compliance of the colon and resting anal pressure, the addition of a posterior levatoroplasty has been suggested. This restoration of the anorectal angle seems to effect an improvement in anal continence (25). Additional benefits of adding the levatoroplasty include a lower rate of recurrence in the short term and therefore also a longer recurrence-free interval (8). Unfortunately, many reported series include levatoroplasty performed at the discretion of the operating surgeon making it difficult to determine the value of levatoroplasty in recent series (1,24).

The surgeons at Cleveland Clinic Florida compared the results of perineal rectosigmoidectomy with and without anterior levatoroplasty in 109 patients (22). Recurrence rates in patients with rectosigmoidectomy alone were 20.6% compared to 7.7% with the addition of a levatoroplasty. In this study, levatoroplasty also increased the mean time to recurrence dramatically from 13.3 months to 45.5 months.

Agachan et al. (8) compared the outcomes of patients undergoing the perineal rectosigmoidectomy alone, with a levatoroplasty and the Delorme procedure. No significant difference in hospital stay was observed among the three groups. All patients experienced an improvement in their incontinence scores, with the greatest improvement seen in patients undergoing the perineal rectosigmoidectomy with levatoroplasty. The recurrence rates were as follows: 38% for the Delorme, 13% for perineal rectosigmoidectomy alone, and 5% for perineal rectosigmoidectomy with levatoroplasty.

STAPLED VERSUS HAND-SEWN ANASTOMOSIS

Historically, bowel was anastomosed with interrupted absorbable sutures, although modification of the anastomotic technique through use of a circular stapling device has been proposed (26–28). When utilizing a circular stapling device, the full thickness resection should begin 2–3 cm proximal to the dentate, since an additional 1 cm will be removed with creation of the anastomosis. Figures 16.6–16.8 illustrate the technique of stapled anastomosis. 0-prolene purse string sutures are placed in the proximal colon and distal rectum. After securing them around the anvil and post of the stapler respectively, the stapler is advanced into the anus and fired.

Figure 16.6

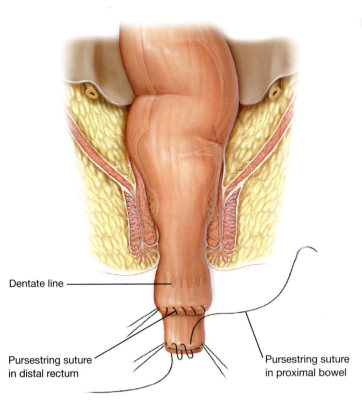

Dentate line

Pursestring suture
in distal rectum

Pursestring suture
in proximal bowel

Figure 16.7

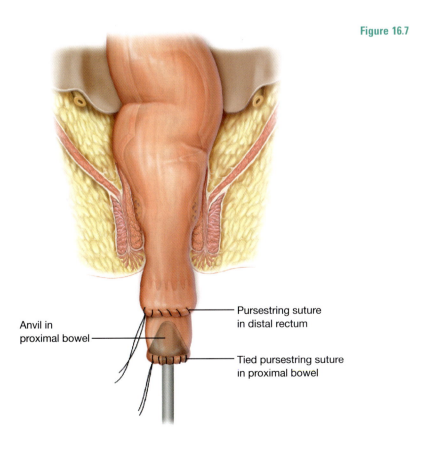

Anvil in
proximal bowel

Pursestring suture
in distal rectum

Tied pursestring suture
in proximal bowel

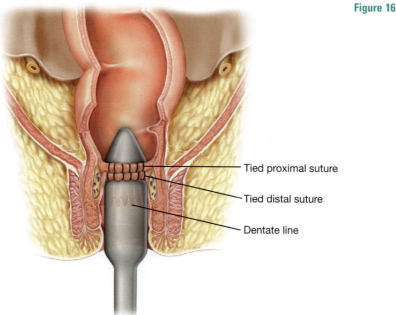

Figure 16.8

Tied proximal suture

Tied distal suture

Dentate line

The application of new technologies in the operating room including next generation instruments for simultaneous cutting and sealing of vessels and the circular stapler have been noted to significantly decrease operative time, blood loss and hospital stay without compromising pain, time to normal activity, morbidity, or mortality (23). Boccasanta et al. published one of the rare randomized control trials in the rectal prolapse literature comparing the use of new technologies, including the circular staples with hand-sewn anastomosis. There was no statistically significant difference in recurrence rates (23). In fact, use of the circular stapling device is included in recent series (1,24), but the recurrence and complication rates for the two anastomotic techniques are not specifically compared. The addition of the circular stapler is a significant time-saving device. Further analysis is needed to determine the safety of the use of this technology in this procedure. There is some concern regarding the significant size discrepancy of the proximal sigmoid colon and the distal rectum. Individual sutures may be better able to accommodate the significantly different luminal caliber of these two pieces of bowel. As technologies continue to advance, the incorporation of new operative techniques and instruments will potentially improve operative outcomes. This benefit should not be overlooked in the patient population served by the perineal rectosigmoidectomy.

More recently, a technique called the perineal stapled prolapse resection for excision of the externally prolapsed rectum utilizing a linear stapler and multiple firings of the curved Contour stapler has been proposed (29). This is not a variation of a true perineal rectosigmoidectomy since it does not address the issue of rectal and colonic redundancy which is part of the pathophysiology of rectal prolapse. The small series of patients (15) and limited follow-up (29) prevent the authors from forming any recommendations regarding this procedure at this time.

 ## COMPLICATIONS

Complications from a perineal proctosigmoidectomy can include anastomotic bleeding and pelvic sepsis from anastomotic leak. Risk of leak can be minimized by taking care not to pull the bowel too tightly (resecting too much) or ligate the mesentery too far proximally, thereby insuring a tension-free, well vascularized anastomosis (6).

The main disadvantage of a perineal proctectomy is the high recurrence rate, with some series reporting recurrences in up to 50–60% of patients (30,31). Not surprisingly, patients undergoing repeat operation for recurrent prolapse have a significantly higher rate of recurrence when the repair is perineal. Steele et al. reported that the abdominal approach continued to have significantly lower recurrence rates (39 vs. 13%; $P < 0.01$) when performed for recurrent rectal prolapse compared with the perineal approach (32). While it was also noted that the patients undergoing perineal repair were significantly older with a mean age of 71.5 years compared to 58.5 years in the abdominal surgery group, the two did not differ significantly in their American Society of Anesthesiologists classification (32). The operative approach for patients with recurrent rectal prolapse after an Altemeier procedure is largely dependent on the amount of redundant bowel remaining. If there is a significant amount of redundant bowel, a repeat Altmeier procedure would be preferred. However, if there is not a significant amount of redundancy, a rectopexy would be indicated if the patient was deemed medically suitable for an abdominal procedure. This strategy allows for removal of the redundant bowel and avoidance of any potential devascularized segment of bowel between two pelvic anastomoses.

Other disadvantages are poor functional results including incontinence, urgency, and soiling secondary to the reduced reservoir capacity of the colon and reduction in the anal sphincter function. To counteract the reduction in reservoir capacity, Baig et al. (33) described a pouch perineal rectosigmoidectomy. There has been some limited suggestion that this may provide better functional results than a straight coloanal anastomosis.

CONCLUSION

Once it has been determined that a perineal approach will be used, the decision of which technique may be largely personal, based on the operating surgeon's training and experience base. Generally speaking, the Delorme procedure is optimally utilized in patients limited to a short segment of full thickness prolapse or with a partial thickness prolapse. In patients who are a poor operative risk, this represents a safe local approach without any violation of the peritoneal cavity. For patients of a more intermediate operative risk, a perineal rectosigmoidectomy with levatoroplasty would certainly be the operation of choice in patients presenting with full thickness rectal prolapse as it has a reduced rate of recurrence and improved functional outcomes relative to the other perineal approaches (34).

Recommended References and Readings

1. Kimmins MH, Everetts BK, Isler J, Billingham R. The Altemeier repair: outpatient treatment of rectal prolapse. *Dis Colon Rectum* 2001;44:565–70.
2. Zbar AP, Takshima S, Hasegawa T, Kitabyashi K. Perineal rectosigmoidectomy (Altemeier's procedure): a review of physiology, technique and outcome. *Tech Coloproctol* 2002;6:109–16.
3. Habr-Gama A, Jacob CE, Jorge JM, et al. Rectal procidentia treatment by perineal rectosigmoidectomy combined with levator ani repair. *Hepatogastroenterology* 2006;53(68):213–17.
4. Williams JG, Rotherberger DA, Madoff RD, Goldberg SM. Treatment of rectal prolapse in the elderly by perineal rectosigmoidectomy. *Dis Colon Rectum* 1992;35:830–4.
5. Senapati A, Nicholls RJ, Thomson JP, Phillips RK. Results of Delorme's procedure for rectal prolapse. *Dis Colon Rectum* 1994;37:456–60.
6. Takesue Y, Yokoyama T, Murakami Y, et al. The effectiveness of perineal rectosigmoidectomy for the treatment of rectal prolapse. *Surg Today* 1999;29:290–3.
7. Prasad MK, Pearl RK, Abcarian H, Orsay CP, Nelson RL. Perineal proctectomy, posterior rectopexy and postanal levator repair for the treatment of rectal prolapse. *Dis Colon Rectum* 1986;29:547–52.
8. Agachan F, Reissman P, Pfeifer J, Weiss EG, Nogueras JJ, Wexner SD. Comparison of three perineal procedures for the treatment of rectal prolapse. *South Med J* 1997;90:925–32.
9. Yakut M, Kaymakciioglu N, Simsek A, Tan A, Sen D. Surgical treatment of rectal prolapse: a retrospective analysis of 94 cases. *Int Surg* 1998;83:53–5.
10. Madoff RD, Mellgren A. One hundred years of rectal prolapse surgery. *Dis Colon Rectum* 1999;42:441–50.
11. Deen KI, Grant E, Billingham C, Keighley MRB. Abdominal resection rectopexy with pelvic floor repair versus perineal rectosigmoidectomy and pelvic floor repair for full-thickness rectal prolapse. *Br J Surg* 1994;81:302–4.
12. Pescatori M, Interisano A, Stolfi VM, Zoffoli M. Delorme's operation and sphincteroplasty for rectal prolapse and fecal incontinence. *Int J Colorectal Dis* 1998;13:223–7.
13. Mikulicz J. Zur operativen betiandlung des prolapsus recti et coli invaginati. *Arch Klin Chir* 1889;38:74–97.
14. Miles WE. Rectosigmoidectomy as a method of treatment for procidentia recti. *Proc R Soc Med* 1933;26:1445–52.
15. Altemeier WA. One-stage perineal surgery for complete rectal prolapse. *Hosp Pract* 1972;7:102.
16. Altemeier WA, Culbertson WR. Technique for perineal repair of rectal prolapse. *Surgery* 1965;58:758.
17. Altemeier WA, Culbertson WR, Schowengardt C, Hunt J. Nineteen years experience with the one-stage perineal repair of rectal prolapse. *Ann Surg* 1971;173:993–1006.
18. Farouk R, Duthie GS. Rectal prolapse and rectal invagination. *Eur J Surg* 1998;164:323–32.
19. Ramanujam PF, Vankatesh KS, Fietz MJ. Perineal excision of rectal procidentia in elderly high-risk patients: a ten-year experience. *Dis Colon Rectum* 1994;37:1027–30.

20. Watts JD, Rotheberger DA, Buls JG, Goldberg SM, Nivatvongs S. The management of procidentia: 30 years' experience. *Dis Colon Rectum* 1985;28:96–102.

21. Kim D-S, Tsang CB, Wong WD, Lowry AC, Goldberg SM, Madoff RD. Complete rectal prolapse: evolution of management and results. *Dis Colon Rectum* 1999;42:460–69.

22. Chun S, Pikarsky A, You S, et al. Perineal rectosigmoidectomy for rectal prolapse: role of levatoroplasty. *Dis Colon Rectum* 2001;44:A5–A26.

23. Boccasanta P, Venturi M, Barbieri S, Roviaro G. Impact of new technologies on the clinical and functional outcome of Altemeier's procedure: a randomized, controlled trial. *Dis Colon Rectum* 2006;49(5):652–60.

24. Altomare DF, Binda GA, Ganio E, De Nardi P, Giamundo P, Pescatori M. Long-term outcome of Altemeier's Procedure for Rectal Prolapse. *Dis Colon Rectum* 2009;52:698–703.

25. Parks AG, Swash M, Urich H. Sphincter denervation in anorectal incontinence and rectal prolapse. *Gut* 1977;18:656–65.

26. Vermeulen FD, Nivatvongs S, Fang DT, Balcos EG, Goldberg SM. A technique for perineal rectosigmoidectomy using autosuture devices. *Surg Gynecol Obstet* 1983;156:84–6.

27. Bennett BH, Geelhoed GW. A stapler modification of the Altemeier procedure for rectal prolapse. *Am Surg* 1985;51:116.

28. Portiz LS. Altemeier using the circular stapler. *Op Tech Gen Surg* 2008;10:194–7.

29. Scherer R, Marti L, Hertzer FH. Perineal stapled prolapse resection: a new procedure for external rectal prolapse. *Dis Colon Rectum* 2008;51:1727–30.

30. Friedman R, Muggia-Sulam M, Freund HR. Experience with the one-stage perineal repair of rectal prolapse. *Dis Colon Rectum* 1983;26:789–91.

31. Hughes ESR. Discussion on rectal prolapse. *Proc R Soc Med* 1949;42:1007–11.

32. Steele SR, Goetz LH, Minami S, Madoff RD, Mellgren AF, Parker SC. Management of recurrent rectal prolapse: surgical approach influences outcome. *Dis Colon Rectum* 2006;49:440–5.

33. Baig MK, Galliano D, Larach JA, Weiss EG, Wexner SD, Nogueras JJ. Pouch perineal rectosigmoidectomy: a case report. *Surg Innov* 2005;12:373–5.

34. Yoshioka K, Ogunbiyi OA, Keighley MR. Pouch perineal rectosigmoidectomy gives better functional results than conventional rectosigmoidectomy in elderly patients with rectal prolapse. *Br J Surg* 1998;85(11):1525–6.

17 Open Lateral Internal Sphincterotomy

S. Alva and Bertram Chinn

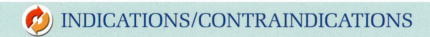

INDICATIONS/CONTRAINDICATIONS

Indications

- Chronic fissures that fail to respond to nonoperative therapy
- Acute fissures with severe pain

Anal fissure is a common disorder that results in bleeding and painful defecation. It is frequently related to the passage of a hard or a constipated bowel movement. A linear tear is noted in the anoderm and is frequently seen with gentle retraction of the buttocks (Fig. 17.1). Approximately 80–90% of fissures are posterior in location with the remainder in the anterior quadrant (1). Occasionally, fissures may be seen in both regions.

Many fissures heal by increasing dietary fiber to soften and bulk the stool, using an emollient suppository and warm sitz baths (2). Over the last decade, topical nifedipine or nitroglycerin ointments and the injection of Botulinum toxin A into the internal sphincter have improved fissure healing by reducing sphincter spasms (3–5).

In chronic conditions, irritation, itching, mucous, and discomfort may be more evident than pain or bleeding. Scarring at the base of the fissure, rolled and indurated edges, a sentinel skin tag, and/or a hypertrophic papilla suggest that the fissure will not heal without surgery (6). A posterior sphincterotomy was once recommended but due to a resultant "keyhole" deformity, Eisenhammer advocated a lateral internal sphincterotomy (LIS) for surgical treatment of fissures (2).

An LIS may also be necessary when pain from an acute fissure is overwhelming.

Contraindications

- Diminished sphincter integrity
- Inflammatory bowel disease
- Infections (tuberculosis and syphilis)
- Leukemia and HIV

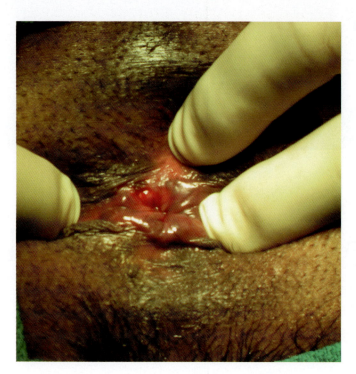

Figure 17.1 Posterior fissure.

When considering an LIS, individuals with diminished sphincter tone or incontinence should be evaluated for their candidacy for alternative therapies. An atypical fissure may suggest the presence of other diseases. Fissures in the lateral quadrants should raise the concern of inflammatory bowel disease, specifically Crohn's disease, tuberculosis, syphilis, leukemia, or HIV. In these situations, treating the underlying disease is recommended instead of performing a sphincterotomy.

 PREOPERATIVE PLANNING

Routine preoperative evaluation and planning that include a history and physical examination with meticulous attention to the anorectal region should be performed. Although a phosphate enema is recommended prior to surgery, discomfort frequently precludes its use. If diminished sphincter tone is suspected or if the patient has had prior anorectal surgery, preoperative anorectal physiology testing may be helpful.

 SURGERY

Positioning

■ Prone jackknife position

The patient is placed in a prone jackknife position. This position allows the surgical team full access to the operative field. Retracting 3-in. silk tape that has been placed on the buttocks and securing it to the sides of the operating table provides exposure. Lithotomy and a left lateral or modified Sims' positions can also be used.

Anesthesia

■ Monitored anesthesia care (MAC)
■ A 0.25% bupivacaine and 1:200,000 epinephrine

Although LIS can be performed under general or regional anesthesia, our preference is MAC and a local block. After initially attaining adequate sedation and comfort under MAC, a local block with bupivacaine and epinephrine is used. This block provides analgesia and allows relaxation of the sphincter to facilitate surgery. The vasoconstrictive effects of epinephrine will decrease vascularity during the surgery and increase the period of postoperative analgesia.

Initially, 10 ml of the local anesthetic is injected circumferentially into the perianal skin and the subcutaneous tissue with a 1.5 in. × 25 gauge needle. A circumferential deeper injection into the sphincter is then performed. Typically, a total of 20–30 ml of the local anesthetic is needed to complete the operation.

Whatever anesthesia is selected, patients may benefit from the use of a local block that contains epinephrine in addition to the analgesic/anesthetic. Procedures performed under general anesthesia still benefit from the additional sphincter relaxation and hemostasis attained with the bupivacaine and epinephrine. The vasoconstrictive effects of epinephrine are also helpful in offsetting the vasodilatory effects of a spinal anesthetic.

Technique

- Confirmation of a fissure and hypertonic/spastic sphincter
- Insertion of a 35-mm Hill-Ferguson retractor with identification of the internal sphincter and intersphincteric groove
- Incision of the perianal skin overlying the intersphincteric groove
- Isolation of the internal sphincter and division under direct vision
- Fissure debridement and excision of a sentinel tag and hypertrophic papilla
- Closure of the sphincterotomy site with interrupted absorbable sutures

After appropriate positioning and anesthesia are attained, the presence of a fissure is confirmed with circumferential examination of the anal canal using a Hirschmann anoscope. A 35-mm Hill-Ferguson retractor provides a consistent measure of the diameter of the anal canal. Resistance during insertion of this retractor confirms the presence of a hypertonic/spastic sphincter and a taught, bank-like internal sphincter is seen (Fig. 17.2). Failure to identify a hypertonic sphincter should prompt further evaluation before a sphincterotomy is performed.

Selection of either the left or the right lateral quadrant for the sphincterotomy is contingent upon where the internal sphincter is best noted and whether hemorrhoidal tissue would interfere with the operative field. An incision is made at the intersphincteric

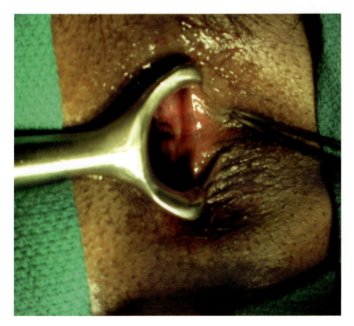

Figure 17.2 Hypertonic internal sphincter.

Part VI: Sphincterotomy—Lateral

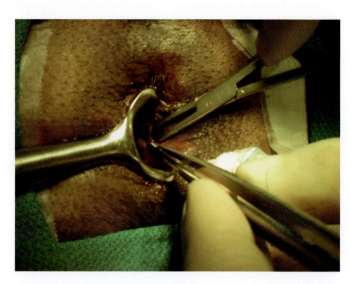

Figure 17.3 Mobilization of anoderm.

groove and extended 1.5–2.0 cm distally to the perianal skin. A fine, curved hemostat is used to mobilize the anoderm off the internal sphincter up to the level of the dentate line (Fig. 17.3). Caution is used to prevent violation of the anoderm since nonhealing of this may result in a fistula. The intersphincteric plane is accessed and the internal sphincter is isolated with the hemostat up to the dentate (Fig. 17.4). Electrocautery may be used to control small points of bleeding.

A Buie scissors is used to divide the internal sphincter under direct vision (Fig. 17.5). Historically, the muscle is divided up to the dentate line. A "tailored" LIS may be performed by dividing the internal sphincter up to the level of the proximal extent of the fissure (7). If there remains resistance to insertion of the Hill-Ferguson retractor, extension

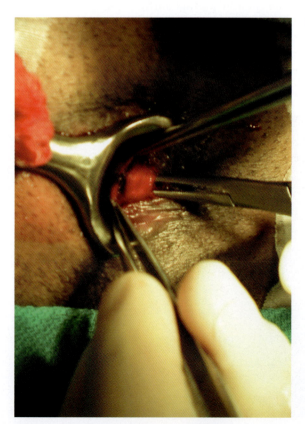

Figure 17.4 Isolation of internal sphincter.

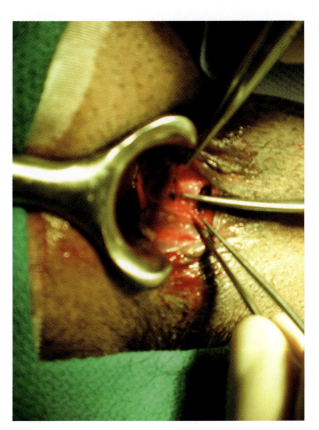

Figure 17.5 Division of internal sphincter.

of the sphincterotomy to the dentate may be needed. Division of the internal sphincter beyond the dentate line is unnecessary and inadvisable.

To facilitate fissure healing, the fibrosis at the base of the fissure is debrided with a curette or by obliquely scraping the fissure with a scalpel. Undermined or rolled edges of the fissure should be excised or saucerized. Excision of a sentinel tag or hypertrophic papillae is performed if present.

After hemostasis is confirmed, the LIS site is closed with two or three interrupted sutures of 3-0 chromic or Vicryl. A topical hemostatic agent may be left at the fissure site.

 ## POSTOPERATIVE MANAGEMENT

Patients begin sitz baths on the evening of surgery; a high-fiber diet and/or fiber supplements are recommended to maintain a soft and bulky stool. Analgesics are provided and patients are informed that postoperative pain typically resolves within 1 week. Patients resume activities as tolerated and are expected to return to normal function within 2 weeks and fissure healing generally occurs within 4 weeks.

 ## COMPLICATIONS

- Abscess
- Fistula-in-ano
- Fecal incontinence
- Recurrent and unhealed fissure

Altered bowel function and continence are not unusual following surgery and are accentuated with the use of a high-fiber diet. Alterations to control are more likely to

TABLE 17.1

| Author | Year | Patient # | Impaired Control | | Fecal Soiling (%) | Persistent Or Recurrent Fissures (%) |
			Flatus (%)	Feces (%)		
Abcarian (8)	1980	150	0	0	0	1.3
Marya et al. (9)	1980	100	0	0	0	2
Ravikumar et al. (10)	1982	60	0	0	5	3.3
Jensen et al. (11)	1984	30	0	0	0	3.3
Frezza et al. (12)	1992	134	0	0	0	0.6
Leong et al. (13)	1994	114	7.9	0	NR	2.6
Pernikoff and Salvati (14)	1994	500	2.8	0.4	4.4	3
Romano G et al. (15)	1994	44	9	4.5	4.5	0
Neufeld DM et al. (16)	1995	112	12.5*	0.9	8.9	2.7
Oh C et al. (17)	1995	1313	1.5*		0	1.3
Usatoff et al. (18)	1995	98	7	1	11	3
Garcia-Aguilar (19)	1996	324	30	12	27	14
Hananel and Gordon (20)	1997	265	0.4	0.4	0.4	1.1
Nyam and Pemberton (21)	1999	487	31*	23*	39*	8
Argov et al. (22)	2000	2108	1.5*		0	1
Richard et al. (23)	2000	38	0	0	0	0
Casillas and Hull (24)	2005	298	4.4	2.8	NR	5.6

*Impaired control reported as temporary.
NR – not reported.

occur with flatus than feces (Table 17.1). These symptoms are expected to resolve during the postoperative period. Persistent and recurrent fissures are also infrequent and depending upon clinical findings, may require an additional limited sphincterotomy on the contralateral side or an advancement flap. Abscess formation is uncommon with an open LIS since any collection of fluid will likely decompresses through the surgical incision. Fistula formation is also uncommon and may be due to incision or compromise of the anoderm.

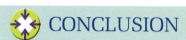 CONCLUSION

Open LIS is a safe surgical option for the treatment of anal fissures. Most are performed due to chronic symptoms despite nonoperative management but occasionally, an LIS is necessary in the acute setting when pain is severe.

References

1. Goligher JC, Duthie HL, Nixon HH. *Surgery of the anus, rectum and colon.* 5th ed. London: Bailliere Tindall, 1984.
2. Eisenhammer S. The surgical correction of chronic internal anal (sphincteric) contracture. *S Afr Med J* 1951;25:486–9.
3. Gorfine SR. Treatment of benign anal disease with topical nitroglycerin. *Dis Colon Rectum* 1995;38:453–6; discussion 6–7.
4. Jost WH, Schimrigk K. Use of botulinum toxin in anal fissure. *Dis Colon Rectum* 1993;36:974.
5. Jonas M, Neal KR, Abercrombie JF, Scholefield JH. A randomized trial of oral vs. topical diltiazem for chronic anal fissures. *Dis Colon Rectum* 2001;44:1074–8.
6. Lock MR, Thomson JP. Fissure-in-ano: the initial management and prognosis. *Br J Surg* 1977;64:355–8.
7. Littlejohn DR, Newstead GL. Tailored lateral sphincterotomy for anal fissure. *Dis Colon Rectum* 1997;40:1439–42.
8. Abcarian H. Surgical correction of chronic anal fissure: results of lateral internal sphincterotomy vs. fissurectomy–midline sphincterotomy. *Dis Colon Rectum* 1980;23:31–6.
9. Marya SK, Mittal SS, Singla S. Lateral subcutaneous internal sphincterotomy for acute fissure in ano. *Br J Surg* 1980;67:299.
10. Ravikumar TS, Sridhar S, Rao RN. Subcutaneous lateral internal sphincterotomy for chronic fissure-in-ano. *Dis Colon Rectum* 1982;25:798–801.

11. Jensen SL, Lund F, Nielsen OV, Tange G. Lateral subcutaneous sphincterotomy versus anal dilatation in the treatment of fissure in ano in outpatients: a prospective randomised study. *Br Med J (Clin Res Ed)* 1984;289:528–30.
12. Frezza EE, Sandei F, Leoni G, Biral M. Conservative and surgical treatment in acute and chronic anal fissure. A study on 308 patients. *Int J Colorectal Dis* 1992;7:188–91.
13. Leong AF, Husain MJ, Seow-Choen F, Goh HS. Performing internal sphincterotomy with other anorectal procedures. *Dis Colon Rectum* 1994;37:1130–2.
14. Pernikoff BJ, Eisenstat TE, Rubin RJ, Oliver GC, Salvati EP. Reappraisal of partial lateral internal sphincterotomy. *Dis Colon Rectum* 1994;37:1291–5.
15. Romano G, Rotondano G, Santangelo M, Esercizio L. A critical appraisal of pathogenesis and morbidity of surgical treatment of chronic anal fissure. *J Am Coll Surg* 1994;178:600–4.
16. Neufeld DM, Paran H, Bendahan J, Freund U. Outpatient surgical treatment of anal fissure. *Eur J Surg* 1995;161:435–8.
17. Oh C, Divino CM, Steinhagen RM. Anal fissure. 20-year experience. *Dis Colon Rectum* 1995;38:378–82.
18. Usatoff V, Polglase AL. The longer term results of internal anal sphincterotomy for anal fissure. *Aust N Z J Surg* 1995;65:576–8.
19. Garcia-Aguilar J, Belmonte C, Wong WD, Lowry AC, Madoff RD. Open vs. closed sphincterotomy for chronic anal fissure: long-term results. *Dis Colon Rectum* 1996;39:440–3.
20. Hananel N, Gordon PH. Lateral internal sphincterotomy for fissure-in-ano–revisited. *Dis Colon Rectum* 1997;40:597–602.
21. Nyam DC, Pemberton JH, Ilstrup DM, Rath DM. Long-term results of surgery for chronic constipation. *Dis Colon Rectum* 1997;40:273–9.
22. Argov S, Levandovsky O. Open lateral sphincterotomy is still the best treatment for chronic anal fissure. *Am J Surg* 2000;179:201–2.
23. Richard CS, Gregoire R, Plewes EA, et al. Internal sphincterotomy is superior to topical nitroglycerin in the treatment of chronic anal fissure: results of a randomized, controlled trial by the Canadian Colorectal Surgical Trials Group. *Dis Colon Rectum* 2000;43:1048–57; discussion 57–8.
24. Casillas S, Hull TL, Zutshi M, Trzcinski R, Bast JF, Xu M. Incontinence after a lateral internal sphincterotomy: are we underestimating it? *Dis Colon Rectum* 2005;48:1193–9.

Part VI: Sphincterotomy—Lateral

18 Sphincter-Sparing Surgical Alternatives in Chronic Anal Fissure

Andrew P. Zbar

Introduction

It is only in the last few years that it has been recognized that conventional open lateral internal anal sphincterotomy (LIS) for chronic anal fissure (CAF) has been associated with a significant incidence of functional impairment adversely affecting the patient's quality of life (1,2). This relatively poor functional result is somewhat unpredictable (3), where definitive preoperative imaging by our group has shown relatively poor coronal internal/external anal sphincter (EAS) overlap in some patients with preexistent EAS atrophy, suggesting that in such selected cases, that conventional open LIS may render the distal anal canal relatively unsupported and lead to expected postoperative fecal seepage (4). This approach towards more routine coronal sphincter imaging in patients with topically resistant CAF is not practical, however, except in selected cases where the clinical impression would be that LIS may particularly render continence at risk. This finding has been coupled with significant concerns regarding the use of routine LIS (however, that is performed) in multiparous patients who present with anterior anal fissures where there may be an expectation of coincident EAS damage, as well as in patients with minimally symptomatic Crohn's-related anal fissures (5).

More recently there has been an improved understanding of the importance of the internal anal sphincter (IAS) in the maintenance of anal continence (6,7), where inherent differences in wave recovery in an IAS-related physiologic function—the rectoanal inhibitory reflex—have been recorded in patients with preexistent EAS atrophy (8). The further importance of the IAS has been shown in observable functional improvement and maintenance of resting anal pressure (a predominantly IAS parameter) when the IAS is preserved in the surgery of high trans-sphincteric anal fistulas (9). Much of this understanding has resulted in the initial widespread use in the management of patients presenting with CAF, of nonoperative topical therapies as well as in selected cases of the utilization of botulinum toxin as a preliminary alternative to sphincterotomy (10,11). Comparative trials have been conducted between these medical alternatives and LIS where in some studies, quite acceptable outcomes are obtained for nonsurgical treatments in terms of fissure healing and quality of life (12–14).

The surgical alternatives to formal LIS include fissurectomy (with or without limited sphincterotomy or anoplasty) (15,16), tailored sphincterotomy (17), pressure-directed sphincterotomy (18), pneumatic sphincter dilatation (19), and anal fissurotomy (20). These alternatives to conventional LIS and available data pertaining to their clinical indications in the current decision making for fissure surgery are discussed in this chapter.

CONTROVERSIES IN THE ASSESSMENT OF CONVENTIONAL LATERAL INTERNAL ANAL SPHINCTEROTOMY

The incidence of significant functional impairment following conventional LIS appears to be underestimated (2,21). This is partly because most evaluations do not assess functional quality-of-life issues such as fecal urgency and seepage. Evidence would also suggest that incontinence to flatus in the post-LIS patient, in particular, is underestimated and is more prevalent as a reported symptom only on direct interview as opposed to the retrospective assessment of continence of the patients' medical files (2). Here, up to 30% of the incontinence initially reported by patients is persistent, particularly when the procedure has been performed in the office under local anesthesia (3,22).

The recent introduction of high-resolution endoluminal imaging of the anal canal has reemphasized the anatomical and clinical importance of the IAS in anal canal anatomy (23). It has become clear that IAS division may be followed by passive incontinence (24); a finding which may be coupled with impaired short- and long-term function following low anterior resection and restorative proctocolectomy in those patients with excessive endoanal manipulation (25). This fact highlights the need for preservation of IAS structure and function (25). Part of the complexity of the response by the IAS to sphincterotomy may be reflected in its known physiology, where continent and incontinent outcomes following partial sphincter division show differential variations in both resting and voluntary squeeze pressure (26) and where minor degrees of incontinence may be present in 28% of patients presenting with a CAF prior to surgery (27).

In the analysis of patients undergoing LIS for CAF, some studies have included the responses to a range of medical and surgical therapies in patients with acute anal fissures without complete characterization of what represents a CAF (28) and in operations where LIS has incorporated additional procedures such as excision of associated hypertrophied anal papillae and sentinel skin tags (29). This literature of CAF management has also been relatively confused with some reports combining nonoperative therapies with a range of different surgeries (30,31). The expanding problem of relatively isolated IAS damage has resulted from an increased use of novel more minimalist techniques in hemorrhoid surgery including Doppler-guided, PPH-stapled, and LigaSure haemorrhoidectomy along with the more widespread availability of endoanal ultrasonography capable of defining the true incidence of postoperative IAS pathology. This knowledge is of considerable clinical relevance given the poor functional results following IAS plication for postoperative fecal seepage deemed primarily to be secondary to IAS damage (32). This problem has recently been somewhat obviated by a range of techniques designed to augment the IAS in postoperative incontinence with varying biomaterials including autologous fat (33), cross-linked collagen (34) and silicone elastomer deployment (35–37), technologies designed to bolster the IAS and anal cushion area such as carbon-bead insertion (38) and radio-frequency application (39) and even sacral nerve stimulation (40). These techniques designed to improve IAS function currently have minimal long-term data and interpretation of outcomes must still be viewed with caution when considering the effects of these therapies, since the mechanisms of incontinence and anal closure differ between the post-LIS and post-haemorrhoidectomy cases so far reported (41). The longer-term continence salvaging data relating to these

TABLE 18.1	Collated Results of Open Lateral Internal Anal Sphincterotomy (LIS) for Chronic Anal Fissure as Referenced in the Chapter					
Author (Ref)	Year	Number	% Healing	% Recurrence	% Incontinence	FU
Garcia-Aguilar et al. (53)	1996	521	96.7	10.9	30.3 (flatus) 26.7 (soiling)	36
Wiley et al. (54)	2004	40	96	–	5	12
Hyman (43)	2004	35	94	Not stated	8.6	3
Casillas et al. (2)	2005	298	Not stated	5.6	30 (flatus)	52
Rotholtz et al. (45)	2005	68	100	–	10.2	66
Menteş et al. (1)	2006	144	Not stated	4.9	2.87 FIQoL	12

FIQoL, fecal incontinence quality of life scale assessment.
FU = Mean follow-up (months).

technologies will have a significant impact on the role of LIS in CAF patients, particularly where currently on clinical grounds, particular cases are deemed to be at relatively higher risk for postoperative incontinence.

Table 18.1 shows some accumulated data concerning outcome following conventional LIS for CAF where data were interpretable for articles referenced in this chapter. Randomized, controlled data have confirmed that such surgical therapy is associated with a very low fissure recurrence rate. In comparison, medically treated patients who have initial success are more likely to experience symptoms over the first year of their assessment and/or to require subsequent surgical therapy over the successive 6 years (42). This result has been accompanied in some series by a high overall satisfaction rate with LIS where over 90% of patients reported that they would again choose the same treatment if the circumstances were the same (43). Such studies are somewhat biased, however, towards single therapies, where variations in reported immediate medical side effects and efficacy will influence initial management decision making. A recent study by Gagliardi and colleagues assessing short- and longer-term medical therapy for CAF with topical high-dose GTN suggests that initially poor responses to such treatment predict for later nonhealing of the fissure and the need for abandonment of the treatment in favour of surgery (28).

Incontinence following LIS is a complex issue due to the sphincterotomy itself rather than showing any linkages to gender, age, other operative procedures combined with sphincterotomy (such as limited haemorrhoidectomy (44)) or previous vaginal delivery history (45). In this respect, prospective endosonographic data have shown that the rostral limit of sphincterotomy performed in a conventional LIS (from dentate line to the anal verge) is often more extensive than intended (46) where overall LIS does not appear to be accompanied by more postoperative complications (such as bleeding, pruritus, mucus discharge, or sepsis) when other anorectal procedures are performed *synchronously* with sphincter division (44,47). The clinical outcome is unaffected in LIS whether the sphincterotomy wound is sutured or is left open (48,49) and patient satisfaction is higher if coincident hypertrophied anal papillae, fibrous anal polyps and sentinel "pile" distal skin tags are excised at the same time (29,50). This data should, however, be evaluated by considering reports which have tried to categorize the sphincterotomy to the apex of the fissure only (rather than to the dentate line), and which claim better continence rates when the sphincterotomy is deemed at operation to have been more limited (51). The standardized terminology of these different operations is, however, somewhat unclear (52). The issues involved in the interpretation of post-LIS outcomes are complex and may be viewed with some scepticism particularly when assessing studies which compare open with closed sphincterotomy techniques where some have claimed continence superiority using the closed method (53,54). In such cases, it is not surprising that reported postoperative quality of life is only improved in patients where both the fissure heals and where continence is fully maintained (55).

Part VI: Sphincterotomy—Lateral

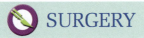

SURGERY

Surgical Alternatives to Conventional Open Lateral Internal Anal Sphincterotomy

Fissurectomy (with or without Advancement Flap)

Functional and healing comparisons of fissure excision with other novel modalities of fissure treatment are shown in Table 18.2. A recent study by Mousavi et al. has shown a slightly higher fissure recurrence and postoperative complication rate with fissurectomy when compared with conventional LIS (15). Other studies have combined fissurectomy with midline posterior sphincterotomy, demonstrating a worse functional continence outcome in the patients presenting with a posterior CAF and reserving its use only for those presenting with coincident posterior anal fistula (56). The reported higher fissure recurrence rate following fissurectomy in some studies is difficult to interpret since patients are often not randomized to these surgeries and as fissurectomy is frequently combined with other procedures, including intersphincteric Botulinum toxin (31,57–59) or Diltiazem administration (60). It would appear in many such studies that these alternatives have been suggested for a select group of patients deemed unsuitable for conventional LIS on clinical rather than functional outcome-based lines.

At present, there are no currently available prospective, randomized data to suggest that preoperative manometry and/or endosonography (for the detection of occult EAS damage) is relevant in directing sphincter-sparing surgery in topically resistant CAF, although this would seem intuitive (61). In this respect, fissurectomy has been proposed specifically in those patients with demonstrated preoperative anal hypotonia and for those fissures located anteriorly (62). Despite this, there has been a moderate rate

				Healing	Incontinence	Other
Author (Ref)	**Year**	**Number**	**Procedure**	**rate (%)**	**(%)**	**complications**
Fissurectomy						
Lambe et al. (66)	2000	37*	Fissurectomy	81	Not stated	Nil recorded
Scholz et al. (57)	2007	40	Fissurectomy + Botulinum	90	Not stated	Nil recorded
Baraza et al. (58)	2008	46	Fissurectomy + Botulinum	50	–	3 Perianal abscesses
Witte et al. (59)	2009	21	Fissurectomy	90	Not stated	Nil recorded
Patti et al. (62)	2009	16	Fissurectomy + advancement flap	100	25	Nil recorded
Mousavi et al. (15)	2009	30	Fissurectomy[†]	96.9	6.2	Nil recorded
Aivaz et al. (31)	2009	19	Fissurectomy[†] + botulinum	74	–	Nil recorded
Flaps						
Kenefick et al. (63)	2002	8	Advancement anoplasty	87.5	–	Nil recorded
Singh et al. (16)	2005	21	Rotation flap	90.4	–	2 Flap dehiscences
Giordano et al. (64)	2009	51	Advancement anoplasty	94.1	–	
Fissurotomy						
Pelta et al. (20)	2007	109	Fissurotomy	98.2	–	Nil recorded

TABLE 18.2   Trials and Studies on Sphincter-Saving Operative Alternatives for Chronic Anal Fissure (CAF)

*Study performed in children.
[†]Controlled randomized trial with LIS.

(12.5%) of continence impairment following fissurectomy and advancement flap anoplasty even in this select group.

The impression from tailored, nonrandomized studies, particularly in the presence of anal sphincter normo- or hypotonia, is that the utilization of either advancement cutaneous flaps or perineal rotation flaps have shown a moderate fissure recurrence rate when these procedures are performed in isolation and when they are unassociated with some form of partial sphincterotomy (16,63,64). In these select cases, local wound flap dehiscence predictably occurs in those patients who have undergone previous mucosal advancements for perirectal sepsis and in this circumstance flap surgery for CAF should probably be avoided. The primary flap approach has, however, been recommended in specific subsets of patients presenting with recalcitrant medically resistant CAF, where acceptable results have been reported in perianal Crohn's disease (5,65) and children (66), although recent data has favoured the more specialist approach of guided Botulinum toxin administration in those children presenting with CAF secondary to chronic constipation and straining (67).

Calibrated Sphincterotomy, Guided Pneumatic Dilatation, and Fissurotomy

As alluded to above, it has been argued that differential therapy may be surgically afforded for patients with CAFs where there is preexistent anal normtonia or hypotonia because of the potential risks of postoperative incontinence (68). This may partly be related to fissure position, where anterior and lateral fissures are more often associated with a normotonic anal pressure profile (69). Rosa and colleagues have described tailoring the extent of sphincterotomy to preoperative anal pressure, where arbitrarily between 20% and 60% of the visible IAS is divided according to preexistent hypertonia (70). In this study, postoperative incontinence was balanced against persistence of the fissure and its symptoms as a retrospective designation case for calibrated sphincter division. This approach has been akin to sphincterotomy performed to the fissure apex, which, when compared with conventional LIS to the dentate line, has been reported to result in sustainably better healing, and less incontinence at the expense of a higher recurrence rate (17,71). This tailored approach is also comparative to a more controlled lateral sphincterotomy (comparing IAS division to the distal end of the fissure, to the dentate line or as a bilateral lateral sphincterotomy), using a calibrated measurement of perceived anal stenosis in relation to the fissure (72). With this more directed approach, in this study, it has been claimed by Cho that postoperative incontinence is eliminated.

The small amount of available data concerning pneumatic dilatation of the anal canal has shown a reduction of postoperative resting anal pressure without either clinical incontinence or endosonographic evidence of IAS disruption (73) and with equivalent fissure healing rates in one prospective, one-sided, endosonographic, manometric and clinical outcome-based assessment (19) and in one prospective, randomized controlled trial comparing dilatation with formal LIS (74). Larger studies of this technique will be required as the postprocedural rates of incontinence appear to be very low and the incidence of painless first defecation after pneumatic dilatation exceeds 80% (19).

One recent alternative for fissure treatment that has been recommended is fissurotomy where a small track in association with the fissure is opened to the level of the dentate line without coincident sphincterotomy. In the only study available of this technique, Pelta and colleagues have reported a success rate of 98.2% in 109 consecutive patients without any alteration in continence (20). This treatment although novel is not particularly supported by the clinical findings or the known etiopathogenesis of fissure where many fissures are not accompanied by associated fistulous tracks and are not generally a feature of medically treated cases that come to surgery (75).

✳ CONCLUSIONS

There is considerable evidence to show that functionally some patients fare badly following conventional LIS for medically resistant CAF. There is a degree of unpredictability relative to postoperative continence so that informed consent is mandatory (76). Given the relatively moderate success of medical therapy alone for this condition (42), it would seem possible that controlled, randomized, prospective outcome studies could be conducted in an effort to answer the question of quality of life-based symptom eradication assessing the surgical alternatives outlined in this chapter in specialized subgroups. It is intuitive that parturient female patients with anterior fissures (77), females with aberrantly located fissures and others with compromised preoperative continence and CAF might benefit from procedures which either do not divide the IAS such as fissurotomy or operations that minimize sphincter division, either as a tailored sphincterotomy or with pneumatic dilatation (whether determined operatively or manometrically). In the absence of available data, we simply do not know the longer-term benefit of these novel methodologies or how preoperative objective sphincter assessments (manometric or imaging-based) influence such decision making.

Currently, we also have little information concerning the prospective effects on IAS function following sphincter-sparing procedures. The author has shown subtle differences in rectoanal inhibition with excessive inhibitory responses on rectal balloon dilatation in those individuals who are incontinent following sphincterotomy when compared with those remaining fully continent (26). These latter patients exhibit an increase in the area under the inhibitory curve with variations in rectoanal inhibitory latency and amplitude, perhaps mirroring the transient IAS relaxations recognized during ambulatory manometry which correlate with patient-reported episodes of leakage in other forms of fecal incontinence (78). Without this complex, prospectively collected data we can only rely on the wealth of information regarding continence outcomes following conventional LIS in unselected patient cohorts where sphincter-sparing procedures are associated with a small risk of recurrence (or persistence) of the fissure balanced against the real risk of incontinence (at least a third of which is persistent) following standard LIS surgery (79).

References

1. Menteş BB, Tezcaner T, Yilmaz U, Leventoğlu S, Oguz M. Results of lateral sphincterotomy for chronic anal fissure with particular reference to quality of life. *Dis Colon Rectum* 2006;49:1045–51.
2. Casillas S, Hull TL, Zutshi M, Trzcinski R, Bast JF, Xu M. Incontinence after a lateral internal sphincterotomy: are we underestimating it? *Dis Colon Rectum* 2005;48:1193–9.
3. Zbar A, Beer-Gabel M, Chiappa AC, Aslam M. Fecal incontinence after minor anorectal surgery. *Dis Colon Rectum* 2001;44:1610–23.
4. Zbar AP, Kmiot WA, Aslam M, et al. Use of vector volume manometry and endoanal magnetic resonance imaging in the adult female for assessment of anal sphincter dysfunction. *Dis Colon Rectum* 1999;42:928–33.
5. Fleshner PR, Schoetz DJ Jr., Roberts PL, Murray JJ, Coller JA, Veidenheimer MC. Anal fissure in Crohn's disease: a plea for aggressive management. *Dis Colon Rectum* 1995;38:1137–43.
6. Sangwan YP, Solla JA. Internal anal sphincter: advances and insights. *Dis Colon Rectum* 1998;41:1297–311.
7. Zbar AP, Jayne DG, Mathur D, Ambrose NS, Guillou PJ. The importance of the internal anal sphincter (IAS) in maintaining continence: anatomical, physiological and pharmacological considerations. *Colorectal Dis* 2000;2:193–202.
8. Zbar AP, Aslam M, Gosling A, Kmiot WA. Parameters of the rectoanal inhibitory reflex in patients with idiopathic fecal incontinence and chronic constipation. *Dis Colon Rectum* 1998;41:200–8.
9. Zbar AP, Ramesh J, Beer-Gabel M, Salazar R, Pescatori M. Conventional cutting vs. internal anal sphincter-preserving seton for high trans-sphincteric fistula: a prospective randomized manometric and clinical trial. *Techn Coloproctol* 2003;7:89–94.
10. Tankova L, Yoncheva K, Kovatchki D, Doytchinova I. Topical anal fissure treatment: placebo-controlled study of mononitrate and trinitrate therapies. *Int J Colorectal Dis* 2009;24:461–4.
11. Madalinski M, Kalinowski L. Novel options for the pharmacological treatment of chronic anal fissure—role of botulin toxin. *Curr Clin Pharmacol* 2009;4:47–52.
12. Mishra R, Thomas S, Maan MS, Hadke NS. Topical nitroglycerin versus lateral internal sphincterotomy for chronic anal fissure: prospective, randomized trial. *ANZ J Surg* 2005;75:1032–5.
13. Iswariah H, Stephens J, Rieger N, et al. Randomized prospective controlled trial of lateral internal sphincterotomy versus injection of botulinum toxin for the treatment of idiopathic fissure in ano. *ANZ J Surg* 2005;75:553–5.
14. Shao WJ, Li GC, Zhang ZK. Systematic review and meta-analysis of randomized controlled trials comparing botulinum toxin injection with lateral internal sphincterotomy for chronic anal fissure. *Int J Colorect Dis* 2009;24:995–1000.
15. Mousavi SR, Sharifi M, Mehdikhah Z. A comparison between the results of fissurectomy and lateral internal sphincterotomy in the surgical management of chronic anal fissure. *J Gastrointest Surg* 2009;13:1279–82.
16. Singh M, Sharma A, Gardiner A, Duthie GS. Early results of a rotational flap to treat chronic anal fissures. *Int J Colorect Dis* 2005;20:339–42.
17. Littlejohn DR, Newstead GL. Tailored lateral sphincterotomy for anal fissure. *Dis Colon Rectum* 1997;40:1439–42.
18. Pescatori M, Maria G, Anastasio G. "Spasm related" internal sphincterotomy in treatment of anal fissure. A randomized prospective study. *Coloproctology* 1991;1:20–2.
19. Renzi A, Izzo D, Di Sarno G, et al. Clinical, manometric and ultrasonographic results of pneumatic balloon dilatation vs. lateral internal sphincterotomy for chronic anal fissure: a prospective, randomized, controlled trial. *Dis Colon Rectum* 2008;51:121–7.
20. Pelta AE, Davis KG, Armstrong DN. Subcutaneous fissurotomy: a novel procedure for chronic fissure-in-ano. A review of 109 cases. *Dis Colon Rectum* 2007;50:1662–7.
21. Nelson R. Operative procedures for fissure in ano. *Cochrane Database Syst Rev* 2005;2:CD002199.
22. Kiyak G, Korukluoğlu B, Kuşdemir A, Sişman IC, Ergül E. Results of lateral internal sphincterotomy with open technique for chronic anal fissure: evaluation of complications, symptom relief, and incontinence with long-term follow-up. *Dig Dis Sci* 2009;54:2220–4.

23. Tan E, Anstee A, Koh DM, Gedroyc W, Tekkis PP. Diagnostic precision of endoanal MRI in the detection of anal sphincter pathology: a meta-analysis. *Int J Colorectal Dis* 2008;23:641–51.

24. Lund JN, Scholefield JH. Aetiology and treatment of anal fissure. *Br J Surg* 1996;83:1335–44.

25. Tuckson W, Lavery I, Fazio VW, Oakley J, Church J, Milsom J. Manometric and functional comparison of ileal pouch anal anastomosis with and without anal manipulation. *Am J Surg* 1991;161:90–6.

26. Zbar AP, Aslam M, Allgar V. Faecal incontinence after internal sphincterotomy for anal fissure. *Techn Coloproctol* 2000;4:25–8.

27. Ammari FF, Bani-Hani KE. Faecal incontinence in patients with anal fissure: a consequence of internal sphincterotomy or a feature of the condition? *Surgeon* 2004;2:225–9.

28. Gagliardi G, Pascariello A, Altomare DF, et al. Optimal treatment of glyceryl trinitrate (GTN) for chronic anal fissure (CAF): results of a prospective randomized trial. *Tech Coloproctol* 2010;14(3):241–8.

29. Gupta PJ, Kalaskar S. Hypertrophied anal papillae and fibrous anal polyps, should they be removed during anal fissure surgery? *World J Gastroenterol* 2004;10:2412–4.

30. Soll C, Dindo D, Hahnloser D. Combined fissurectomy and botulinum toxin injection. A new therapeutic approach for chronic anal fissures. *Gastroenterol Clin Biol* 2008;32:667–70.

31. Aivaz O, Rayhanabad J, Nguyen V, Haigh PI, Abbas M. Botulinum toxin A with fissurectomy is a viable alternative to lateral internal sphincterotomy for chronic anal fissure. *Ann Surg* 2009;75:925–8.

32. Leroi AM, Kamm MA, Weber J, Denis P, Hawley PR. Internal anal sphincter repair. *Int J Colorectal Dis* 1997;12:243–5.

33. Shafik A. Perianal injection of autologous fat for treatment of sphincteric incontinence. *Dis Colon Rectum* 1995;38:583–7.

34. Kumar D, Benson MJ, Bland JE. Glutaraldehyde cross-linked collagen in the treatment of faecal incontinence. *Br J Surg* 1998;85:978–9.

35. Tjandra JJ, Lim JF, Hiscock R, Rajendra P. Injectable silicone biomaterial for fecal incontinence caused by internal anal sphincter dysfunction is effective. *Dis Colon Rectum* 2004;47:2138–46.

36. de la Portilla F, Fernández A, León E, et al. Evaluation of the use of PTQ implants for the treatment of incontinent patients due to internal anal sphincter dysfunction. *Colorectal Dis* 2008;10:89–94.

37. de la Portilla F, Vega J, Rada R, et al. Evaluation by three-dimensional anal endosonography of injectable silicone biomaterial (PTQ) implants to treat fecal incontinence: long-term localization and relation with the deterioration of the continence. *Tech Coloproctol* 2009;13:195–9.

38. Aigner F, Conrad F, Margreiter R, Oberwalder M; Coloproctology Working Group. Anal submucosal carbon bead injection for treatment of idiopathic fecal incontinence: a preliminary report. *Dis Colon Rectum* 2009;52:293–8.

39. Ruiz D, Pinto RA, Hull TL, Efron JE, Wexner SD. Does the radiofrequency procedure for fecal incontinence improve quality of life and incontinence at 1-year follow-up? *Dis Colon Rectum* 2010;53:1041–6.

40. Dudding TC, Parès D, Vaizey CJ, Kamm MA. Sacral nerve stimulation for the treatment of faecal incontinence related to dysfunction of the internal anal sphincter. *Int J Colorect Dis* 2010;25:625–30.

41. Zbar AP. Measurement of anal cushions in idiopathic faecal incontinence. *Br J Surg* 2009;96:1373–4.

42. Brown CJ, Dubreuil D, Santoro L, et al. Lateral internal sphincterotomy is superior to topical nitroglycerin for healing chronic anal fissure and does not compromise long-term fecal continence: six-year follow-up of a multicenter, randomized, controlled trial. *Dis Colon Rectum* 2007;50:442–8.

43. Hyman N. Incontinence after lateral internal sphincterotomy: a prospective study and quality of life assessment. *Dis Colon Rectum* 2004;47:35–8.

44. Syed SA, Waris S, Ahmed E, Saeed N, Ali B. Lateral internal sphincterotomy for anal fissure: with or without associated anorectal procedures. *J Col Physicians Surg Pak* 2003;13:436–9.

45. Rotholtz NA, Bun M, Mauri MY, Bosio R, Peczan CE, Mezzadri NA. Long-term assessment of fecal incontinence after lateral internal sphincterotomy. *Techn Coloproctol* 2005;9:115–8.

46. Sultan AH, Kamm MA, Nicholls RJ, Bartram CI. Prospective study of the extent of internal anal sphincter division during lateral sphincterotomy. *Dis Colon Rectum* 1994;37:1031–3.

47. Leong AF, Husain MJ, Seow-Choen F, Goh HS. Performing internal sphincterotomy with other anorectal procedures. *Dis Colon Rectum* 1994;37:1130–2.

48. Aysan E, Aren A, Ayar E. A prospective, randomized, controlled trial of primary wound closure after lateral internal sphincterotomy. *Gastrointest Endosc* 2003;57:483–91.

49. Kang GS, Kim BS, Choi PS, Kang DW. Evaluation of healing and complications after lateral internal sphincterotomy for chronic anal fissure: marginal suture of incision vs. open left incision: prospective, randomized, controlled study. *Dis Colon Rectum* 2008;51:329–33.

50. Gupta PJ, Kalaskar S. Removal of hypertrophied anal papillae and fibrous anal polyps increases patient satisfaction after anal fissure surgery. *Tech Coloproctol* 2003;7:155–8.

51. Elsebae MM. A study of fecal incontinence in patients with chronic anal fissure: prospective, randomized, controlled trial of the extent of internal anal sphincter division during lateral sphincterotomy. *World J Surg* 2007;31:2052–7.

52. Pernikoff BJ, Eisenstat TE, Rubin RJ, Oliver GC, Salvati EP. Reappraisal of partial lateral internal sphincterotomy. *Dis Colon Rectum* 1994;37:1291–5.

53. Garcià-Aguilar J, Belmonte C, Wong WD, Lowry AC, Madoff RD. Open vs. closed sphincterotomy for chronic anal fissure: long-term results. *Dis Colon Rectum* 1996;39:440–3.

54. Wiley M, Day P, Rieger N, Stephens J, Moore J. Open vs. closed lateral internal sphincterotomy for idiopathic fissure-in-ano: a prospective, randomized, controlled trial. *Dis Colon Rectum* 2004;47:847–52.

55. Ortiz H, Marzo J, Armendariz P, De Miguel M. Quality of life assessment in patients with chronic anal fissure after lateral internal sphincterotomy. *Br J Surg* 2005;92:881–5.

56. Abcarian H. Surgical correction of chronic anal fissure: results of lateral internal sphincterotomy vs. fissurectomy – midline sphincterotomy. *Dis Colon Rectum* 1980;23(1):31–6.

57. Scholz T, Hetzer FH, Dindo D, Demartines N, Clavien PA, Hahnloser D. Long-term follow-up after combined fissurectomy and Botox injection for chronic anal fissures. *Int J Colorect Dis* 2007;22:1077–81.

58. Baraza W, Boereboom C, Shorthouse A, Brown S. The long-term efficacy of fissurectomy and botulinum toxin injection for chronic anal fissure in females. *Dis Colon Rectum* 2008;51:239–43.

59. Witte ME, Klaase JM, Koop R. Fissurectomy combined with botulinum toxin A injection for medically resistant chronic anal fissures. *Colorectal Dis* 2010;12:e163–9.

60. Arthur JD, Makin CA, El-Sayed TY, Walsh CJ. A pilot comparative study of fissurectomy/diltiazem and fissurectomy/botulinum toxin in the treatment of chronic anal fissure. *Techn Coloproctol* 2008;12:331–6.

61. Zbar AP. The role of functional evaluation before anorectal surgery. *SICCR (Societa Italiana di Chirurgia ColoRettale)* 2005;9:74–83.

62. Patti R, Famà F, Barrera T, Migliore G, Di Vita G. Fissurectomy and anal advancement flap for anterior chronic anal fissure without hypertonia of the internal anal sphincter in females. *Colorectal Dis* 2010;12(11):1127–30.

63. Kenefick NJ, Gee AS, Durdey P. Treatment of resistant anal fissure with advancement anoplasty. *Colorectal Dis* 2002;4:463–6.

64. Giordano P, Gravante G, Grondona P, Ruggiero B, Porrett T, Lunniss PJ. Simple cutaneous advancement flap anoplasty for resistant chronic anal fissure: a prospective study. *World J Surg* 2009;33:1058–63.

65. Wolkomir AF, Luchtefeld MA. Surgery for symptomatic haemorrhoids and anal fissures in Crohn's disease. *Dis Colon Rectum* 1993;36:545–7.

66. Lambe GF, Driver CP, Morton S, Turnock RR. Fissurectomy as a treatment for anal fissures in children. *Ann R Coll Surg Engl* 2000;82:254–7.

67. Keshtgar AS. Ward HC, Clayden GS. Transcutaneous needle-free injection of botulinum toxin: a novel treatment of childhood constipation and anal fissure. *J Pediatr Surg* 2009;44:1791–8.

68. Menteş BB, Güner MK, Leventoglu S, Akyürek N. Fine-tuning of the extent of lateral internal sphincterotomy: spasm-controlled vs. up to the fissure apex. *Dis Colon Rectum* 2008;51:128–33.

Part VI: Sphincterotomy—Lateral

69. Bove A, Balzano A, Perrotti, Antropoli C, Lombardi G, Pucciani F. Different anal pressure profiles in patients with anal fissure. *Techn Coloproctol* 2004;8:151–7.

70. Rosa G, Lolli P, Piccinelli D, et al. Calibrated lateral internal sphincterotomy for fissure. *Techn Coloproctol* 2005;9:127–32.

71. Menteş BB, Ege B, Leventoglu S, Oguz M, Karadag A. Extent of lateral internal sphincterotomy: up to the dentate line or up to the fissure apex? *Dis Colon Rectum* 2005;48:365–70.

72. Cho DY. Controlled lateral sphincterotomy for chronic anal fissure. *Dis Colon Rectum* 2005;48:1037–41.

73. Renzi A, Brusciano L, Pescatori M, et al. Pneumatic balloon dilatation for chronic anal fissure: a prospective, clinical, endosonographic and manometric study. *Dis Colon Rectum* 2005;48:121–5.

74. Yucel T, Gonullu D, Oncu M, Koksoy FN, Ozkan SG, Aycan O. Comparison of controlled-intermittent anal dilatation and lateral internal sphincterotomy in the treatment of chronic anal fissures: a prospective, randomized study. *Int J Surg* 2009;7:228–31.

75. Zbar AP. Sphincter-sparing surgical alternatives for chronic anal fissure: the place of fissurotomy. *Dis Colon Rectum* 2008;51:1299.

76. Beck DE. Medicolegal aspects of coloproctologic practice. In: Wexner SD, Zbar A, Pescatori M, eds. *Complex Anorectal Disorders: Investigation and Management*. London: Springer, 2005:767–78.

77. Pascual M, Pares D, Pera M, et al. Variation in clinical, manometric and endosonographic findings in anterior chronic anal fissure: a prospective study. *Dig Dis Sci* 2008;53:21–6.

78. Bannister JJ, Read NW, Donnelly TC, Sun WM. External and internal anal sphincter responses to rectal distension in normal subjects and in patients with idiopathic faecal incontinence. *Br J Surg* 1989;76:617–21.

79. Garcia-Granero E, Sanahuja A, Garcia-Botello SA, et al. The ideal lateral internal sphincterotomy: clinical and endosonographic evaluation following open and closed internal anal sphincterotomy. *Colorectal Dis* 2009;11:502–7.

19 Technical Considerations in the Surgical Management of Presacral Tumors

Najjia Mahmoud and Robert Fry

Presacral tumors, whether benign or malignant, represent a very small proportion of neoplasms encountered in clinical practice. Estimates of incidence vary and are difficult to precisely obtain, but in U.S. adults, patients with retrorectal tumors are thought to present to major referral centers two to six times per year (1). A study from the Mayo clinic reported that retrorectal tumors accounted for one in 40,000 hospital admissions (2).

Presacral masses are classified into categories that tend to reflect the histologically heterogeneous nature of the presacral space itself. These masses may be congenital, neurogenic, inflammatory, osseous, and "miscellaneous" (Table 19.1). Undoubtedly, the most challenging issue for surgeons is the location of these malignancies. The small, confined space defined by the framework of the lower bony pelvis houses nerves, vessels, muscles, and genitourinary and gastrointestinal organs within millimeters of one another. An invasive mass in this area represents special technical challenges and almost always portends the loss of function and form, either from surgery or the neoplasm itself. The most important preoperative decision when treating to cure or palliate is the creation of a multidisciplinary team appropriate for the location of the mass. Clearly, these rare tumors require careful preoperative planning for best short- and long-term outcomes. This chapter serves to categorize these tumors, discuss preoperative planning, and offer technical approaches and insights into surgical extirpation and reconstruction.

ANATOMY

The pelvis is defined by the confines of its bony structure—the sacrum posteriorly, pubic bone anteriorly, and the sacral rami laterally. It is invested by the endopelvic fascia called the "presacral fascia" anterior to the sacrum (Fig. 19.1). Along the presacral fascia run the hypogastric nerves as they branch laterally and anteriorly to coalesce with their parasympathetic counterparts to form the sacral plexus. Laterally, the internal

TABLE 19.1	Classification of Retrorectal Masses			
Congenital	**Inflammatory**	**Neurogenic**	**Osseous**	**Miscellaneous**
Developmental cysts	Inflammatory bowel disease	Neurofibroma	Osteoma	Metastatic disease
Epidermoid cyst	Perirectal abscess (cryptoglandular)	Neurolemmoma	Osteogenic sarcoma	Lymphangioma
Dermoid cyst	Pelvirectal abscess (descending, e.g., diverticulitis)	Ependymoma	Sacral bone cyst	Desmoid tumor
Tailgut cyst	Tuberculosis/Pott's disease	Ganglioneuroma	Ewing's tumor	Leiomyoma
Teratoma		Neurofibrosarcoma	Giant cell tumor	Fibrosarcoma
Chordoma			Chondromyxosarcoma	Endothelioma
Anterior meningocele				
Rectal duplication				
Adrenal rest tumors				

Modified with permission from *Dis Colon Rectum* 1975;18:581.

and external iliac vessels and the ureters run along the retroperitoneum anterior to the iliopsoas muscle and the bony framework of the true pelvis. Retrorectal masses may reside between the fascia propria of the rectum posteriorly and the presacral fascia. The space is actually a potential one, bound by the rectum (and mesorectum) anteriorly, the presacral fascia posteriorly, and the endopelvic fascia (lateral ligaments) laterally. The inferior border is Waldeyer's fascia overlying the perineal muscles and the superior boundary is the peritoneal reflection. These masses may also arise from neural or osseous elements located posterior to this. The retrorectal space contains elements derived embryologically from the hindgut, notochord, and neuroectoderm; consequently, tumors that arise are heterogeneous.

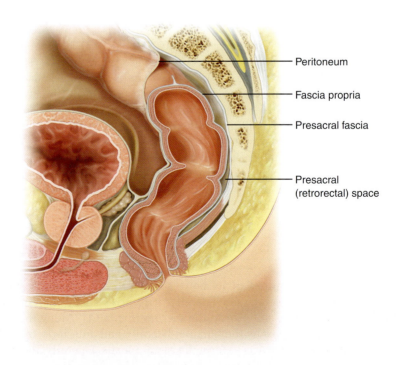

Figure 19.1 Boundaries of the presacral space. The boundaries of the retrorectal space are the fascia propria of the mesorectum anteriorly, the presacral fascia posteriorly, the peritoneal reflection superiorly, and Waldeyer's fascia overlying the levator ani muscles inferiorly. (Adapted from Nicholls J, Dozios RR, eds. Surgery of the Colon and Rectum. Edinburgh: Churchill Livingstone, 1997.)

Peritoneum

Fascia propria

Presacral fascia

Presacral (retrorectal) space

Congenital Lesions

Congenital lesions constitute two-thirds of all lesions found in the retrorectal space and represent the persistence and eventual growth of embryologic elements (3). Developmental cysts, anterior meningoceles, chordomas, rectal duplications and tailgut cysts, and adrenal rest tumors all derive from persistent embryologic elements and are considered congenital in nature. In adults, cystic congenital tumors are typically benign and solid ones are usually malignant.

Developmental Cysts

Developmental cysts constitute two-thirds of the retrorectal tumors encountered in clinical practice and are almost always benign (4). They have a prominent female preponderance of approximately 5:1 in most series (4). They can arise from any embryonic cell layer. Epidermoid, dermoid, or teratoma tumors are the three most common entities and are comprised of one, two, and three embryologically distinct cell layer origins, respectively (Fig. 19.2). Tailgut cysts are included in the developmental cyst group, although they are quite rare, and are derived from mesodermal tissue of the embryonic gastrointestinal tract. Tailgut cysts are considered retrorectal cystic hamartomas and result from failure of regression of the embryonic tail (5,6). Rectal duplication cysts are similarly rare and frequently harbor a secretory gut epithelial lining as well as all of the layers of the rectal wall. Like intestinal duplication cysts elsewhere, they may share a common wall with the true rectum. Dermoid and epidermoid cysts often contain dermal elements and are commonly filled with a sebaceous-like material secreted from glands within the cyst wall. Dermoid cysts are the most commonly encountered retrorectal mass in clinical practice, and a simple posterior juxtasacral incision to excise is frequently all that is required because they are so distally located and easily accessible. Teratomas often feature mature embryologic elements comprised of all three embryonic layers. Teeth, hair, sebaceous material, and bone can be found. They can be either cystic or solid or have elements of both and are often noted to be firmly adherent to the coccyx even when benign. As with ovarian teratomas, approximately 5–10% will undergo malignant degeneration (5).

All of these lesions are most often completely asymptomatic. They can (rarely) present with obstructed labor when large or alternatively be detected on a prenatal ultrasound or physical examination. Routine gynecologic examinations result in detection of some lesions, and others present with a vague, dull "pressure" sensation that calls attention to their presence (7). The most sensitive and specific test for diagnosis is magnetic resonance imaging (MRI) (8). The goals of imaging for any presacral mass

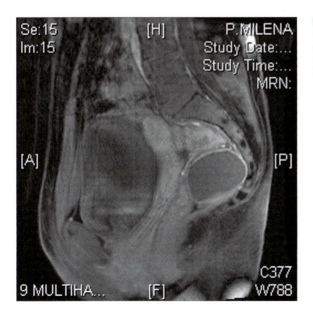

Figure 19.2 Sagittal view of dermoid cyst on magnetic resonance imaging. Presacral dermoid cyst in a young female. (Courtesy of Najjia N. Mahmoud, University of Pennsylvania.)

Part VII: Presacral Tumors

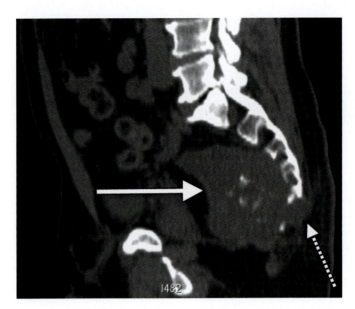

Figure 19.3 Sagittal computed tomographic (CT) image of a chordoma. Sagittal reformatted CT image shows the mass arising from the sacrum, with large presacral (*solid arrow*) and smaller postsacral (*dotted arrow*) soft-tissue components. (Farsad K, et al. *Radiographics* 2009;29: 1525–1530, with permission.)

lesion are delineation of anatomy, characterization of the lesion, and assessment of adjacent tissue involvement. Preoperative biopsy of these discrete lesions is contraindicated to avoid infecting the lesion resulting in an inflammatory reaction or infection and increasing the technical difficulty involved in excision. Elective excision is recommended, particularly with teratomas, where malignant degeneration, as mentioned, is a possibility. Otherwise, prognosis following successful resection of these lesions is 100%.

Chordomas

Chordomas are the most common malignant lesion in the presacral space and the second most common variety of retrorectal tumor (Fig. 19.3). It arises from the embryonic notochord and has a predilection for male gender 2:1 (3). Chordomas typically present in males aged 40–60. Patients present with symptoms implying neurologic involvement characterized by pain, urinary incontinence or retention, and impotency or erectile dysfunction. Lower extremity paralysis tends to be uncommon unless the tumor is located in the lumbar or thoracic vertebrae. Thirty to fifty percent of chordomas are located in the sacrococcygeal region (9). The radical surgery typically required to clear the tumor's lateral margins frequently results in motor and sensory dysfunction. Chordomas are quite resistant to chemotherapy and are radiation-insensitive. Radical resection represents the only chance for cure. Survival rates after chordoma resection have been rising. In the 1970s, recurrence rates were reported in excess of 90% and survival was less than 20% following diagnosis (10). Advances in imaging, surgery, and reconstruction have been credited with improving survival four-fold. Even so, recurrence rates at 5 years are as high as 40–70%. Survival after local recurrence is rare (11).

Anterior Sacral Meningocele

Anterior sacral meningocele (ASM) is a rare developmental lesion with a slight female predominance precipitated by a congenital defect representing an area of sacral agenesis through which the dura herniates. ASM is associated with the Currarino syndrome or triad, an autosomal dominant condition that includes findings of presacral mass, sacral deformity, and anorectal malformation (12). It is most commonly, an isolated finding. The associated sac is filled with cerebrospinal fluid. Patients frequently complain of headaches, pressure, lower back pain, and urinary difficulty. Headache during defecation or obstructed defecation can result as well. Diagnosis is typically made by imaging studies such as computed tomography or MRI, but a classic, often mentioned finding on plain film is the "scimitar sign" associated with the herniation of the dural

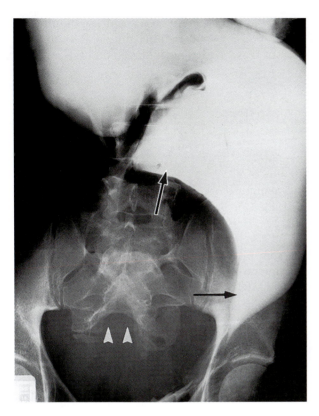

Figure 19.4 Barium enema demonstrating an anterior sacral meningocele. Anterior sacral meningocele in a 43-year-old man with a history of headache, meningitis, and chronic constipation. Frontal image from a barium enema examination shows a rectal stenosis due to extrinsic compression (*arrows*) with a distended proximal colon. Note the sacral bone defect (the scimitar sign) (*arrowheads*). (Dahan H, et al. *Radiographics* 2001;21:575–84, with permission.)

sac (13) (Fig. 19.4). Biopsy of this lesion is absolutely contraindicated as it can cause cerebrospinal fluid leak and meningitis (13).

Other Congenital Lesions

Other rare retrorectal masses include adrenal rest tumors, which are exceedingly uncommon and typically excised taking precautions similar to those employed when removing pheochromocytomas in other locations. Rectal duplication cysts may share a common wall with the rectum and can be difficult to excise (14). They contain secreting mucosa and a fully formed wall with smooth muscle and a separate feeding vessel. They may fill with mucous and exert pressure on surrounding structures causing pain and discomfort. Although their malignant potential is unknown, excision of duplication cysts is recommended. Surveillance is difficult if not impossible (14).

Osseous and Neurogenic Lesions

Osseous lesions are rare and comprise 5–10% of retrorectal lesions. Osteomas, sacral bone cysts, giant cell tumors, Ewing's sarcoma, and chondrosarcomas reflect the large range of benign and malignant possibilities. Complete excision (for cure if malignant and to prevent recurrence if benign) is encouraged (2,15). Neurogenic lesions include neurofibromas that may be associated with the diagnosis of neurofibromatosis, ganglioneuromas, neurolemmomas, and neurofibrosarcomas. As with all retrorectal tumors, complete excision is the rule and diagnosis is often made afterwards to avoid risk of infection and perforation of the mass with tumor seeding that may complicate biopsy or fine-needle aspiration (2,15).

Inflammatory

Inflammatory lesions typically affect the retrorectal space as a result of an infectious process adjacent to the area. Pain, fever, drainage, history of anal fistula, congenital cyst, prior rectal resection or surgery, or Crohn's diagnosis should raise suspicion of infection or inflammation. Tuberculosis can rarely present as a draining presacral sinus with infected bone (Pott's disease). Treatment of these symptoms is directed at the underlying cause.

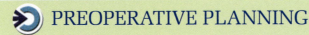

PREOPERATIVE PLANNING

Diagnosis and Planning

A high index of suspicion prompted by symptoms of pressure, pain, pelvic neuropraxia or neuropathies, fever, headache, obstructed or difficult defecation should initiate a workup that considers a retrorectal source. A digital rectal examination will nearly always identify most congenital cysts such as dermoids. Computed tomography with and without rectal and IV contrast is very useful at delineating cystic from solid masses. MRI, however, is imperative in the preoperative planning process. Many retrorectal tumors have very characteristic findings on MRI that make identification possible in the absence of tissue. MRI can delineate soft tissue planes identifying precise areas of invasion thereby enabling surgical planning. Specifically, extent of neurologic, vascular, rectal, and bony invasion can be adequately and accurately assessed. For patients with sacral meningocele, specific identification of the level of the connection between the cyst and the thecal sac can be made. Preoperative counseling and surgical team scheduling can proceed on this basis. Finally, direct examination of the rectal mucosa should be completed to exclude fistulizing or invasive lesions. Colonoscopy, flexible sigmoidoscopy, or proctoscopy serves this purpose and can help better characterize the nature of the lesion prior to a major procedure.

As previously mentioned, the role of biopsy or FNA for diagnosis of these lesions is rarely required and mostly detrimental (16). Since treatment of most retrorectal masses consists of complete excision, and preoperative chemotherapy and radiation is almost never indicated, the information from a biopsy is infrequently needed to aid in decision-making and treatment planning. For some lesions, such as dermoid cysts, the physical findings are unmistakable and diagnosis based on physical examination and MRI is typical. Preoperative biopsy only serves to cause inflammation that makes excision more difficult and dangerous. Biopsy of anterior meningocele carries a 30% mortality rate from meningitis and is absolutely contraindicated (13). If it is felt that biopsy is imperative, then it may be acceptable to biopsy via an organ or tissue that is to be included in the resection (rectum, sacrum) to avoid tumor seeding along the tract.

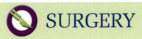

SURGERY

Treatment

Operative approaches to retrorectal masses are predicated on several key factors: location of the mass, involvement of adjacent structures, malignant potential, and patient performance status. Tumors can be approached several ways: via an anterior or abdominal approach, through a posterior or transsacral approach, or using both methods. Typically, if a lesion can be palpated through the anus on rectal examination and the upper extent of the lesion is appreciated, a posterior-only approach is effective.

Preoperative imaging data will guide the need for additional specialist involvement in the procedure. Anterior sacral meningocele resection will require a team that includes a neurosurgeon and cases that involve sacral or other bony resection, which will mandate involvement of either a neurosurgeon or an orthopedic surgeon with experience in sacral or vertebral resection, pelvic stabilization, and neurologic or dural surgery.

Excision of dermoid, epidermoid, and teratomas can typically be accomplished via a small juxtasacral (longitudinal) incision extending from just above the anal sphincter

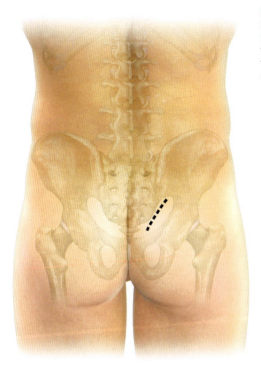

Figure 19.5 Schematic representation of a juxtasacral incision for a presacral dermoid cyst excision. The incision (dotted lines) follows the side of the sacrum from just superior to the anal sphincter mechanism to the cranial extent of the retrorectal cyst. The incision should be on the side of the sacrum that the cyst most closely approximates.

(Fig. 19.5). Alternatively, a transverse incision may be made overlying the coccyx, but exposure more proximally for larger lesions may be compromised (17). A preoperative bowel preparation the day before surgery is advised. The dissection is undertaken through the lumbosacral fascia to the levators. A finger in the rectum helps to push the mobile structure to the side of the incision and define the margins of the mass. The cyst wall is frequently found to push up through the levator musculature and attenuate it somewhat so that the muscle itself is "draped" over the structure and must be dissected or transected off the cyst wall at this point. The cyst is then reflected off of the posterior rectal wall. A very apparent plane is nearly always observed between the cyst and the rectum. If adherent to the coccyx, then the coccyx is simply taken en bloc with the cyst. Transection of the anococcygeal ligament facilitates exposure of the coccyx. It can then be transected by a Mayo scissors, bone rongeur, or electrocautery device. The surgeon should avoid violating the rectum as well as the cyst wall to minimize chance of fistula and infection. Complete excision of the cyst wall is felt to be necessary to avoid recurrence. Closure of the space occupied by the cyst in layers with absorbable suture over a small drain brought out laterally is advisable. Skin closure can be done with a small caliber absorbable monofilament such as Biosyn™.

Survival after resection of benign developmental cysts is 100% (1). Recurrence, particularly after excision of teratomas, may be related to failure to resect the coccyx, where nests of totipotential cells may reside. En bloc resection of the coccyx with the recurrence (or at the initial resection) is the solution to this problem. Larger tumors extending above S3–S4 may require an abdominal approach alone or a combination approach. Dissection of the benign lesion may begin in the lithotomy position or the lateral decubitus position to allow access to the retrorectal space via both a juxtasacral as well as an abdominal approach.

Since chordomas comprise the most common class of invasive retrorectal cysts, there is more information regarding chordoma resection techniques, complications, and functional perturbations than with other less common malignancies. Most of the following discussion is derived from experience with radical chordoma resection but can be generalized to any low- to moderate-grade invasive tumor. The surgeon should have an understanding preoperatively, based on imaging, physical examination, and preoperative symptoms, what structures may be compromised and which specialists may be needed. Functional compromise must be planned for as well, based on the expected extent of resection. Preoperative counseling regarding the need for a stoma, the need to self-catheterize the urinary bladder, or the possibility of lower extremity motor dysfunction should be anticipated.

Larger tumors extending above the level of S3-S4 or involving structures such as dura or bone will almost always require a combined abdominoperineal approach to resection. The combined approach has the advantage of allowing good visualization of structures such as ureters and nerves and adequate control of vessels during the resection. For invasive tumors like chordomas requiring sacral resection at or above the level of S3, several technical considerations must be made. Positioning can be challenging. Depending upon tumor involvement of additional organs, the resection may begin with the patient in lithotomy position and can be started with mobilization of the rectum off of the tumor if possible or resection of bowel if invaded. Closure of the pelvis with a rectus flap is an option when approaching the sacral resection from the anterior position (Fig. 19.6 and Fig. 19.7). If preferred for better exposure, the patient can be transitioned into the lateral decubitus or prone position for completion of the partial or total

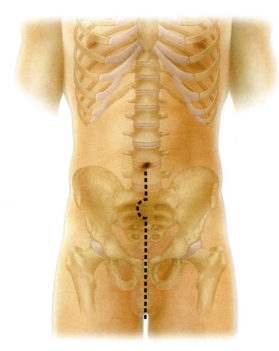
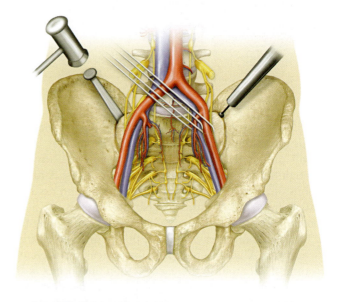
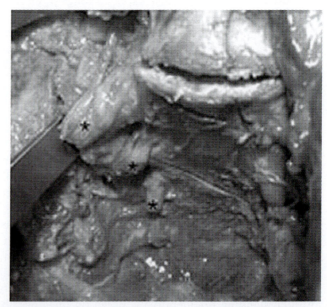

Figure 19.6 High lesions or those involving resection of intra-abdominal organs are better resected via an anterior or combined approach. (Zhang HY, Thangtrangan I, Balabhadra RS, et al. Surgical techniques for total sacrectomy and spinopelvic reconstruction. *Neurosurg Focus* 2003;15(2):E5, with permission.)

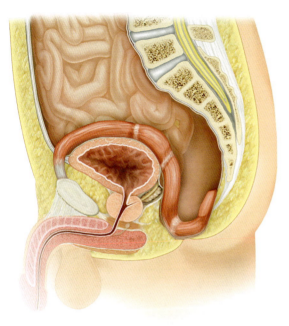

Figure 19.7 A rectus flap may be a good choice to fill the pelvis and the spaces previously occupied by the sacrum and pelvic structures. (Zhang HY, Thangtrangan I, Balabhadra RS, et al. Surgical techniques for total sacrectomy and spinopelvic reconstruction. *Neurosurg Focus* 2003;15(2):E5, with permission.)

sacrectomy. Alternatively, maturation of stomas and closure of the abdomen with complete transition to the prone jackknife position afterwards for better visualization of the sacral foramina and nerves is also an option. In this case, the entire specimen is taken en bloc with the sacrum from the posterior position and gluteal or latissimus flaps are used to close the defect. If no other organs are involved in the resection, then doing the entire sacrectomy in the prone position is an option. Exposure and visualization is quite good (Fig. 19.8–Fig. 19.11). Anticipation of closure of the large sacral defect with soft tissue

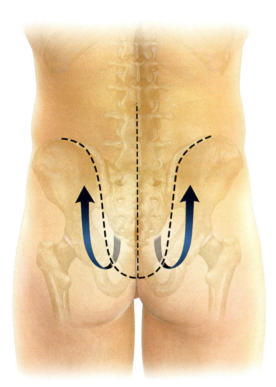

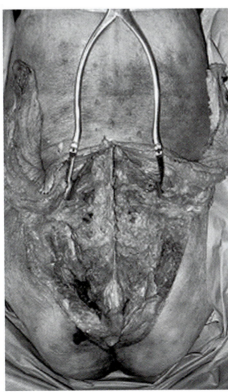

Figure 19.8 Posterior sacrectomy, posterior approach. The posterior approach is shown here with the patient in the prone position. The incision is midline, with both skin and potential biopsy sites resected en bloc with the sacrum. (Zhang HY, Thangtrangan I, Balabhadra RS, et al. Surgical techniques for total sacrectomy and spinopelvic reconstruction. *Neurosurg Focus* 2003;15(2):E5, with permission.)

Figure 19.9 Division of the sacrospinous muscles and ligaments laterally facilitates bony resection. (Zhang HY, Thangtrangan I, Balabhadra RS, et al. Surgical techniques for total sacrectomy and spinopelvic reconstruction. *Neurosurg Focus* 2003;15(2):E5, with permission.)

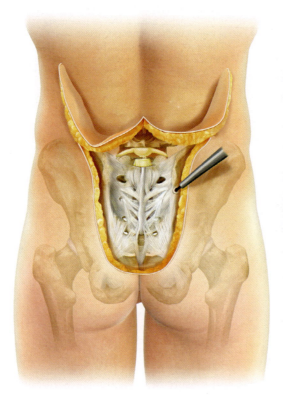
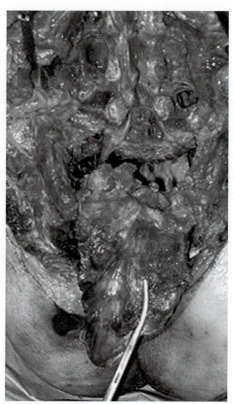

flaps, either local (gluteal) or from the abdomen (rectus) or latissimus dorsi, is part of the preoperative planning (Fig. 19.12, Fig. 19.13). Because gluteal flaps are often used for reconstruction, some authors advocate preservation of the internal iliac vessels if possible to preserve good blood supply to these tissues (18). Alternatively, if the vessels must be sacrificed during the resection, consideration for another flap should be made. If the sacral resection is below the level of S4, then the entire resection may be done in the lithotomy or lateral decubitus position. Resection of the sacrum above the S3

Figure 19.10 The postsacrectomy pelvis. (Zhang HY, Thangtrangan I, Balabhadra RS, et al. Surgical techniques for total sacrectomy and spinopelvic reconstruction. *Neurosurg Focus* 2003;15(2):E5, with permission.)

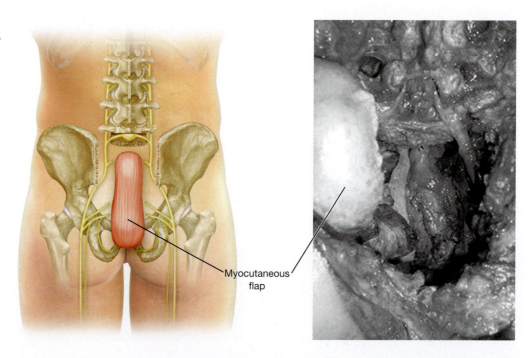

Myocutaneous flap

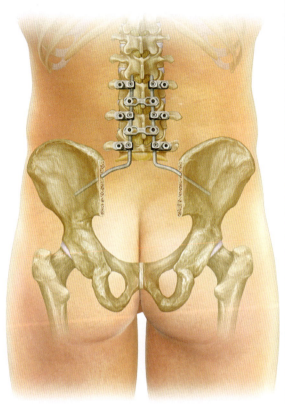

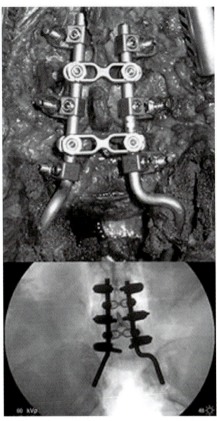

Figure 19.11 Sacral reconstruction and stabilization must be completed with hardware if a total sacrectomy is done. Preservation of S1 or most of the body of S1 reduces sacral strength, but probably does not require a fixation device. (Zhang HY, Thangtrangan I, Balabhadra RS, et al. Surgical techniques for total sacrectomy and spinopelvic reconstruction. *Neurosurg Focus* 2003;15(2):E5, with permission.)

level involves sacrifice of the sacroiliac joint and need for pelvic stabilization with fixation provided by bone screws, allograft, and use of fixation devices (Fig. 19.14). Subtotal sacral resection distal to the mid-S1 vertebral body does not completely destabilize the pelvis (13). Total sacrectomy, however, produces unacceptable destabilization of the spine and pelvis and requires reconstruction and reinforcement of the pelvic ring. Studies focused on biomechanics and stress have shown that sacroiliac stability is minimally affected by sacral resection distal to S3, with preservation of the sacroiliac joint. Division of the sacrum between the S1 and S2 vertebral bodies weakens the pelvis by 30%. When the sacrum caudal to the midpoint of the S1 body is removed, the

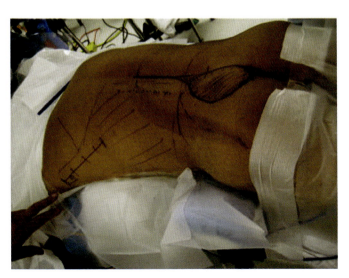

Figure 19.12 Prone positioning for en bloc sacral resection. The posterior approach to en bloc sacral resection is facilitated by prone positioning. Markings for potential flaps (latissimus dorsi, in this example) can also be contemplated. (Newman CB, Keshavarzi S, Aryan HE. En bloc sacrectomy and reconstruction: technique modification for pelvic stabilization. *Surg Neurol* 2009;72:752–6, with permission.)

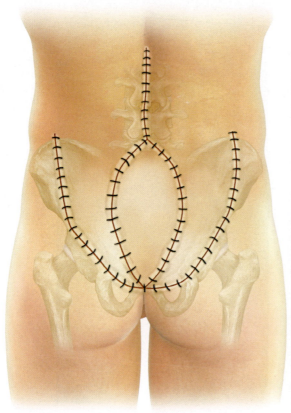
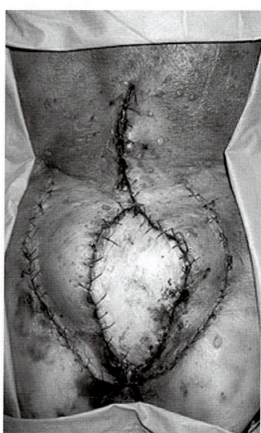

Figure 19.13 A number of local rotational and pedicle flaps can be utilized when sacrectomy is completed via a completely posterior approach to avoid repositioning the patient. (Zhang HY, Thangtrangan I, Balabhadra RS, et al. Surgical techniques for total sacrectomy and spinopelvic reconstruction. *Neurosurg Focus* 2003;15(2):E5, with permission.)

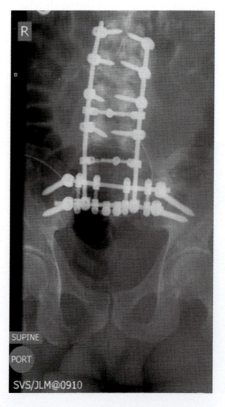

Figure 19.14 Sacral fixation hardware radiograph. (Newman CB, Keshavarzi S, Aryan HE. En bloc sacrectomy and reconstruction: technique modification for pelvic stabilization. *Surg Neurol* 2009;72:752–6, with permission.)

ring weakens by 50%; however, in clinical studies, patients who retain at least 50% of the S1 body do not demonstrate instability and are typically not stabilized using biomechanical prostheses (19–22). Various techniques for pelvic ring reconstruction after total sacrectomy have been described. Many surgeons have taken advantage of a Galveston-type cross-pelvis technique using an L5 pedicle screw to join L5 and the ilium. Modifications using a transiliac rod to bridge these structures is thought to improve biomechanical stabilization (20,21).

Consideration of the functional impairment caused by sacral nerve root disruption or resection must be made preoperatively. Bilateral nerve transection above the level of S2 or S3 is associated in all series with serious and permanent impairment of fecal continence and severe bladder and sexual dysfunction. While unilateral nerve sparing at the S2 level and below is shown to preserve function fairly well in most series, some authors have proposed, based on clinical data, that bilateral S2 preservation with unilateral S3 sparing is associated with less functional disruption and better predictability (3).

ASM repair requires dural resection and closure and involves identification and ligation of the herniated dural stalk. The approach to this lesion depends on the level of the meningocele. Sacral defects below S3 may be approached via a posterior incision, whereas those cranial to this level may be more readily accessed from the abdomen. The defect is always anteriorly located. The rectum is mobilized laterally and the stalk is ligated and oversewn. The area may be reinforced with a patch of autologous tissue or fat to help avoid a dural leak.

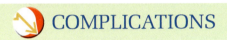 COMPLICATIONS

Complications and Function

Complications associated with simple dermoid or epidermoid cyst excision are rare. Wound infection and hematoma are most common. Less than 3% of cases are complicated by rectal fistula, and this complication can be avoided by careful identification and preservation of the posterior rectal wall (4). Complications from radical chordoma resection are more common and severe, variable in nature, and depend upon the structures involved. Most series are retrospective and involve limited numbers of patients. Loss of bowel and bladder control when sacral resection proceeds with sacrifice of nerves above the S2 level is universally reported (22–25). By far, the most common immediate complication is some degree of wound breakdown occurring in most series in about 40% of patients and treated with debridement, hyperbaric oxygen, antibiotics, and avoidance of weight bearing (23). Some authors advocate routine use of omental flaps in addition to keeping small bowel out of the postresectional pelvis. Because of the high rate of local recurrence, salvage radiotherapy is often used. Omental flaps may be a way to mitigate the effects of radiation on the small bowel and bladder.

In summary, retrorectal tumors are uncommon, but most surgeons can expect to encounter at least one case in their career, and far more if at a large tertiary referral center. Familiarity with the use of imaging for diagnosis and the ability to carefully plan are essential. Preoperative tissue biopsy should, in most cases, be avoided. Although most dermoid and epidermoid cysts are fairly easily excised via a posterior approach by a surgeon familiar with the technique, clearly lesions such as ASMs and chordomas require a much higher level of planning and multiple surgical specialists who must approach the case as a team.

Acknowledgments

Dr. Mahmoud acknowledges 3M, Inc. for ongoing clinical trial funding. (A Randomized Double-Blind Study of 2% Chlorhexidine Gluconate/70% Isopropyl Alcohol vs. Iodine Povacrylex [0.7% Available Iodine]/74% Isopropyl Alcohol for Perioperative Skin Preparation in Open Elective Colorectal Surgery).

Recommended References and Readings

1. Uhlig BE, Johnson RL. Presacral tumors and cysts in adults. *Dis Colon Rectum* 1975;18:581–9.
2. Jao SW, Beart RW Jr, Spencer RJ, et al. Retrorectal tumors. Mayo Clinic experience, 1960–1979. *Dis Colon Rectum* 1985;28:644–52.
3. Hobson KG, Ghaemmaghami V, Roe JP, et al. Tumors of the retrorectal space. *Dis Colon Rectum* 2005;48(10):1964–74.
4. Freier DT, Stanley JC, Thompson N. Retrorectal tumors in adults. *Surg Gynecol Obstet* 1971;132(4):681–6.
5. Bullard Dunn K. Retrorectal Tumors. *Surg Clin N Am* 2010;90: 163–71.
6. Hjermstad BM, Helwig EB. Tailgut cysts. Report of 53 cases. *Am J Clin Pathol* 1988;89:139–47.
7. Sobrado CW, Mester M, Simonsen OS, et al. Retrorectal tumors complicating pregnancy. Report of two cases. *Dis Colon Rectum* 1996;39(10):1176–9.
8. Yang BL, Gu YF, Shao WJ, et al. Retrorectal tumors in adults: magnetic resonance imaging findings. *World J Gastroenterol* 2010;16(46):5822–9.
9. McMaster ML, Goldstein AM, Bromley CM, et al. Chordoma: incidence and survival patterns in the United States, 1973–1995. *Cancer Causes Control* 2001;12(1):331–46.
10. Gray SW, Singhabhandhu B, Smith RA, et al. Sacrococcygeal chordoma: report of a case and review of the literature. *Surgery* 1975;78:573–82.
11. Bergh P, Kindblom LG, Gunterberg B, Remotti F, Ryd W, Meis-Kindblom JM. Prognostic factors in chordoma of the sacrum and mobile spine: a study of 39 patients. *Cancer* 2000;88: 2122–34.
12. Isik N, Elmaci I, Gokben B, et al. Currarino triad: surgical management and follow up results of four cases. *Pediatr Neurosurg* 2010;46(2):110–19.
13. Oren M, Lorber B, Lee SH, Truex RC Jr, Gennaro AR. Anterior sacral meningocele: report of five cases and review of the literature. *Dis Colon Rectum* 1977;20:492–505.
14. Shivnani AT, Small W Jr, Benson A III, et al. Adenocarcinoma arising in a rectal duplication cyst: case report and review of the literature. *Am Surg* 2004;70(11):1007–9.
15. Stewart RJ, Humphreys WG, Parks TG. The presentation and management of presacral tumours. *Br J Surg* 1986;73:153–5.
16. Verazin G, Rosen L, Khubchandani IT, Sheets JA, Stasik JJ, Riether R. Retrorectal tumor: is biopsy risky? *South Med J* 1986; 79:1437–9.
17. Abel ME, Nelson R, Prasad ML, et al. Parasacrococcygeal approach for the resection of retrorectal developmental cysts. *Dis Colon Rectum* 1985;28:855–8.
18. Newman CB, Keshavarzi S, Aryan HE. En bloc sacrectomy and reconstruction: technique modification for pelvic stabilization. *Surg Neurol* 2009;72:752–6.
19. Gunterberg B, Romanus B, Stener B. Pelvic strength after major amputation of the sacrum: an experimental study. *Acta Orthop Scand* 1976;47:635–42.
20. Stener B, Gunterberg B. High amputation of the sacrum for extirpation of tumors. Principles and technique. *Spine* 1978;3: 351–66.
21. Fuchs B, Yaszemski MJ, Sim FH. Combined posterior pelvis and lumbar spine resection for sarcoma. *Clin Orthop* 2002;397: 12–18.
22. Gallia GL, Haque R, Garonzik I, et al. Spinal pelvic reconstruction after total sacrectomy for en bloc resection of giant sacral chordoma. *J Neurosurg Spine* 2005;3:501–6.
23. York JE, Kaczaraj A, Abi-Said D, et al. Sacral chordoma: 40-year experience at a major cancer center. *Neurosurgery* 1999;44:74–9; discussion 9–80.
24. Bergh P, Gunterberg B, Meis-Kindblom JM, et al. Prognostic factors and outcome of pelvic, sacra, and spinal chondrosarcomas: a center-based study of 69 cases. *Cancer* 2001;91:1201–12.
25. Hsieh PC, Xu R, Sciubba DM, et al. Long-term clinical outcomes following en bloc resections for sacral chordomas and chondrosarcomas: a series of twenty consecutive patients. *Spine* 2009; 34(20):2233–9.

20 Standard Transanal

Steven R. Hunt

 INDICATIONS/CONTRAINDICATIONS

Transanal excision is appropriate for adenomas, carcinoids, and favorable early-stage rectal cancers within 8 cm of the anal verge. While it is sometimes possible to remove tumors above 8 cm with this technique, consideration should be given to alternative means, such as transanal endoscopic microsurgery or a low anterior resection of the rectum.

Only the most favorable adenocarcinomas should be considered for transanal excision. Favorable characteristics include the following:

- Size <4 cm
- Freely mobile
- Well to moderate differentiation
- No lymphovascular invasion
- Ultrasound T1
- Ultrasound N0

Mucinous and signet-cell pathologies are relative contraindications for transanal excision, as they have a high risk of recurrence.

If a patient has comorbid conditions that would preclude radical surgery, less favorable tumors can be transanally excised. In such cases, patients may benefit from neoadjuvant or adjuvant radiation to sterilize the lymphatics.

 PREOPERATIVE PLANNING

Before performing a transanal excision, the tumor must be carefully evaluated to confirm that it is amenable to local treatment. Examination in the office should consist of a careful digital rectal examination to determine the location of the tumor and its mobility. The examination should also include anoscopy or rigid proctoscopy to determine the distance of the tumor from the anal verge and to assess the feasibility of transanal excision. The laterality and anterior–posterior localization of the tumor is important in the positioning of the patients for the procedure. A transrectal ultrasound or magnetic resonance imaging should be performed to stage the tumor. While it is often difficult to differentiate between an adenoma and a superficial T1 tumor on ultrasound, it is important to exclude deeper invasion, as more advanced tumors should be managed with proctectomy in medically fit patients. All biopsy results of any tumors that are considered for local excision should be carefully reviewed. If transanal excision is to be performed for cancer, a staging assessment consisting of a CT scan, CEA, chest x-ray, and complete colonoscopy should be done.

It is our practice to prepare each patient with a sodium phosphate enema on the day of surgery. We do not routinely use antibiotic or DVT prophylaxis at the time of surgery.

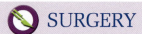 SURGERY

Clinical Anatomy

In transanal excision, the relevant anatomy consists of the anal canal and rectum within 10 cm of the anal verge, as more proximal tumors are very difficult to remove by conventional transanal techniques. Important anatomical landmarks include the anal verge, which is the distal end of the anal canal with the buttocks effaced. The dentate line is a visible irregular line that separates the columnar epithelium of the rectum from the stratified epithelium of the anal canal whose location within the anal canal is variable. The anal canal refers to the area from the anal verge to the top of the anal sphincter complex. The upper edge of the anal canal is defined by the anorectal ring. Above the anorectal ring, the rectum becomes much more capacious. The anal canal is of varying length depending on the habitus of the patient and can vary in length from 2 to 4 cm. The muscularis propria of the rectum consists of inner circular smooth muscle fibers and an outer layer of longitudinal smooth muscle fibers. The internal anal sphincter is an extension of the circular smooth muscle of the rectum. The distal end of the internal anal sphincter is palpable at the anal verge and defines the inner aspect of the intersphincter plane.

Posteriorly and laterally, the mesorectal fat surrounds the rectum. In women, the vagina is immediately anterior to the muscularis propria above the anal canal. In men, the prostate gland and seminal vesicles are encountered anteriorly above the anal verge. The anterior peritoneal reflexion varies between men and women and can vary according to the habitus of the patient. In general, the anterior peritoneal reflexion lies somewhere between 6 and 9 cm above the anal verge anteriorly and anterolaterally to the rectum.

Positioning

Patient positioning is dependent on the location of the lesion. Anterior and lateral lesions are best approached with patients in the prone jackknife position. The patient's buttocks should be pulled laterally with tape to partially efface the anus (Fig. 20.1). Patients with posterior lesions should be placed in the dorsal lithotomy position; the buttocks should be taped apart.

Technique

The choice of anesthesia is dependent on surgeon preference as it is possible to perform a local excision under MAC/local, spinal, or general anesthesia. The anus is effaced with a Lone Star retractor (Fig. 20.2). Visualization is best accomplished with a lighted anoscope. It may be necessary to place stay sutures at the lateral margins of higher tumors to provide traction and deliver the tumor into view. The tumor itself should not be handled with instruments. The default procedure should be a full-thickness excision, unless the tumor is assuredly benign, in which case, a submucosal excision is acceptable.

A 1-cm margin is scored around the tumor with the cautery. In scoring the margin, it is necessary to create a char rather than mere blanching of the mucosa, as visualization of this margin in the latter portions of the procedure can become difficult due to

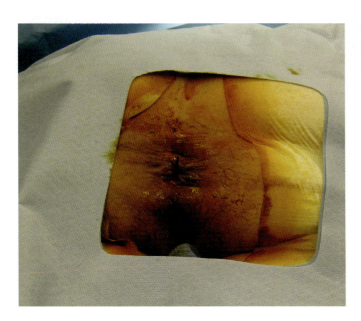

Figure 20.1 With the patient in the prone jackknife position, the buttocks are taped apart to efface the anus.

blood. After the margins have been circumferentially scored, the full-thickness excision should begin. It is easiest to start the excision at the distal margin of the tumor. During this incision, the operator should take note of each layer as it is crossed including the submucosa, the muscularis layer, and the exposure of the perirectal fat. There may be a paucity of perirectal fat around distal lesions, and the levator muscles may become immediately visible upon full incision of the muscularis propria. Anteriorly, there is also scant mesorectal fat and the vagina or Denonvilliers' fascia of the prostate may be encountered immediately after incising through the rectal wall.

After a full-thickness incision has been made, the incision should be extended laterally around the tumor. Placing an Allis–Adair clamp or sutures on the margins of the specimen facilitates visualization (Fig. 20.3). Dissection in the mesorectal fat should then commence underneath the tumor to leave a wide margin of mesorectal fat on the specimen. Finally, the remaining superior rectal wall is divided. While we use the electrocautery for the majority of our dissection, vessel-sealing devices can also be used to obtain hemostasis during the dissection.

Once the tumor has been excised, it should be removed and oriented for the pathologists by suturing or pinning it to a board. The defect should be inspected and irrigated with saline, and meticulous hemostasis should be obtained with electrocautery (Fig. 20.4).

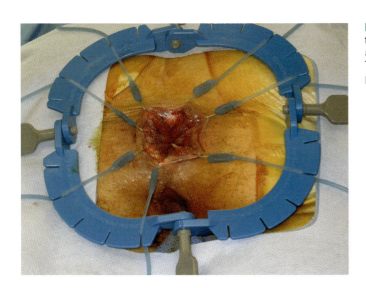

Figure 20.2 The Lone Star retractor is used to further efface the anus and provide better exposure. The hooks of the retractor are placed at the dentate line.

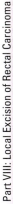

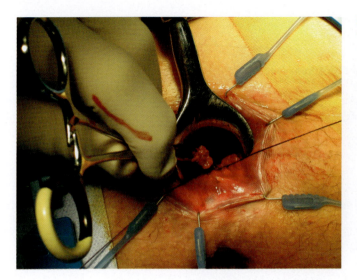

Figure 20.3 An Allis clamp is used to grasp the edge of the polyp during excision, while lateral stay sutures are used to provide better exposure during dissection of the upper borders of the polyp.

The defect is transversely closed with running absorbable sutures. For large defects, it is helpful to orient the transverse closure by starting with a single suture in the center to approximate the two edges and orient the line of closure.

Following closure, the suture line should be inspected and interrogated for any defects. The rectal lumen above the line of closure should also be inspected to confirm that the rectal lumen has not been obliterated by the closure.

In many cases, closure of the wound is difficult or results in significant narrowing of the rectal lumen. In these cases, it is safe to leave these wounds open to heal by secondary intention; however, in our experience, these patients have significantly more pain postoperatively.

In the rare cases of a pedunculated or extremely mobile rectal polyp, it is sometimes possible to evert the polyp through the anal canal and excise the lesion with an Endo-GIA stapler.

While more proximal rectal polyps often must be excised by transanal endoscopic microsurgery or low anterior resection, it is possible to excise lesions using an operating proctoscope and a transanal snare. As this is not a full-thickness excision, it should be reserved for benign tumors. When attempting to remove a lesion with the snare, great care must be taken with anterior and anterolateral tumors to avoid entering the peritoneal cavity. Larger lesions should be excised in a piecemeal fashion as an en bloc snare excision can often result in a full-thickness injury to the rectal wall.

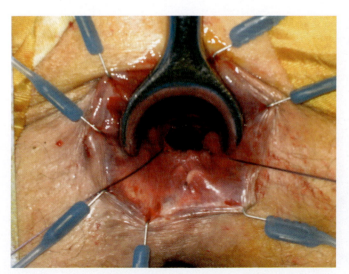

Figure 20.4 Meticulous hemostasis of the excision bed is important prior to transverse closure.

POSTOPERATIVE MANAGEMENT

The majority of patients can be treated in the outpatient setting. As urinary retention is a common postoperative complication, patients should be able to void prior to discharge. In our practice, patients who have an open wound are discharged on 7 days of oral antibiotics. Patients should be given an ample supply of pain medications and stool softeners. Sitz baths may provide some relief for patients with low lesions that extend down into the anal canal.

 COMPLICATIONS

Complications with transanal excisions are similar to those of other anorectal procedures and include urinary retention and bleeding. While pelvic sepsis is rare, it should be considered in patients who develop fever, worsening pain, or delayed urinary retention. If sepsis is suspected, the patient should be taken to the operating room expeditiously for an examination under anesthesia. Rectal or anal stenosis after a transanal excision is a rare complication that is usually corrected with simple dilation.

 CONCLUSIONS

Transanal excision is a minimally invasive means by which to remove a rectal tumor, but it is by no means a simple procedure. The key to the surgery lies in adequate exposure and lighting. While appropriate for benign distal rectal lesions, careful selection should be used for malignant lesions that are to be treated with local excision alone.

Suggested Readings

Bleday R, Breen E, Jessup JM, et al. Prospective evaluation of local excision for small rectal cancers. *Dis Colon Rectum* 1997;40:388–92.

Bonnen M, Crane C, Vauthey JN, et al. Long-term results using local excision after preoperative chemoradiation among selected T3 rectal cancer patients. *Int J Radiat Oncol Biol Phys* 2004;60:1098–105.

Borschitz T, Heintz A, Junginger T. The influence of histopathologic criteria on the long-term prognosis of locally excised pT1 rectal carcinomas: results of local excision (transanal endoscopic microsurgery) and immediate reoperation. *Dis Colon Rectum* 2006;49:1492–506; discussion 500–5.

Gordon P, Nivatvong S, eds. Neoplasms of the Colon, Rectum, and Anus. New York: Informa Healthcare, 2007:328–39.

Gordon P, Nivatvong S, eds. Principles and Practice of Surgery for the Colon, Rectum, and Anus. New York: Informa Healthcare, 1999:491–9.

Madbouly KM, Remzi FH, Erkek BA, et al. Recurrence after transanal excision of T1 rectal cancer: should we be concerned? *Dis Colon Rectum* 2005;48:711–9; discussion 9–21.

Nascimbeni R, Burgart LJ, Nivatvongs S, Larson DR. Risk of lymph node metastasis in T1 carcinoma of the colon and rectum. *Dis Colon Rectum* 2002;45:200–6.

Nastro P, Beral D, Hartley J, Monson JR. Local excision of rectal cancer: review of literature. *Dig Surg* 2005;22:6–15.

Rothenberger D, Garcia-Aguilar J. Rectal cancer: local treatment. In: Fazio V, Church J, Delaney C, eds. Current Therapy in Colon and Rectal Surgery. Philadelphia, PA: Elsevier Mosby, 2005:179–84.

Saclarides TJ. TEM/local excision: indications, techniques, outcomes, and the future. *J Surg Oncol* 2007;96:644–50.

21 Transanal Endoscopic Microsurgery

Theodore John Saclarides

Transanal endoscopic microsurgery (TEM) was first developed by Professor Gerhard Buess (1) and manufactured by the Richard Wolf Company almost 30 years ago. Several modifications have been proposed by others since the 1980s, which are all based upon Buess's original vision of improving the visibility and reach of transanal surgery by employing superior optics, carbon dioxide (CO_2)-induced rectal distention, and longer instruments. The number of TEM manuscripts published since the 1980s has greatly increased and training courses have become available at a number of centers across the globe. Indeed, most of the early publications were authored by Buess himself and in these he described his personal journey of first using the instruments on an animal model (2). He then reported his clinical experience on an ever-increasing volume of human patients at a time when the concept of minimally invasive surgery, which he called "minimally aggressive but accurate," was capturing the attention of all surgeons. As more surgeons learned and practiced TEM, the number of publications increased, but it has been slow to catch on. Buess's training courses were spread over several days, taking the students through a step-by-step process of cutting and sewing felt cloth, to an open bovine model, and then finally to a closed but distended segment of bovine bowel. Time was needed to master the technique since the initial participants had minimal experience in endoscopic or laparoscopic surgery. In contrast, today's TEM students learn the techniques and master the learning curve much more quickly because of laparoscopic and video skills acquired early during their surgical career.

TEM represents a unique blend between the old and the new. Although transanal excision of rectal tumors has been part of the surgeon's armamentarium for almost a century, surgeons have been somewhat restricted by the suboptimal exposure and limited reach afforded by conventional instruments. TEM circumnavigates these restrictions, however, having the technology is not license to use it inappropriately. While virtually any adenoma can be removed with TEM, strict selection criteria must be used when addressing malignant lesions in order to not compromise cure and adversely affect patient outcome. By virtue of its longer reach, better exposure, and enhanced visibility, TEM has placed itself in the category of minimally invasive surgical procedures. Some lesions in the mid and upper rectum, which may have required a laparotomy and radical resection for removal, may now be addressed with a less invasive approach. As such, less postoperative pain, shorter recovery period, and a faster return to normal function are real and attainable goals. This is especially so when one considers the high morbidity associated with the Mason and Kraske procedures where wound infection and fecal fistulas can be disastrous for the patient.

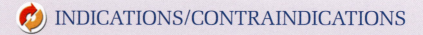

INDICATIONS/CONTRAINDICATIONS

Indications

As stated above, most adenomas regardless of size, location, and degree of circumferential involvement can be removed with TEM instrumentation. Provided the lesion can be reached with a rigid scope and is visible in its entirety, it can be removed. If the lesion extends around the rectosigmoid junction or if the curvature of the sacrum prohibits passage of a rigid scope up to the lesion, then perhaps TEM is not the best approach. Lesions which encompass 360 degrees of the wall circumference can be successfully removed with TEM and intestinal continuity reestablished with a hand-sewn end-to-end anastomosis performed transanally.

Proper patient selection must be followed when considering TEM for malignant lesions. These selection criteria require that the lesion have only superficial penetration of the rectal wall (preoperative staging with either endorectal ultrasound or magnetic resonance imaging (MRI) is essential), well to moderately well differentiation, lack perineural and lymphovascular invasion, and perhaps also lack a mucinous component, although this last feature is controversial. Budding tumor cells at the leading edge of the lesion has also been considered an ominous feature and a potential contraindication for transanal excision. If these criteria are not met, the risk of lymph node metastases is increased and such nodes would potentially go untreated by any method that locally removes a tumor and does not incorporate mesorectal excision in its plan. Large tumor size (greater than 3–4 cm) has been considered a relative contraindication for transanal excision of rectal cancer, primarily because difficult exposure with conventional instruments could lead to inadequate removal, positive resection margins, and higher recurrence rates. TEM, however, eliminates larger size as a contraindication for transanal excision. If one is contemplating TEM for a rectal cancer, previous endoscopic biopsies should be reviewed with an experienced pathologist for the above features and the lesion should be imaged to determine the depth of penetration and the presence of nodal metastases. If favorable histologic features are present, there is no evidence of enlarged lymph nodes, and the lesion does not penetrate beyond the submucosa, then one can consider TEM. The surgeon, however, should adopt the mentality that such an excision is in reality an excisional biopsy, and that further therapy may be indicated after histologic review of the entire lesion has been performed. If, in fact, the lesion is a pT1 tumor, then many would consider TEM sufficient treatment; however, local excision alone is not an appropriate treatment for any tumor that has penetrated into the muscularis propria or beyond. This will be discussed elsewhere in this chapter.

There are instances when TEM can be used to treat cancer even though cure may not be possible or as readily obtained. Palliation of a tumor can be considered in instances where diffuse systemic metastases are present. Unfortunately, most primary tumors in these instances are large and may not be amenable to transanal excision. If the patient is medically unfit to undergo conventional surgery because of multiple comorbid factors, TEM may be considered if used in conjunction with radiation and chemotherapy. Experience in this regard is limited, therefore, caution should be exercised. Adjuvant therapy combined with TEM may also be considered for those patients who are emotionally unwilling to undergo conventional surgery that may involve a stoma. The use of TEM combined with adjuvant or neoadjuvant therapy will be discussed elsewhere in this chapter.

There are extended applications in the literature for TEM; however, for many of these conditions, experience is limited to anecdotal case reports or small series. Theoretically, TEM can be used to treat complex, supra-sphincteric or extra-sphincteric fistulas with advancement flaps. The flap should consist of mucosa, submucosa, and a portion of the muscularis; its base should be several times the width of its apex, and there should be sufficient cephalad mobilization to avoid tension as the flap is advanced caudally. TEM has been used to treat rectovaginal fistulas (3) as well as rectourethral fistulas (4–6) with varying success. The author has tried using TEM instrumentation to correct circular stapler-induced rectovaginal fistulas following low anterior resection. In this regard, all three cases so attempted failed primarily because diminished rectal capacity secondary to radiation and prior resection lead to limited visibility and access. Strictureplasty can be performed with TEM instrumentation as well, the operation being done with single or multiple longitudinal incisions closed transversely or with a 180 or 270 degree transverse excision of the stricture followed by transverse closure of the defect. Such efforts are best done in the lateral and posterior portions of the extra-peritoneal rectum (7,8). TEM has been used to repair an anastomotic leak (9) and to excise retrorectal tumors (10,11).

PREOPERATIVE PLANNING

Preoperative Assessment and Patient Preparation

If the goal of treatment is cure, then accurate preoperative staging is paramount. Assessment begins with a digital rectal examination, which may reveal fixation or bulky extramural adenopathy. All patients must also undergo either a colonoscopy or a double contrast barium enema to evaluate for synchronous lesions. To determine local extent of disease, as previously stated, endorectal ultrasound or MRI can be used. A meta-analysis by Bipat et al. analyzed 90 studies comparing ultrasound, CT, and MRI from 1985 to 2002. Ultrasound was found to be the most accurate for determining depth of penetration, being over 90% sensitive in detecting invasion of the muscularis propria and perirectal tissue. MRI frequently over-staged T1 lesions (12). Ultrasound accuracy may decrease when used to evaluate more advanced and circumferential tumors (13). Ultrasound, CT, and MRI have comparably low sensitivities when ruling out perirectal lymph node metastases (67%, 55%, 66%, respectively) (12). The definition of what constitutes a metastatic lymph node has varied among operators and researchers. For example, one study considered any oval or circular structure greater than 5 mm to be malignant while others use 10 mm as the threshold; others have stated that any detectable node should be considered metastatic regardless of size (13). Certainly, the positive predictive value of a hypoechoic node detected within the mesorectum increases with increasing size, but it is probably best to overtreat rather than undertreat the patient and to consider any detectable node suspicious. Abdominal CT scans are usually not necessary for early, superficial cancers or adenomatous lesions, as the likelihood for distant metastases is low (14).

If a patient is referred to a surgeon for possible TEM, rigid proctosigmoidoscopy must be performed by the surgeon in order to determine the level of the lesion in the rectum and whether a rigid scope can access the lesion and reveal it in its entirety. Moreover, the exact spatial orientation of the lesion (anterior vs. posterior, right lateral vs. left lateral) must be determined as this will dictate patient position on the operating table. Informed consent should be obtained with the following considerations in mind. If bleeding is encountered or if a lesion cannot be removed, conversion to a transabdominal approach may be necessary. In addition, for anteriorly located lesions, one may inadvertently enter the peritoneal cavity. Although such an occurrence may be repaired with transanal suturing techniques, conversion to an abdominal approach may be required. Although bowel cleansing is not required for colectomy, it is still essential for TEM in order to ensure visibility and reduce the risk of infection. Moreover, if the effects of general anesthesia decline midway during the operation and the patient strains or coughs, residual stool, if present, may appear at a most inopportune time. Bowel cleansing may be accomplished with oral cathartics, enemas, or lavage solutions. General or regional anesthesia is required. Patients are positioned on the operating room table such that the lesion is at the bottom of the optical field, for example, lithotomy for a posterior lesion. Most cases can be done on an outpatient basis or with a single overnight stay. Some patients may experience anesthesia-related nausea, urinary retention, or may require observation for bleeding. Pain is generally not an issue and patients do not usually require parenteral medications.

Equipment

TEM utilizes a closed endoscopic system that allows for the instillation and retention of CO_2 gas; this creates constant rectal distention, which facilitates exposure and visualization of the lesion, excision of the tumor, control of bleeding, and subsequent closure of the wound defect. Other distinguishing features of TEM are the long reach of the instruments and the unique stereoscopic magnified image. A combined multifunctional endosurgical unit regulates suction, irrigation, intrarectal pressure, and gas insufflation. Suction removes fluid, blood, waste, and smoke. Irrigation helps maintain a relatively clean operative field and can rinse the end of the scope. CO_2 insufflation maintains distention of the rectum throughout the procedure and flow can be increased as high as 6 l/minute. The intrarectal pressure is set at a desired level (usually 10–15 cm H_2O) and the four functions mentioned above are regulated to achieve a constant steady state at that level. The surgeon may choose at various times during the operation to increase the suction; when this occurs, the endosurgical unit will increase flow of CO_2 to maintain a steady state. If intrarectal pressure does not rise or if the rectum does not distend, there is likely a leak in the system and the surgeon should be able to systematically check the set up for air leaks. This is probably the most frequently encountered problem that the surgeon must learn to troubleshoot.

The operating rectoscopes are beveled and are approximately 4 cm in diameter. A straight, nonbeveled rectoscope is also available and may be preferable for the very distal lesions where the lower lip of a beveled scope could slip exterior to the patient allowing for the escape of CO_2 and collapse of the operative field. Since the end of a beveled scope must face downward at the lesion, patients are variably positioned, depending upon where the lesion is located along the anterior–posterior dimensions of the rectal wall. For example, if a patient has an anterior lesion, he or she should be placed in the prone position with the legs spread apart to permit close access to the perineum. After the legs are placed upon and secured to long and well-padded long-arm boards, the foot of the table is dropped to allow the surgeon to sit close to the patient. Alternatively, stirrups placed parallel to the floor and coming off the end of the table can be used to support the legs in the prone position. For a posterior lesion, the patient is placed in the lithotomy position and if the lesion is laterally located, the patient is placed in the appropriate lateral decubitus position. The end of the rectoscope is covered with a sealed facepiece, which has airtight rubber seals and sealed working ports through which the long-shafted instruments necessary for the dissection are inserted. The suction catheter can be electrified and in this way a bleeding vessel can be coagulated while the blood is being aspirated. In a similar way, the tissue graspers can be electrified for control of a bleeding vessel. Vision is obtained through a binocular stereoscopic eyepiece, which provides a unique image yet magnifies at the same time. An accessory scope may be inserted for video recording and transmission of the image to a video monitor for viewing by surgical assistants, medical students, and surgical residents. The binocular eyepiece provides 6× magnification and has a 50 degree downward view and a 75 degree lateral field of view. In contrast, the accessory scope has a 40 degree downward view and a reduced lateral view. Because of the discrepancy, the image seen through the accessory scope and the video monitor is reduced in its scope relative to the binocular eyepiece.

Most of the bleeding occurring during full-thickness TEM dissections is encountered when one traverses the mesorectum. The standard TEM cautery may be insufficient in stemming the flow of brisk bleeding, the surgeon may then have to work with a tissue grasper in each hand, working them in a hand-over-fist manner to get to the bleeding vessel, grasp it, and then coagulate it. This can be somewhat cumbersome. At those points during an operation when bleeding is likely to occur, the surgeon may chose to use an alternative energy device for hemostasis such as a harmonic scalpel (15). Studies have shown that a harmonic scalpel reduces operative time and bleeding. Ayodeji et al. compared harmonic dissection with the standard TEM cautery unit in a nonrandomized fashion, correcting for differences in tumor size between the two groups. The harmonic dissector reduced operative time by 26%; however, in 50% of the harmonic group, the surgeon used a hybrid approach and used cautery for portions of the case (16). Hermsen et al. showed that when the long harmonic shears are used, a further reduction in operative time can be achieved as well as a significant reduction in blood loss (17). Caution should be exercised. In rare instances, pelvic sepsis has occurred following cases, which used the harmonic dissectors possibly as a result of prolonged application of energy to the tissue. When cautery is used to traverse the mesentery, the energy is imparted in short bursts at very focal and precise areas. In contrast, when a harmonic dissector is used, tissue is grasped and energy imparted over a longer period of time until the tissue separates.

The TEM needle holder is self-righting. The needle can be grasped when in an inverted position, yet the needle holder will automatically place it in the upright position when the locking mechanism is activated. Sutures are started and finished with silver shots applied to the thread with a specially designed applicator. Traditional instrument knot tying is too tedious to perform on a constant basis.

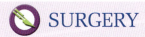

SURGERY

Technique

Once the anesthetic has been administered, the patient is positioned according to the location of the tumor. The buttocks and perineum are washed with antiseptic solution, sterile drapes are placed, and the rectoscope is inserted up to the lesion under direct vision aided by the manual insufflations of air. The scope is then secured to the operating room table with the adjustable, double-jointed Martin arm and the facepiece is locked into place on the end of the scope. The Martin arm is moved multiple times during the procedure in order to keep the lesion and the area of dissection in the center of the optical field. Rubber sleeves, covered by rubber caps with a hole in their center are placed onto the working ports of the facepiece. The long shafted instruments are inserted and the tubing necessary for CO_2 insufflation, saline irrigation, and pressure monitoring are connected. The binocular eyepiece and the accessory scope are inserted.

The technique of excision will vary according to preoperative histology, suspicion that a "benign" lesion may contain an occult cancer, and the location of the lesion within the rectum. Small adenomas may be removed by dissecting within the submucosal plane; this is especially appropriate for an anterior lesion in a woman where the anterior peritoneal reflection is unpredictable in its location and a full-thickness excision may be hazardous. For a submucosal excision of a small adenoma, a 5-mm margin of normal appearing mucosa is marked around the lesion, the mucosal edge is lifted with the tissue grasper, and the lesion is excised without entering the muscularis. Larger adenomas may contain invasive cancer and are excised using a full-thickness technique whereby the dissection is taken down into the mesorectal fat. If the peritoneum is violated, it should be repaired promptly and the operation completed as planned, conversion to laparotomy is not necessary. Before the patient is extubated, the abdomen should be examined in the event a large pneumoperitoneum needs needle decompression. Cancers are removed with a full-thickness excision after a 1-cm margin has been marked around the lesion. To help orient the pathologist to the deep and lateral margins, the specimen should be sutured or pinned to a flat surface such as cork board or a piece of Telfa paper. Wounds are closed transversely with a 3-0 running monofilament suture and SH needle. TEM surgeons frequently debate whether or not the wound needs to be closed. Small submucosal excisions can certainly be left open; however, larger open wounds are more likely to cause a longer period of tenesmus, bleeding, and mucous discharge during the days or weeks

Part VIII: Local Excision of Rectal Carcinoma

after surgery. Ramirez prospectively randomized TEM patients into a group that underwent wound closure and a group that did not. Wound closure extended surgery by 16 minutes but this was not significantly significant. In fact, no significant differences were noted with respect to intraoperative bleeding, length of stay, and early or late complications (18). This author's belief is that closure should be attempted in all mainly to maintain one's skills in suturing. There will be instances where suturing is mandatory such as in cases of peritoneal entry or following excision of circumferential lesions.

Technical pearls are as follows:

1. Sutures of short length are preferable in order to be able to pull the suture tight yet stay within the narrow confines of the rectum.
2. Crossover of instruments should be avoided, rather, they should be manipulated in parallel.
3. One should avoid dropping the needle. It is far better to pass it from instrument to instrument otherwise time will be wasted looking for the needle.
4. One should avoid high-power settings on the cautery unit as excessive heat will fog the lens and create unnecessary smoke. Moreover, the end of the scope should be kept at a distance from the lesion in order to avoid splatter and debris from hitting the lens.
5. The surgeon should become adept at knowing where air leaks in the system are likely to occur and how to fix them.
6. The scope should be repositioned several times during the course of the dissection in order to keep the operative field in the center of the optical field.
7. All of the instruments including the shaft of the eyepiece should be lubricated with mineral oil to facilitate passage and reduce wear and tear on the rubber seals of the facepiece.
8. For large wound defects, one should use multiple sutures of short length. When closure is complete, one should be sure that the rectal lumen has not been inadvertently closed by passing a rigid proctoscope through the area.

 ## COMPLICATIONS

TEM complications occur less frequently compared to other resection methods. Buess reported a minor complication rate of 16% and a major complication rate of 9% (19). Complications occurring intraoperatively include conversion to open or laparoscopic surgery because of technical difficulty, equipment failure, difficulty in extubating the patient, bleeding, and entry into the peritoneal cavity. Postoperative complications include urinary retention (5%), abdominal or rectal pain (1%), bleeding (1%), fluid overload (1%), suture line dehiscence (1%), perirectal abscess (<1%), and stricture (1%) (20). Bignell et al. reported on 262 consecutive TEM cases and noted that pelvic sepsis occurred in 3% of patients and was more common when the lesion was located within 2 cm of the dentate line. Hemorrhage was noted in another 3% but was noted less often when the harmonic scalpel was used (21). Rectovaginal fistulas have also been noted (22).

Wound dehiscence probably occurs more commonly than is thought, the exact incidence is not known because most surgeons do not routinely inspect the wound during the first 2 weeks after TEM. The addition of neoadjuvant radiation therapy does impair wound healing. Marks et al. found that radiation significantly increased the incidence of wound complications, 26% of patients so treated experienced varying degrees of wound separation. Although most instances were successfully treated with outpatient antibiotics, one patient did require a diverting stoma (23).

Peritoneal entry does not mandate conversion to an open approach and is not associated with an increase in postoperative complications (24–26). The defect can be repaired immediately and the operation completed as planned. If there are concerns about the adequacy of closure, the wound can be inspected laparoscopically and additional sutures placed. The incidence of peritoneal entry varies in the literature, ranging from 2% to 10% (24–26), and in the authors experience (unpublished data) it has occurred in 1.2%. Baatrup et al. pooled data from several TEM databases from the UK,

Germany, Denmark, and Norway and found 22 instances of perforation into the peritoneal cavity in 888 cases (2%). All perforations were treated endoscopically, and there were no deaths or severe complications noted in this group (25).

Incontinence to feces and flatus are concerns because of the wide diameter of the scope, the long duration of many of the TEM cases, and the frequent need to reposition the scope during surgery. Solanas et al. studied anal manometry in 40 TEM patients. Patients who had previous anal surgery and preoperative defects were excluded from evaluation. There was a global fall in anal resting pressure and maximal squeeze pressure; however, at 6 months, patients remained continent. Fifteen percent had rupture of their internal sphincter, producing variable degrees of incontinence, which resolved after 6 months in 67% of patients so affected (27). Operative time, tumor size, age, and gender did not seem to influence outcome (28), although Herman et al. have postulated that a resection of more than 50% of the circumference might contribute to persistent anal dysfunction (29). Wang et al. studied patients with manometry at 2 weeks, 6 weeks, 3 months, and 1 year after TEM. Lower resting pressures, squeeze pressures, and maximum tolerable volumes were noted early after surgery but normal values were recovered by the 1-year time point (30). Jin et al. used manometry and an incontinence survey to study patients at 2 weeks, 3 months, and 6 months after TEM. Squeeze pressures were depressed at 2 weeks but returned to normal by 3 months. Resting pressures and maximum tolerable volumes were significantly depressed at 3 months but returned to normal by 6 months. Ultrasound of the sphincter muscle was used to determine whether injuries to the muscle were sustained; no patients had an injury to the external sphincter; however, 14% of patients were found to have defects in the internal sphincter, 80% of these were incontinent of flatus (31). Incontinence after TEM has been shown to be mild and self-limiting. Cataldo et al. focused less on the changes in sphincter physiology and more on the quality of life as assessed using scores measuring lifestyle, coping, depression, and embarrassment. No change was noted between preoperative and postoperative scores. TEM did not produce any deterioration in the ability to defer defecation or the number of bowel movements in a 24-hour period (32).

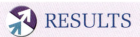

RESULTS

Comparing TEM with Conventional Local Excision

It is not likely that there will ever be a randomized prospective study comparing TEM with conventional transanal excision, which requires that surgeons enroll their own patients to either technique. Once the TEM technique is learned, it will be difficult for a surgeon to revert to a method accompanied by poor visibility, difficult reach, and doubt about the adequacy of the margins. Furthermore, TEM and transanal excision using conventional instruments are not the same operation, so a direct comparison is faulted. There are several published reports comparing TEM with other methods of local excision within a given institution in a retrospective manner. Moore and Cataldo studied 171 patients, 89 of which underwent conventional transanal excision and the remaining 82 underwent TEM. The number of postoperative complications was similar (15% and 17% for TEM and conventional excision, respectively); however, the conventional group had more major complications that included fistula, anastomotic leak, and bleeding. TEM was more likely to produce clear margins, cause less specimen fragmentation, and have a lower recurrence rate (33).

Lin et al. compared TEM patients treated at their institution with a group of patients who underwent a posterior transsphincteric approach (Mason's operation) at another institution. In this study, 31 patients underwent TEM between 1995 and 2003 and were compared to patients who underwent Mason's operation between 1995 and 2004. There were no differences noted in operative time or blood loss. The median hospital stay and time until resumption of food intake were shorter in the TEM group. In the Mason group, wound infections and fecal fistulas developed in 3.9% of patients each. One patient required a transverse colostomy for the fistula to heal. Incontinence to flatus or liquid stool occurred in 31.4% of the Mason group while 6.5% of the TEM group had incontinence for flatus only. Both groups showed complete recovery of continence, although the Mason group took almost a week longer to recover. There were no recurrences noted in the TEM group, whereas a 3.9% recurrence rate was noted in the Mason group at 30 months follow-up (34).

In a study of excision of adenomas alone, de Graaf et al. compared transanal excision (n = 43) with TEM (n = 216). Although the study was not randomized, the lesions were matched for tumor size and distance from the anal verge. Significant differences were noted in favor of TEM with respect to operative time (35 vs. 47 minutes), complication rates (5% vs. 10%), ability to achieve negative margins (88% vs. 50%), cause less tissue fragmentation (1.4% vs. 24%), and recurrence rates (6% vs. 29%). The authors concluded that TEM is superior to conventional transanal excision for rectal adenomas (35). Christoforidis et al. retrospectively studied only early rectal adenocarcinomas excised with either TEM (n = 42) or conventional instruments (n = 129) between 1997 and 2006. Metastatic, recurrent, previously irradiated, and snare excised tumors were excluded from the analysis. TEM was more likely to achieve clear margins (2% vs. 16%, P = 0.017). In this study, tumor margin status was an independent predictor of local recurrence and disease-free survival (36). These studies underscore the distinct differences between TEM and other methods of locally excising rectal neoplasms; they are not the same operation and the differences suggest that TEM is the preferred approach. Because of the constant rectal distention, the magnified image, its longer reach, a more precise excision and wound closure is possible. This leads to better specimen handling, namely less tissue fragmentation and a higher likelihood of obtaining negative margins, which in turn will lead to lower recurrence rates.

Follow-up and Treatment of Cancer Recurrence

Most experts agree that properly selected, favorable pT1 cancers do not require additional treatment after TEM. Favorable histologic features include well or moderately well differentiation, lack of lymphovascular invasion, lack of tumor budding at the leading edge, and lack of a mucinous component (controversial). The presence of unfavorable features should lead one to consider additional treatment even if the lesion is confined to the submucosa. Borschitz et al. studied the influence of histopathologic criteria on long-term prognosis following TEM excision of pT1 rectal cancers. Low-risk tumors, that is, those with favorable features, had a local recurrence rate of 6%. In contrast, high-risk pT1 cancers had a local recurrence rate of 39%. In this study, some patients with high-risk pT1 cancers underwent immediate radical surgery, a local recurrence rate of 6% was noted in this subgroup and the 10-year cancer-free survival was 93% (37). These data suggest that performing TEM prior to radical surgery does not adversely affect outcome, a finding confirmed on reviewing outcome in the UK database from 21 regional centers (38). Moreover, the submucosa has been divided into three layers based on thickness and are classified as SM1, SM2, and SM3. Penetration into the deepest submucosal layer has been considered an indication for additional treatment; however, not all pathologists espouse this subdivision citing concerns about tangential cuts through the tumor yielding misleading information. In a study of a national data base from the UK, the outcomes of 487 patients treated with TEM for cancer were evaluated. TEM was found to produce long-term outcomes comparable to those published for radical total mesorectal excision when TEM was applied for properly selected, favorable tumors. Prompt radical surgery for those with adverse features appears safe for certain pT1 and pT2 cancers, that is, cure is not compromised by the patient having undergone TEM prior to radical surgery (38). If radical surgery is deemed necessary, one should allow sufficient time for the wound and cavity to heal (at least 1 month) following TEM. TEM alone, or any method of local excision, is not an appropriate treatment for a cancer that penetrates into the muscularis propria or beyond because of unacceptably high recurrence rates, probably from untreated nodal metastases within the mesentery. Borschitz et al. showed that even for low-risk pT2 lesions (completely excised with negative margins, well differentiation, no lymphovascular invasion), recurrence rates of 29% were noted (39).

Follow-up after TEM should include frequent proctoscopic examinations (every 3 months for the first 2 years), and in the case of cancer, ultrasound to inspect for enlarging adenopathy. Since the anatomy may be distorted by TEM, one should refrain from making any conclusions based on a single ultrasound examination. Rather, one should look for changes on serial ultrasounds performed over time. A colonoscopy should be performed at 1 year. Recurrence of an adenoma may be treated with endoscopic fulguration or with repeat TEM, but the recurrence rate should be 10% or less. Recurrence rates following TEM excision of pT1 cancers vary in the literature, most range from 0% to 12.5%, with an occasional report citing rates from 20% to 25% (40,14). Assuming negative margins were obtained, recurrence of a pT1 cancer occurs by one of two mechanisms, either the tumor was incorrectly staged at the onset and nodal metastases were present at the initial diagnosis or exfoliated cancers cells were implanted and grew in the wound defect. In either case, the mesorectum is at risk and should be treated accordingly with neoadjuvant chemotherapy and radiation prior to radical surgery.

Doornebosch et al. evaluated the management and outcome of local recurrence after TEM for pT1 rectal cancers. Of 88 patients treated in this fashion, recurrences were noted in 18 (20.5%), the time to detection of the recurrence was 10 months. Of the 18 patients, 2 did not undergo surgery because of systemic metastases, and the remaining 16 underwent salvage surgery. A complete, margin-free excision was possible in 15 patients, 1 subsequently experienced local recurrence, whereas 7 developed distant recurrence. At 3 years, cancer-related survival was 58% (41). It is arguable that distant recurrence may or may not be a consequence of the original treatment. Furthermore, none of the patients received neoadjuvant radiation or chemotherapy prior to salvage surgery, a point of contention in light of the potential mechanisms proposed to explain recurrence of a pT1 lesion mentioned above. That local recurrence (without systemic disease) can be successfully salvaged was shown in a study by Patey et al. Thirty-four patients developed recurrence after TEM, of whom 17 were considered surgical candidates. The remainder were either unfit for surgery or had systemic disease and died at a mean of 1.1 years. Of the patients undergoing salvage for local recurrence, 82% were successfully treated (42).

TEM Followed by Adjuvant Radiation Therapy

Occasionally, TEM excision of a suspected adenoma or T1 cancer yields a pathology report showing the tumor was more advanced than originally thought. Although most clinicians would advise radical surgery in these instances, a patient may be medically unfit or unwilling to do so. Ramirez et al. removed a series of rectal carcinomas with TEM and then enrolled 28 patients in a study of postoperative radiation if a pT1 cancer had unfavorable features or if the lesion was staged pT2. Local recurrence was noted in three (11%) of these patients. Five-year overall survival was 94%, and cancer-specific survival was 96% (43). Duek et al. reported a series of 12 patients with pT2 cancers removed with TEM who then underwent radiation therapy. At a median follow-up of 3 years, there were no local recurrences. In contrast, local recurrence was noted in 50% of the patients who did not receive radiation (44).

Radiation Therapy Followed by TEM

Lezoche treated 35 patients with a full course of pelvic radiation (5,040 Gy) followed by full-thickness TEM excision of the lesions, which were pT2 after histologic assessment. After a median follow-up of 38 months, there was one local recurrence. The probability of surviving 8 years was 83% (45). In another study by Lezoche, 100 patients with rectal cancer underwent preoperative imaging with ultrasound; there were 54 uT2 and 46 uT3 cancers. All patients underwent preoperative radiation followed by TEM excision. Definitive histologic examination revealed 9 pT1, 54 pT2, and 19 pT3 cancers. A complete pathologic response was noted in three patients; only microscopic tumor was noted confined to the mucosa and submucosa in another 15 patients. At a median follow-up of 55 months, local recurrence was noted in 5% and distant metastases were noted in 2%. At 90 months, the cancer-specific survival was 89% (46). In a study of 137 patients with rectal cancer treated with preoperative radiation followed by TEM, Guerreri found a local recurrence rate of 5%, almost half of these patients succumbed to systemic metastases at a median follow-up of 46 months. A disease-free survival rate of 100% was noted in 55 patients with either pT0 or pT1 cancers, 81% in 59 patients with pT2 cancers, and 59% in 23 patients with pT3 cancers (47).

Neoadjuvant Chemotherapy and Radiation Followed by TEM

Significant downstaging can be achieved with preoperative chemotherapy and radiation, some patients will have an apparent complete clinical response, and maybe even a complete pathologic response. Although the standard of care is to proceed with radical surgery regardless of response to treatment, perhaps there is a subset of patients for whom radical treatment is not necessary. There is no reliable imaging or endoscopic test capable of selecting such patients, however. There are several reports investigating whether local excision alone is adequate treatment for cancers which are pT0 after neoadjuvant chemoradiation. Tulchinsky et al. reported on 97 consecutive patients treated with neoadjuvant chemoradiation followed by radical surgery. Seventeen (18%) patients had no residual tumor at the primary site in the rectal wall, of these, only one had positive lymph nodes (48). The results would suggest that the vast majority of patients without mural disease do not need radical surgery and lymphadenectomy. Kim et al. performed full-thickness local excisions on 22 patients who were apparent complete *clinical* responders to neoadjuvant therapy. Seventeen (65%) had no residual disease within the rectal wall, no further surgery was done, and none developed local recurrence after a short mean follow-up of 24 months (49). Mohiuddin also achieved a very low recurrence rate in a similar group of patients (50). Schell et al. reported on 11 patients downstaged with neoadjuvant therapy who underwent transanal excision and were followed for a median of 48 months. None developed local recurrence, however, one patient had systemic metastases (51). Bonnen performed local excision on 26 patients, 54% had a complete local pathologic response, and 35% had microscopic residual disease. Two patients developed local recurrence at a mean follow-up of 46 months. Five-year actuarial overall survival rates was 86% (52).

Lezoche et al. staged 135 patients with rectal cancer with endorectal ultrasound, MRI, or CT and enrolled them in a study. Those patients staged with T2N0 lesions ($n = 84$) received neoadjuvant therapy and then underwent TEM, those with T1N0 lesions ($n = 51$) underwent TEM alone. For the former group, local recurrence developed in 5% and at a median follow-up of 97 months, disease-free survival was 93%. For the patients staged with T1N0 cancers, local recurrence was 0% and disease-free survival was 100%. Final pathology revealed that there were 24 (18%) complete pathologic responders, 66 (49%) pT1 cancers, and 45 (33%) pT2 cancers. All of the recurrences occurred in the patients who had been staged as having T2 cancers and were still ypT2 after neoadjuvant therapy (53). Caricato et al. treated 30 patients with neoadjuvant chemoradiation followed by TEM for the patients ($n = 8$) who had a good clinical response and open surgery for those ($n = 22$) with evident residual disease noted endoscopically or with imaging studies. After a mean follow-up of 47 months, the TEM group had a disease-free survival rate of 100%, and the open group had a disease-free survival rate of 77% (54).

Borschitz et al. performed an online search and accumulated data from seven different studies on 237 patients with clinical T2 and T3 cancers who underwent neoadjuvant chemoradiation followed by local excision. None of the patients with ypT0 cancers developed local recurrence. Recurrence rates were as follows: 0–6% for ypT1 cancers, 6–20% for ypT2 cancers, and up to 42% for ypT3 cancers (55).

Studies Comparing TEM with Radical Surgery

In a nonrandomized study, De Graaf et al. compared 80 patients treated with TEM to 75 treated with total mesorectal excision. All patients had pT1 cancers and negative margins. The TEM group had shorter operative times, less bleeding, shorter hospital stays, fewer complications, and lower reoperation rates. At 5 years, overall survival and cancer-specific survival rates were comparable. Local recurrence developed in 24% of the TEM group and 0% of the TME group, yet survival was not affected (56). Ptok et al. reported a nonrandomized retrospective German multicenter trial involving 282 hospitals and 479 patients with low-risk pT1 cancers treated for cure. Eighty-five patients were treated with conventional transanal excision and 35 patients underwent TEM. Collectively, local recurrence developed in 6% of this group at a mean follow-up of 44 months. Of the 359 patients treated with radical surgery, local recurrence developed in 2% ($P = 0.05$); however, tumor-free survival did not differ between the groups (57). Lee et al. compared TEM and radical surgery, also in a nonrandomized fashion, for patients with pT1 and pT2 cancers. No chemotherapy or radiation was administered. There was no significant difference in local recurrence rates for patients with pT1 cancers treated with TEM or radical surgery. For T2 cancers, however, local recurrence developed in 19.5% of the TEM patients and 9.4% of those undergoing radical surgery ($P = 0.04$). There were no significant differences between the two groups in terms of 5-year disease-free survival rates. The authors concluded that further treatment is warranted for a pT2 cancer removed by TEM (22).

In a randomized, prospective trial with a minimum of 3 years of follow-up, Lezoche randomized 40 patients into a TEM group ($n = 20$) and a total mesorectal laparoscopic resection group ($n = 20$) following neoadjuvant therapy. Final pathology in the TEM group revealed that there were seven pT0 cancers, six pT1 cancers, and seven pT2 cancers. For the mesorectal excision group, there were seven pT0 cancers, four pT1 cancers, and seven pT2 cancers. Significant downstaging occurred in both groups. At a mean follow-up of 56 months, one local recurrence and one distant recurrence developed in each group. The probability of local or distant failure was 10% for TEM and 12% for laparoscopic resection, whereas the probability of survival was 95% for TEM and 83% for laparoscopic resection. The authors conclude that the results were comparable between the two study arms in terms of failure and survival (58). Lezoche updated his series to include 35 patients in each arm and the results have held up; similar results were noted in each treatment arm with respect to local failure and probability of survival (59).

⚙ CONCLUSIONS

TEM is a safe technique with a broad range of applications including the excision of rectal neoplasms, treatment of complex rectal fistulas, and strictureplasty. Virtually, any adenoma can be removed with this technique; however, caution should be exercised regarding its use with rectal cancer. The standard against which it will be compared is level-appropriate mesorectal excision. Most would agree that TEM excision of favorable, low-risk pT1 cancers is acceptable. It should not be used as the sole form of therapy for pT2 or deeper cancers. There is considerable interest in combining TEM with post-operative radiation or neoadjuvant chemotherapy and radiation for these locally advanced tumors. Publications investigating combined therapy all have small sample sizes and few prospectively randomize patients, nevertheless, the results are compelling. These papers show the following: TEM excision of favorable pT1 cancers is safe, TEM does not compromise outcome if prompt radical surgery is considered necessary because of unfavorable histology, and many patients do not require radical surgery and lymphadenectomy if neoadjuvant therapy produces a complete histologic response at the primary site in the rectal wall. TEM may play an expanding role in the future based on these findings, that is, local excision of the post treatment scar or ulcer before subjecting the patient to radical and disfiguring surgery. Future use of TEM may even include transanal lymph node sampling or dissection with or without the use of sentinel lymph node technology. In fact, Buess himself had alluded to the potential for node retrieval in the 1980s. Technical modifications are likely in the future to make the equipment more affordable, as such, TEM will likely gain in popularity.

References

1. Buess G, Theiss R, Hutterer F, et al. Transanal endoscopic surgery of the rectum—testing a new method in animal experiments. *Leber Magen Darm* 1983;13(2):73–7.

2. Kipfmuller K, Buess G, Naruhm M, Junginger T. Training program for transanal endoscopic microsurgery. *Surg Endosc* 1988;2(1):24–7.

3. Vavra P, Dostalik J, Vavrova M, et al. Transanal endoscopic microsurgery: a novel technique for the repair of benign rectovaginal fistula. *Surgeon* 2009;7(2):126–7.

4. Quinlan M, Cahill R, Keane F, et al. Transanal endoscopic microsurgical repair of iatrogenic recto-urethral fistula. *Surgeon* 2005;3(6):416–17.

5. Andrews EJ, Royce P, Farmer KC. Transanal endoscopic microsurgery repair of rectourethral fistula after high-intensity focused ultrasound ablation of prostate cancer. *Colorectal Dis* 2011;13(3):342–3.

6. Bochove-Overgaauw DM, Beerlage HP, Bosscha K, Gelderman WA. Transanal endoscopic microsurgery for correction of rectourethral fistulae. *J Endourol* 2006;20(12):1087–90.

7. Baatrup G, Svensen R, Ellensen VS. Benign rectal strictures managed with transanal resection—a novel application for transanal endoscopic microsurgery. *Colorectal Dis* 2010;12(2):144–6.

8. Kato K, Saito T, Matsuda M, et al. Successful treatment of a rectal anastomotic stenosis by transanal endoscopic microsurgery (TEM) using the contact Nd:YAG laser. *Surg Endosc* 1997;11(5):485–7.

9. Beunis A, Pauli S, Van Cleemput M. Anastomotic leakage of a colorectal anastomosis treated by transanal endoscopic microsurgery. *Acta Chir Belg* 2008;108(4):474–6.

10. Zoller S, Joos A, Dinter D, et al. Retrorectal tumors: excision by transanal endoscopic microsurgery. *Rev Esp Enferm Dig* 2007;99(9):547–50.

11. Serra Aracil X, Gomez Diaz C, Bombardo Junca J, et al. Surgical excision of retrorectal tumor using transanal endoscopic microsurgery. *Colorectal Dis* 2010;12(6)594–5.

12. Bipat S, Glas AS, Slors FJ, et al. Rectal cancer: local staging and assessment of lymph node involvement with endoluminal US, CT, and MR imaging—a meta-analysis. *Radiology* 2004;232:773–83.

13. Huh JW, Park YA, Jung EJ, et al. Accuracy of endorectal ultrasonography and computer tomography for restaging rectal cancer after preoperative chemoradiation. *J Am Coll Surg* 2008;207(1):7–12.

14. Saclarides TJ. TEM/local excision: indications, techniques, outcomes, and the future. *J Surg Oncol* 2007;96:644–50.

15. Druzijanic N, Perko Z, Kraljevic D, et al. Harmonic scalpel in transanal microsurgery. *Hepatogastroenterology* 2008;55(82–83):356–8.

16. Ayodeji ID, Hop WC, Tetteroo GW, et al. Ultracision Harmonic Scalpel and multifunctional tem400 instrument complement in transanal endoscopic microsurgery: a prospective study. *Surg Endosc* 2004;18(12):1730–7.

17. Hermsen PE, Ayodeji ID, Hop WH, et al. Harmonic long shears further reduce operation time in transanal endoscopic microsurgery. *Surg Endosc* 2009;23(9):2124–30.

18. Ramirez JM, Aguilella V, Arribas D, Martinez M. Transanal full-thickness excision of rectal tumours: should the defect be sutured? A randomized controlled trial. *Colorectal Dis* 2002;4(1):51–5.

19. Buess G, Mentges B, Manncke K, et al. Technique and results of transanal endoscopic microsurgery in early rectal cancer. *Am J Surg* 1992;163(1):63–70.

20. Ganai S, Kanumuri P, Rao RS, Alexander IA. Local recurrence after transanal endoscopic microsurgery for rectal polyps and early cancers. *Ann Surg Oncol* 2006;13(4):547–56.

21. Bigness MB, Ramwell A, Evans JR, et al. Complications of transanal endoscopic microsurgery (TEMS): a prospective audit. *Colorectal Dis* 2010;12(7 Online):e99–103.

22. Lee W, Lee D, Choi S, Chun H. Transanal endoscopic microsurgery and radical surgery for T1 and T2 rectal cancer. *Surg Endosc* 2003;17(8):1283–7.

23. Marks JH, Valsdottir EB, DeNittis A, et al. Transanal endoscopic microsurgery for the treatment of rectal cancer: comparison of wound complication rates with and without neoadjuvant radiation therapy. *Surg Endosc* 2009;23(5):1081–7.

24. Gavagan JA, Whiteford MH, Swanstrom LL. Full-thickness intraperitoneal excision by transanal endoscopic microsurgery does not increase short-term complications. *Am J Surg* 2004;187(5):630–4.

25. Baatrup G, Borschitz T, Cunningham C, Qvist N. Perforation into the peritoneal cavity during transanal endoscopic microsurgery for rectal cancer is not associated with major complications or oncological compromise. *Surg Endosc* 2009;23(12):2680–3.

26. Koebrugge B, Bosscha K, Ernst MF. Transanal endoscopic microsurgery for local excision of rectal lesions: is there a learning curve? *Dig Surg* 2009;26(5):372–7.

27. Gracia Solanas JA, Ramirez Rodriguez JM, Aguilella Diago V, et al. A prospective study about functional and anatomic consequences of transanal endoscopic microsurgery. *Rev Esp Enferm Dig* 2006;98(4):234–40.

28. Doornebosch PG, Gosselink MP, Neijenhuis PA, et al. Impact of transanal endoscopic microsurgery on functional outcome and quality of life. *Int J Colorectal Dis* 2008;23:709–13.

29. Herman RM, Richter P, Walega P, Popiela T. Anorectal sphincter function and rectal barostat study in patients following transanal endoscopic microsurgery. *Int J Colorectal Dis* 2001;16(6):370–6.

30. Wang HS, Lin JK, Yang SH, et al. Prospective study of the functional results of transanal endoscopic microsurgery. *Hepatogastroenterology* 2003;50(53):1376–80.

31. Jin Z, Yin L, Xue L, Lin M, Zheng Q. Anorectal functional results after transanal endoscopic microsurgery in benign and early malignant tumors. *World J Surg* 2010;34(5):1128–32.

32. Cataldo PA, O'Brien S, Osler T. Transanal endoscopic microsurgery: a prospective evaluation of functional results. *Dis Colon Rectum* 2005;48(7):1366–71.

33. Moore JS, Cataldo PA, Osler T, Hyman HN. Transanal endoscopic microsurgery is more effective than traditional transanal excision for resection of rectal masses. *Dis Colon Rectum* 2008;51(7):1026–31.

34. Lin GL, Meng WC, Lau PY, Qiu HZ, Yip AW. Local resection for early rectal tumours: comparative study of transanal endoscopic microsurgery (TEM) versus posterior trans-sphincteric approach (Mason's operation). *Asian J Surg* 2006;29(4):227–32.

35. de Graaf EJ, Burger JW, van Ijsseldijk AL, et al. Transanal endoscopic microsurgery is superior to transanal excision of rectal adenomas. *Colorectal Dis* 2011;13(7):762–7.

36. Christoforidis D, Cho HM, Dixon MR, et al. Transanal endoscopic microsurgery versus conventional transanal excision for patients with early rectal cancer. *Ann Surg* 2009;249(5):776–82.

37. Borschitz T, Heintz A, Junginger T. The influence of histopathologic criteria on the long-term prognosis of locally excised pT1 rectal carcinomas: results of local excision (transanal endoscopic microsurgery) and immediate reoperation. *Dis Colon Rectum* 2006;49(10):1492–506; discussion 1500–5.

38. Bach SP, Hill J, Monson JR, et al. A predictive model for local recurrence after transanal endoscopic microsurgery for rectal cancer. *Br J Surg* 2009;96(3):280–90.

39. Borschitz T, Heintz A, Junginger T. Transanal endoscopic microsurgical excision of pT2 rectal cancer: results and possible indications. *Dis Colon Rectum* 2007;50(3):292–301.

40. Sengupta S, Tjandra JJ. Local excision of rectal cancer: what is the evidence? *Dis Colon Rectum* 2001;44:1345–1361.

41. Doornebosch PG, Ferenschild FT, de Wilt JH, et al. Treatment of recurrence after transanal endoscopic microsurgery (TEM) for T1 rectal cancer. *Dis Colon Rectum* 2010;53(9):1234–9.

42. Paty PB, Nash GM, Baron P, et al. Long-term results of local excision for rectal cancer. *Ann Surg* 2002;236(4):522–30.

43. Ramirez JM, Aguilella V, Valencia J, et al. Transanal endoscopic microsurgery for rectal cancer. Long-term oncologic results. *Int J Colorectal Dis* 2011;26(4):437–43.

44. Duek SD, Issa N, Hershko DD, Krausz MM. Outcome of transanal endoscopic microsurgery and adjuvant radiotherapy in patients with T2 rectal cancer. *Dis Colon Rectum* 2008;51(4):379–84; discussion 384.

45. Lezoche E, Guerrieri M, Paganini AM, Feliciotti F. Long-term results of patients with pT2 rectal cancer treated with radiotherapy

and transanal endoscopic microsurgical excision. *World J Surg* 2002;26(9):1170–4.

46. Lezoche E, Guerrieri M, Paganini AM, et al. Long-term results in patients with T2-3 N0 distal rectal cancer undergoing radiotherapy before transanal endoscopic microsurgery. *Br J Surg* 2005;92(12):1546–52.

47. Guerrieri M, Feliciotti F, Baldarelli M, et al. Sphincter-saving surgery in patients with rectal cancer treated by radiotherapy and transanal endoscopic microsurgery: 10 years' experience. *Dig Liver Dis* 2003;35(12):876–80.

48. Tulchinsky H, Rabau M, Shacham-Shemueli E, et al. Can rectal cancers with pathologic T0 after neoadjuvant chemoradiation (ypT0) be treated by transanal excision alone? *Ann Surg Oncol* 2006;13:347–52.

49. Kim CJ, Yeatman TJ, Coppola D, et al. Local excision of T2 and T3 rectal cancers after downstaging chemoradiation. *Ann Surg* 2001;234:352–8.

50. Mohiuddin M, Marks G, Bannon J. High-dose preoperative radiation and full-thickness local excision: a new option for selected T3 distal rectal cancers. *Int J Radiat Oncol Biol Phys* 1994;30:845–9.

51. Schell SR, Zlotecki RA, Mendenhall WM, et al. Transanal excision of locally advanced rectal cancers downstaged using neoadjuvant chemoradiotherapy. *J Am Coll Surg* 2002;194: 584–90.

52. Bonnen M, Crane C, Vauthey JN, et al. Long-term results using local excision after preoperative chemoradiation among selected T3 rectal cancer patients. *Int J Radiat Oncol Biol Phys* 2004; 60:1098–105.

53. Lezoche G, Guerrieri M, Baldarelli M, et al. Transanal endoscopic microsurgery for 135 patients with small nonadvanced low rectal cancer (iT1-iT2, iN0): short- and long-term results. *Surg Endosc* 2011;25:1222–9.

54. Caricato M, Borzomati D, Ausania F, et al. Complementary use of local excision and transanal endoscopic microsurgery for rectal cancer after neoadjuvant chemoradiation. *Surg Endosc* 2006;20(8):1203–7.

55. Borschitz T, Wachtlin D, Mohler M, et al. Neoadjuvant chemoradiation and local excision for T2-3 rectal cancer. *Ann Surg Oncol* 2008;15(3):712–20.

56. De Graaf EJ, Doornebosch PG, Tollenaar RA, et al. Transanal endoscopic microsurgery versus total mesorectal excision of T1 rectal adenocarcinomas with curative intention. *Eur J Surg Oncol* 2009;35(12):1280–5.

57. Ptok H, Marusch F, Meyer F, et al; Colon/Rectal Cancer (Primary Tumor) Study Group. Oncological outcome of local vs. radical resection of low-risk T1 rectal cancer. *Arch Surg* 2007;142(7):649–55; discussion 656.

58. Lezoche E, Guerrieri M, Paganini AM, et al. Transanal endoscopic versus total mesorectal laparoscopic resections of T2-N0 low rectal cancers after neoadjuvant treatment: a prospective randomized trial with a 3-years minimum follow-up period. *Surg Endosc* 2005;19(6):751–6.

59. Lezoche G, Baldarelli M, Guerrieri M, et al. A prospective randomized study with a 5-year minimum follow-up evaluation of transanal endoscopic microsurgery versus laparoscopic total mesorectal excision after neoadjuvant therapy. *Surg Endosc* 2008;22(2):352–8.

22 Transvaginal

G. Willy Davila

Introduction

Rectocele repair represents one of the most commonly performed gynecologic pelvic reconstructive procedures. Both gynecologists and colorectal surgeons treat rectoceles on a frequent basis by itself or in conjunction with other reconstructive procedures. Dysfunction of the posterior compartment may be very differently managed by different specialists as there is a lack of consensus about indications, surgical techniques, and outcome assessment.

The restoration of normal anatomy to the posterior vaginal wall is referred to as a posterior repair or colporrhaphy. Although frequently used interchangeably with the term "rectocele repair," the two operations may have vastly different treatment goals. While rectocele repair focuses on repairing a herniation of the anterior rectal wall into the vaginal canal due to a weakness in the rectovaginal septum, a posterior colporrhaphy is designed to correct a rectal bulge, as well as normalize vaginal caliber by restoring structural integrity to the posterior vaginal wall and introitus.

This chapter will cover various aspects of the gynecologic approach to rectocele repair, including symptoms, anatomy, physical examination, indications for repair, surgical techniques, and treatment outcomes.

SYMPTOMS

Posterior vaginal support defects can occur with or without symptoms. Posterior wall weakness typically entails pelvic and perineal pressure, a vaginal bulge, associated lower back pain, and/or defecatory dysfunction including a sense of incomplete emptying, tenesmus, need to splint, or use digitalization for defecation.

Defecatory Function

Weber et al. described defecatory dysfunction in association with pelvic organ prolapse > stage I. In this study, 92% reported bowel movements at least every other day, 63% needed to strain, 29% required digitation of the rectum during bowel movement, and

14% reported fecal incontinence. Many women need to digitally reduce or splint the posterior vaginal bulge or the perineum in order to initiate or complete a bowel movement. Accumulation of stool within the rectocele reservoir leads to increasing degrees of perineal pressure and obstructive defecation. In the absence of digital reduction, women will note incomplete emptying, which leads to a high degree of frustration. A vicious cycle of increasing pelvic pressure, need for stronger Valsalva efforts, enlargement of the rectocele bulge, and increasing perineal pressure ensues. Rectal digitation is not commonly self-reported by patients with a symptomatic rectocele unless asked by their physicians.

Patients very commonly have associated complaints of constipation. The symptom of constipation is not clearly understood by all gynecologists. Its vague nature, coupled with a poor understanding of the complexity of colonic function, frequently results in an incomplete evaluation of the symptom of constipation by the gynecologist. Unfortunately, this may result in surgical treatment of abnormal bowel function via a rectocele repair when conservative therapy for constipation may have been satisfactory. The persistence of abnormal defecation symptoms postoperatively may be responsible for the high rectocele recurrence rate.

Sexual Dysfunction

This disorder has a significant prevalence in pelvic organ prolapse (POP). Prolapse in general has been associated with sexual complaints in several studies. Common sexual symptoms about female sexual dysfunction in relation with pelvic organ prolapse include dyspareunia, decreased sexual desire, and anorgasmia. An enlarging rectocele will widen the levator hiatus and increase vaginal caliber. In addition, women with increasing degrees of prolapse have progressively larger genital hiatuses (4), which may lead to sexual difficulties including symptoms of vaginal looseness and decreased sensation during intercourse. Whether this is due to the enlargement of the vaginal introitus and levator hiatus or coexistent damage to the pudendal nerve supply to the pelvic floor musculature is unclear. Some theoretical explanations for sexual dysfunction due to posterior wall pelvic organ prolapse can be due to the loss or damage to pudendal terminal nerve endings, caused either by loss of support of the perineum and distal vagina, by surgical dissection, or by a vasculogenic factor (diminished pelvic blood flow) causing hypoxia, mucosal dryness, and dyspareunia.

Rectocele, Enterocele, and Perineal Descent

The vaginal epithelium can provide clear signs about the location of the rectovaginal fascia tears because the rugation pattern is frequently lost above the defect. Rectoceles can be caused by transverse, lateral, central, distal, or superior fascial tears (2). In general, enteroceles and most rectoceles are caused by superior tears at the cervical or vaginal cuff level, with very thin, unrugated epithelium noted overlying the defect. Denervation of the pelvic diaphragm results in opening of the genital hiatus and separation of the anterior and posterior vaginal walls, loss of muscular tone, and laxity in the rectovaginal fascia. As such, pressure applied to the anterior and posterior vaginal walls must be counteracted upon by the connective tissue alone. The connective tissue response to constant pressure is attenuation or tearing of the rectovaginal fascia. A large enterocele or rectocele may extend beyond the hymeneal ring. Once exteriorized, the patient is at risk for vaginal mucosal erosion and ulceration. Normally, the perineum should be located at the level of the ischial tuberosities or within 2 cm of this landmark. A perineum found below this level either at rest or with straining represents perineal descent and is usually caused by a detachment of the rectovaginal fascia from the vaginal apex/uterus or less commonly from the perineal body. It translates to a widening of the genital hiatus and perineal body and flattening of the intergluteal sulcus. Excessive perineal descent can be related to as little as a 20% elongation of the pudendal nerve fibers.

PREOPERATIVE PLANNING

Anatomy

The anatomy of the posterior vaginal wall cannot be clearly conceptualized apart from the anatomical support of the rest of the vagina. Vaginal support arises from several interactions between pelvic musculature and connective tissue.

Rectoceles result from defects in the integrity of the posterior vaginal wall and rectovaginal septum and subsequent herniation of the posterior vaginal wall and anterior rectal wall into the vaginal lumen through these defects.

The normal posterior vagina is lined by squamous epithelium that overlies the lamina propria, a layer of loose connective tissue. A fibromuscular layer of tissue composed of smooth muscle, collagen, and elastin underlies this lamina propria and is referred to as the rectovaginal fascia. This is an extension of the endopelvic fascia that surrounds and supports the pelvic organs and contains blood vessels, lymphatics, and nerves that supply and innervate the pelvic organs.

The layer of tissue between the vagina and the rectum, or rectovaginal fascia, was felt to be analogous to the rectovesical septum in males and became known as Denonvilliers' fascia or the rectovaginal septum in the female. Others described the rectovaginal septum as a support mechanism of the pelvic organs, and they were successful in identifying this layer during surgical and autopsy dissections (13,19,21). It is unclear whether this fascial layer extends from the vaginal cuff to the perineum or is only present along the distal vaginal wall from the levator reflection to perineum.

The normal vagina is stabilized and supported on three levels. Superiorly, the vaginal apical endopelvic fascia is attached to the cardinal–uterosacral ligament complex. Laterally, the endopelvic fascia is connected to the arcus tendineus fasciae pelvis, with the lateral posterior vagina attaching to the fascia overlying the levator ani muscles. Inferiorly, the lower posterior vagina connects to the perineal body, comprised of the anterior external anal sphincter, transverse perineum, and bulbous cavernosus muscles. The cervix (or vaginal cuff in the women following hysterectomized woman) is considered to be the superior attachment site or "superior tendon," and the perineal body the inferior attachment site or "inferior tendon." The endopelvic fascia extends between these two sites comprising the rectovaginal septum (Fig. 22.1). A rectocele results from a stretching or actual separation or tear of the rectovaginal fascia, leading to a bulging of the posterior vaginal wall noted on examination during a Valsalva maneuver. Trauma from vaginal childbirth commonly leads to transverse defects above the usual location of the connection to the perineal body (Fig. 22.2). In addition, patients may present with lateral, midline, or high transverse fascial defects. Separation of the rectovaginal septum fascia from the vaginal cuff results in the development of an enterocele as a hernia sac without fascial lining and filled with intraperitoneal contents (Fig. 22.2).

Vaginal muscular support is provided by the interrelation among the pelvic diaphragm, the levator ani muscles (puborectalis, pubococcygeus, and ileococcygeus), and the coccygeus muscles. The levator musculature extends from the pubic bone to the coccyx and provides support for the change in vaginal axis from vertical to horizontal along the mid-vagina creating a U-shaped sling. A rectocele typically develops at, or below, the levator plate, along the vertical vagina, weakening the fascial condensation of the attachments of the perineal musculature (Fig. 22.3).

PHYSICAL EXAMINATION

Pelvic examination allows the surgeon to define the grade of prolapse and determine the integrity of the connective tissue and muscular support of the posterior vaginal wall. The typical finding in a woman with a symptomatic rectocele is a lower posterior

Figure 22.1 Diagrammatic representation of the rectovaginal
septum including its attachment
from vaginal apex to perineal body.

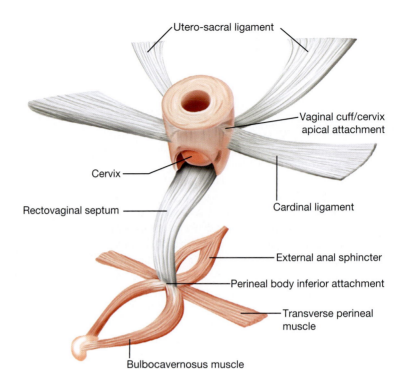

Utero-sacral ligament

Vaginal cuff/cervix
apical attachment

Cervix

Cardinal ligament

Rectovaginal septum

External anal sphincter

Perineal body inferior attachment

Transverse perineal
muscle

Bulbocavernosus muscle

vaginal wall bulge noted on physical examination in a dorsal lithotomy position. It may
superiorly extend to weaken the support of the upper, posterior vaginal wall, leading
to an enterocele, or to the vaginal apex, leading to vaginal vault prolapse. In an isolated
rectocele, the bulge extends from the edge of the levator plate to the perineal body. As
the rectocele enlarges, the perineal body may further distend and lose its bulk, leading
to an evident perineocele; enteroceles and rectoceles frequently coexist. The physical

Figure 22.2 Fascial tears of the
rectovaginal (RV) septum can
occur superiorly or inferiorly at
sites of attachment to a central
tendon.

Rectovaginal septum tear at apex

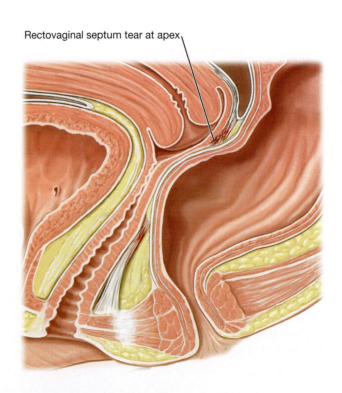

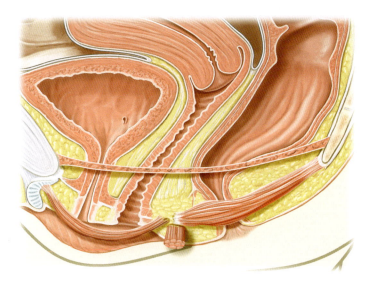

Figure 22.3 Rectoceles develop at or below the levator muscles, splaying the perineal musculature attachments.

examination should include not only a vaginal examination but must also include a rectal examination, as the perineocele may not be evident on vaginal examination. At times, it can be identified only upon digital rectal examination where an absence of fibromuscular tissue in the perineal body anterior to the rectum is confirmed.

The gynecologic preoperative evaluation of a symptomatic posterior vaginal bulge typically includes only history and physical examination. Gynecologists have not adopted the performance of defecography or other functional evaluation techniques to assess rectoceles. While 80% of colorectal surgeons use defecography, only 6% of gynecologists use it (3,9,14). In addition, differentiation between the enterocele and rectocele components of posterior vaginal wall prolapse is typically performed on a clinical and intraoperative basis. It is unclear at this time whether surgical therapy outcomes are negatively impacted by the lack of a preoperative evaluation beyond history and physical examination. Patients presenting with defecatory dysfunction should also have a gastrointestinal evaluation including a barium enema or colonoscopy to exclude colorectal malignancy. If the patient has any other suspected anorectal pathology such as internal hemorrhoids, internal rectal prolapse, or rectal ulcer, an anoscopy or proctosigmoidoscopy should be performed.

Typically, gynecologists consider rectocele repair for treatment of obstructive defecation symptoms, lower pelvic pressure and heaviness, prolapse of posterior vaginal wall, and pelvic relaxation with enlarged vaginal hiatus. However, one should be cautioned that although repair of rectoceles may correct abnormal anatomy symptoms, including constipation, other symptoms may persist.

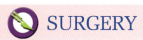 SURGERY

Surgery to Correct a Rectocele

There are several goals of surgery to repair a rectocele: endopelvic fascial integrity from the apex to the perineum and levator plate integrity should be re-established. Anterior rectal wall support should be re-established and the perineal body should be reinforced; the end result should be a vagina of normal caliber and length.

Posterior Colporrhaphy Technique

Posterior colporrhaphy is the most common gynecologic type of rectocele repair and is commonly performed in conjunction with a perineoplasty to address a relaxed perineum

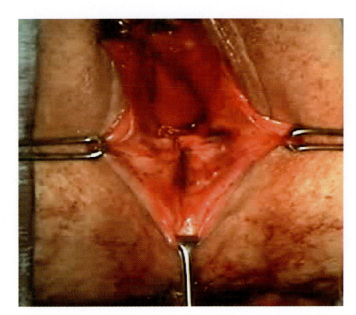

Figure 22.4 Multiple interrupted sutures are used to approximate the endopelvic fascia at the perineal body apex in the midline.

and widened genital hiatus. Preoperatively, the severity of the rectocele is assessed, as well as the desired final vaginal caliber. The original technique included plication of the pubococcygeus muscles along with plication of the posterior vaginal wall and reconstruction of the perineal body. Allis clamps are placed on the inner labia minora/hymeneal remnants bilaterally and then approximated in the midline. The resultant vagina should loosely admit two to three fingers. A triangular incision over the perineal body is made between the Allis clamps and a midline vertical incision is extended to the superior edge of the rectocele. Lateral sharp dissection is performed to separate the posterior vaginal mucosa from the underlying rectovaginal fascia.

The dissection extends laterally to the lateral vaginal sulcus and to the medial margins of the puborectalis muscles. The rectovaginal fascia with or without the underlying levator ani muscles is then plicated with interrupted sutures beginning at the level of the levator plate while depressing the anterior rectal wall with the nondominant hand (Fig. 22.4). Typically, thick, absorbable sutures using #1 Vicryl are placed along the length of the rectocele until plication to the level of the perineal body is complete. Excess vaginal mucosa is carefully trimmed and then reapproximated. A concomitant perineoplasty may be performed by plicating the bulbocavernosus and transverse perineal muscles in the midline with #1 Vicryl. This reinforces the perineal body and provides enhanced support to the corrected rectocele.

Most published studies report a greater than 75% improvement in anatomical outcome or bulge and the need to splint the perineum to defecate. However, the studies suggest that there is at least a 15% incidence of de novo dyspareunia after posterior colporrhaphy, with or without levator plication. Patients with symptoms of slow-transit constipation have little improvement in defecation dysfunction. Kahn and Stanton reported 24% of recurrent rectocele (mean follow-up 42.5 months); Mellgren in a prospective study found recurrent rectocele in 20%. Weber and colleagues (25) found dyspareunia in 25% of women after posterior colporrhaphy. Dyspareunia is dependent not only on the caliber of the vagina; it can also result from excessive mucosal trimming, loss of vaginal depth, scar tissue formation, or levator spasm.

Discrete Fascial Defect Repair Technique

Discrete tears or breaks in the rectovaginal fascia or rectovaginal septum have been described and may contribute to the formation of rectoceles (Fig. 22.2). Similarly to other hernia repairs the technique involves identifying the discrete fascial tears, reducing the hernia, and then closing the defect (6,10,16,18). The surgical dissection is similar to the traditional posterior colporrhaphy, whereby the vaginal mucosa is dissected off the underlying rectovaginal fascia to the lateral border of the levator muscles. This dissection must be very careful to avoid creating iatrogenic fascial defects. Instead of plicating the fascia and levator muscles in the midline, however, the fascial tears are identified, and the edges are reapproximated with interrupted permanent sutures. Richardson describes anteriorly pushing with a finger in the rectum to identify areas of rectal muscularis that are not covered by the rectovaginal septum (19). Thereby, the operator can locate fascial defects, identify fascial margins, and reapproximate them. A perineoplasty may be necessary if a widened vaginal hiatus is present. The discrete fascial defect repair or site-specific fascial repair may also be used to correct enteroceles by attaching torn endopelvic fascia to its apical attachment site at the cervix or cardinal–uterosacral ligament complex with interrupted sutures.

Modifications of the Rectocele Repair

The posterior colporrhaphy and the discrete fascial defect repair may be combined. After dissecting the rectovaginal fascia off the overlying vaginal mucosa, all fascial tears are identified and the edges are reapproximated with permanent suture, such as silk. The levator ani muscles can then be plicated in the midline, anterior to the rectovaginal fascia, using absorbable sutures in the traditional fashion. This technique, especially when a commonly found apical transverse fascial defect is identified and repaired, is our preferred technique due to proven longevity and high success rates. It is illustrated in the accompanying video on transvaginal rectocele repair.

Grafts Use in Posterior Vaginal Wall Repair

Reconstructive pelvic surgeons have increasingly reported reinforcement of prolapse repairs with synthetic and biologic prostheses. Synthetic type I polypropylene mesh is widely used for anti-incontinence surgery and abdominal sacrocolpopexy to repair vaginal vault prolapse. Although high success rates have been reported, mesh erosion through the vaginal mucosa and mesh contraction with resultant dyspareunia may occur with reported rates ranging from 1 to 20% (1,7). Autologous grafts and allograft prostheses, including fascia lata, rectus sheath, and dermal grafts, have been employed for these surgeries as well, with much lower complication rates. Few complications have been associated with these biologic grafts, but dyspareunia rates can range from 1 to 10%. Xenograft materials, including bovine pericardium and porcine skin and small intestinal mucosa, have also been used to reinforce these repairs (26). However, only a few reports detailing complications and success rates exist.

When using graft material to reinforce a rectocele repair, the graft may be apically as well as bilaterally sutured to the lateral posterior vaginal sulcus using absorbable or permanent suture. The graft should be trimmed prior to placement so that it lies as a flat layer between the vaginal mucosa and the newly repaired rectovaginal fascia (Fig. 22.5). There is no evidence that soaking the graft material in antibiotic solution prior to placement decreases the incidence of vaginal infection or erosion.

Few prospective comparative studies have reported on the use of graft materials to reinforce posterior compartment defects. Sand reported on 132 women undergoing either standard rectocele repair or rectocele repair reinforced with Polyglactin 910 mesh (an absorbable mesh) and found no difference in recurrence rates between the two groups (20). Two small observational studies on the use of Marlex mesh for rectocele repair did not include any erosions or any recurrence (17,22).

The use of biological grafts in posterior vaginal wall repair is not superior to native tissue repair for anatomic or symptomatic outcomes. The use of synthetic absorbable grafts does not improve anatomic outcomes over posterior colporrhaphy.

Maher et al. in a Cochrane database systematic reviews of posterior vaginal wall prolapse repair showed that vaginal approach was associated with a lower rate of recurrent rectocele and/or enterocele than the transanal approach (RR = 0.24, 95% CI = 0.09–0.64),

Figure 22.5 Posterior vaginal wall reinforcement graft in place from vaginal apex to perineum. Biologic graft attached to vaginal cuff.

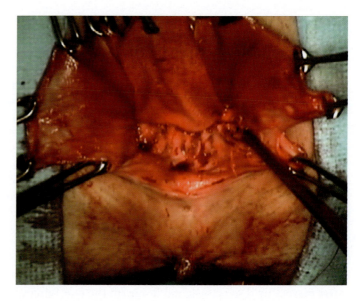

although there was a higher blood loss and greater need for postoperative narcotic use (24). However, data on the effect of surgery on bowel symptoms and the use of polyglactin mesh inlay or porcine small intestine graft inlay on the risk of recurrent rectocele were insufficient for meta-analysis.

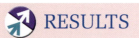 RESULTS

Although commonly performed, posterior colporrhaphy has been described as "among the most misunderstood and poorly performed" gynecologic surgeries (15). Although many authors have reported satisfactory anatomic results, conflicting effects on postoperative bowel and sexual function have been noted. Several authors have reported high sexual dysfunction rates of up to 50% of women reporting dyspareunia or apareunia after posterior colporrhaphy (5). Some authors caution the performance of rectocele repair in patients with preoperative abnormal colonic transit studies secondary to continued constipation postoperatively (12). Other authors performed preoperative defecography on all patients and found that the grade of rectocele emptying did not influence long-term outcome. In addition, pre- and postoperative defecography was reported to show an increase in maximal anal resting pressure postoperatively, suggesting that it may be due to levator plication (Table 22.1) (11).

Many authors have suggested that the significant rate of postoperative dyspareunia may be due to the plication of the levator ani muscles and has led several authors to the popularization of the discrete fascial defect repair (8,23). Several authors have reported a similar anatomic cure rate with this surgery, along with significant improvement in quality of life measures. Unlike the traditional posterior colporrhaphy, all of these series report less postoperative dyspareunia. The authors noted significant improvement in

TABLE 22.1	Outcomes for Posterior Colporrhaphy	
	Preoperative (%)	Postoperative (%)
POP symptoms	64	31
Constipation	22	33
Fecal incontinence	4	11
Sexual dysfunction	18	27
Anatomic defect	100	24

POP= pelvic organ prolapse.
231 surgeries over 5 years: 61% examined, 71% questioned.

splinting, vaginal pressure, and stooling difficulties. However, rates of fecal incontinence and constipation were postoperatively unchanged. These studies show promising anatomical and functional results; however, prospective long-term studies are warranted. We have not found a high rate of dyspareunia with a combination of site-specific repair and high perineoplasty. The multiple goals of restoration of anterior rectal support and normalization of vaginal hiatus size are achieved without significant negative consequence.

CONCLUSIONS

Gynecologic indications for rectocele repair are numerous because gynecologists primarily address vaginal symptoms when repairing a rectocele. Obstructive defecation symptoms are included among many others in a list of accepted indications. Preoperative evaluation by gynecologists typically includes clinical assessment gained from the history and physical examination only, and gynecologists rarely depend on defecography to plan a reconstructive procedure for rectocele. Overall, surgical correction success rates are quite high when using a vaginal approach for rectocele correction. Vaginal dissection results in good visualization and access to the endopelvic fascia and levator musculature, which theoretically allows for a more anatomic correction than does transanal repair. More comprehensive data collection is necessary to better understand the effect of various surgical techniques on vaginal, sexual, and evacuatory symptoms.

Recommended References and Readings

1. Birch C, Fynes MM. The role of synthetic and biological prostheses in reconstructive pelvic floor surgery. *Curr Opin Obstet Gynecol* 2001;14:527–35.
2. Cundiff GW, Weidner AC, Visco AG, Addison WA, Bump RC. An anatomic and functional assessment of the discrete defect rectocele repair. *Am J Obstet Gynecol* 1998;179:1451–7.
3. Davila GW, Ghoniem GM, Kapoor DS, Contreras-Ortiz O. Pelvic floor dysfunction management practice patterns: a survey of members of the international urogynecological association. *Int Urogynecol J* 2002;13:319–25.
4. Delancey JOL, Hurd WW. Size of the urogenital hiatus in the levator ani muscles in normal women and women with pelvic organ prolapse. *Obstet Gynecol* 1998;91:364–8.
5. Francis WJ, Jeffcoate TN. Dyspareunia following vaginal operations. *J Obstet Gynaecol Br Emp* 1961;68:1–10.
6. Glavind K, Madsen H. A prospective study of the discrete fascial defect rectocele repair. *Acta Obstet Gynecol Scand* 2000;79:145–7.
7. Iglesia CB, Fenner DE, Brubaker L. The use of mesh in gynecologic surgery. *Int Urogynecol J* 1997;8:105–15.
8. Kahn MA, Stanton SL. Posterior colporrhaphy: its effects on bowel and sexual function. *Br J Obstet Gynaecol* 1997;104:82–6.
9. Kapoor DS, Davila GW, Wexner SD, Ghoniem GM. Posterior compartment disorders: survey of colorectal surgeons practice patterns and review of the literature. *Int Urogynecol J* 2001;12:S53.
10. Kenton K, Shott S, Brubaker L. Outcome after rectovaginal reattachment for rectocele repair. *Am J Obstet Gynecol* 1999;181:1360–3.
11. Lopez A, Anzen B, Bremmer S, et al. Durability of success after rectocele repair. *Int Urogynecol J Pelvic Floor Dysfunct* 2001;12:97–103.
12. Mellgren A, Anzen B, Nilsson BY, et al. Results of rectocele repair. A prospective study. *Dis Colon Rectum* 1995;38:7–13.
13. Milley PS, Nichols DH. A correlative investigation of the human rectovaginal septum. *Anat Rec* 1969;163:443–52.
14. Mizrahi N, Kapoor D, Baig MK, et al. A gynecologic perspective of posterior compartment defects. *Colorectal Dis* 2002;4:68.
15. Nichols DH. Posterior colporrhaphy and perineorrhaphy: separate and distinct operations. *Am J Obstet Gynecol* 1991;164:714–21.
16. Paraiso MF, Weber AM, Walters MD, Ballard LA, Piedmonte MR, Skibinski C. Anatomic and functional outcome after posterior colporrhaphy. *J Pelvic Surg* 2001;7:335–9.
17. Parker MC, Phillips RKS. Repair of rectocele using Marlex mesh. *Ann R Coll Surg Eng* 1993;75:193–4.
18. Porter WE, Steele A, Walsh P, Kohli N, Karram MM. The anatomic and functional outcomes of defect-specific rectocele repairs. *Am J Obstet Gynecol* 1999;181:1353–8.
19. Richardson AC. The rectovaginal septum revisited: Its relationship to rectocele and its importance in rectocele repair. *Clin Obstet Gynecol* 1993;36:976–83.
20. Sand PK, Koduri S, Lobel RW. Prospective randomized trial of Polyglactin 910 mesh to prevent recurrences of cystoceles and rectoceles. *Am J Obstet Gynecol* 2001;184:1357–64.
21. Uhlenhuth E, Wolfe WM, Smith EM, Middleton EB. The rectogenital septum. *Surg Gynecol Obstet* 1948;86:148–63.
22. Watson SJ, Loder PB, Halligan S. Transperineal repair of symptomatic rectocele with Marlex mesh: a clinical, physiological and radiological assessment of treatment. *J Am Coll Surg* 1996;183:257–61.
23. Cundiff GW, Fenner D. Evaluation and treatment of women with rectocele: focus on associated defecatory and sexual dysfunction. *Obstet Gynecol* 2004;104(6):1403–21.
24. Maher C, Baessler K, Glazener CM, Adams EJ, Hagen S. Surgical management of pelvic organ prolapse in women. *Cochrane Database Syst Rev* 2007;(3):CD004014. DOI:10.1002/14651858.CD004014.pub3.
25. Weber AM, Walters MD, Ballard LA, Booher DL, Piedmonte MR. Posterior vaginal prolapse and bowel function. *Am J Obstet Gynecol* 1998;179:1446–9.
26. Paraiso MF, Barber M, Muir T, Walters MD. Rectocele repair: A randomized trial of three surgical techniques including graft augmentation. *Am J Obstet Gynecol* 2006;195:1762–71.

23 Transanal

Sthela M. Murad-Regadas and Rodrigo A. Pinto

Functional evaluation of the pelvic floor helps identify all anatomical defecatory disorders, which facilitate the choice of treatment options. Some studies have shown that the application of a complete functional investigation of the pelvic floor can modify the surgical management in up to 30–40% of cases (1,2). Specific indications for surgical repair of rectoceles depends on the patients' symptoms, physical examination findings, results of physiological tests as well as failure of medical management including dietary modifications, fiber supplements, laxatives, and biofeedback.

SURGICAL TECHNIQUES

Various preoperative bowel preparation techniques maybe used. While some surgeons advocate sodium phosphate enemas, others recommend bowel cleansing with polyethylene glycol or oral sodium phosphate preparation. Preoperative parenteral antibiotic prophylaxis is frequently used. The transanal approach is preferred by most colorectal surgeons, as they are experienced with transanal surgery. Patients are positioned in the prone jackknife or lithotomy positions depending on the surgeon's preference.

The transanal repair involves excising the distal redundant anterior rectal mucosa, followed by longitudinal or transverse plication of the muscularis propria layer of the rectum and rectovaginal septum (3,4). While plicating the muscular layer using interrupted or continuous absorbable stitches, special care must be taken to not include the posterior vaginal wall, which could lead to subsequent formation of a rectovaginal fistula (4–7). All of the hand-sewn methods have some basic principles in common: to excise the rectocele and the excessive anterior mucosa layer; to firmly reapproximate the anterior rectal wall by plication of the submucosa and muscularis; and to induce submucosal fibrosis through surgical manipulation (3,4,6).

Block (5) developed the closed obliterative suture technique in 1986, which consists of a tightly drawn continuous lock-stitch suture that strangulates the mucosa, submucosa, and muscularis layers of the rectocele without opening the rectum, allowing the repair to heal faster. Advantages of this technique include the short operative time that results from not having to dissect all layers of the rectal wall for repair, which also minimizes tissue trauma.

RESULTS AND COMPLICATIONS

Patients usually have a short hospital stay after rectocele repair (1 to 2 days). The symptomatic defecatory improvement using the transanal approach ranges from 30–90% (5–12). However, most of the series report unsatisfactory evacuation in 10–30% of patients (13,14). The causes for unsuccessful repairs are usually multifactorial, including inadequate repair, inappropriate patient selection and other coexisting undiagnosed or occult evacuation disorders.

The overall complication rate has been reported as up to 9% (6,8,12,15), and includes bleeding from the dissected mucosa (≤9%) (12,15), infection, wound breakdown (≤8%) (8,11,16), and rectovaginal fistulas (<1%) (5–7,16). Tjandra et al. (9) noted postoperative complications in 3% of patients excluding local sepsis or rectovaginal fistulas using the transanal technique. The low morbidity rate has been attributed to meticulous dissection, adequate hemostasis, use of prophylactic antibiotics, and accurate placement of sutures during the plication of the muscularis propria of the rectum. Paradoxical puborectalis contraction is associated with symptomatic rectoceles in 20–70% of cases (17–20), and some studies have shown that this association worsened overall postoperative results, despite some postoperative improvement in constipation and quality of life (9,15,16). Tjandra et al. (9) reported improvement of evacuation in patients without anismus in 93% as compared to 38% in patients with associated anismus. Accordingly, all patients with anismus should be submitted to biofeedback prior to rectocele repair (21). Postoperative decreased anal sphincter pressures have been reported and fecal incontinence is found in 3–34% of patients (6,8). Ho et al. (22) noticed impaired mean resting and squeeze pressures 6 months after the transanal technique in 21 females. Nevertheless, no patients were postoperatively incontinent and all had improved outlet obstruction symptoms. Heriot et al. (23), alternatively, failed to find any changes in either resting or squeeze pressures after the operation in 45 patients. Results of anorectal physiological analysis following rectocele repair is inconsistent, whether assessed by anal manometry or by pudendal nerve terminal motor latency (24,25).

Long-term results of transanal repair decrease with time (10,13,16,26). Abbas et al. (26) reviewed 150 females who had undergone an anterior Delorme's operation in the management of symptomatic rectocele. One hundred seven patients at a mean follow-up of 4 years (range 2–11) had significant improvement of the obstructed defecation as defined by the Rome II criteria (14). There was also significant reduction in each of the following symptoms of outlet obstruction: straining, incomplete emptying, feeling of blockage, and digitations. Patients with incontinence had also significant reduction in their symptoms after transanal repair. Conversely, Roman & Michot (13) found 35 recurrences in 71 patients after a mean follow-up of 74 months. Persistence of symptoms 2 months after surgery was a predictive factor in rectocele recurrence, and preoperative clinic, defecographic, and manometric parameters are not helpful in predicting recurrence. Similarly Arnold et al. (10) reported continued symptoms of constipation (54%), sexual dysfunction (21%), and rectal pain (4%) in a follow-up period of 2–5 years after transanal and transvaginal approaches. However, 83% of the patients noted symptomatic improvement in constipation after surgery despite these reported symptoms. Van Dam et al. (16) reported good or excellent functional results in 67.6% patients after a median follow-up of 58 months. Therefore, it seems that there is no evidence of deterioration of the functional results of transanal repair with time (Table 23.1).

A potential drawback of this procedure is its inability to treat circumferential mucosal prolapse and/or rectoanal intussusceptions. However, as mentioned earlier, rectoceles, mucosal prolapse, hemorrhoids, and perineal descent are different processes that consequently require management (27). Transanal repair of rectocele is a safe alternative as it provides amelioration of symptoms, reflected by anatomical improvement with an acceptable risk profile.

TABLE 23.1	Long-Term Success of Transanal Nonstapled Approach			
Author	Year	No. of patients	Success (%)	Follow-up (months)
Sullivan (3)	1968	151	79.5	18.5
Sehapayak (5)	1985	204	84.5	3–72
Murthy (8)	1996	26	92	31
Van Dam (16)	1997	74	67.6	58
Abbas (26)	2003	107	72	48
Heriot (23)	2004	45	93.3	24
Roman & Michot (13)	2005	71	50.7	74

Recommended References and Readings

1. Thompson JR, Chen AH, Pettit PMD, Bridges MD. Incidence of occult rectal prolapse in patients with clinical rectoceles and defecatory dysfunction. *Am J Obstet Gynecol* 2002;187:1494–500.
2. Kaufman HS, Buller JL, Thompsom JR, et al. Dynamic pelvic magnetic resonance imaging and cystocolpoproctography alter surgical management of pelvic floor disorders. *Dis Colon Rectum* 2001;44:1575–84.
3. Sullivan ES, Leaverton GH, Hardwick CE. Transrectal perineal repair: an adjunct to improved function after anorectal surgery. *Dis Colon Rectum* 1968;11:106–14.
4. Sarles JC, Arnaund A, Selezeneff I, Olivier S. Endorectal repair of rectocele. *Int J Colorectal Dis* 1989;4(3):167–71.
5. Sehapayak S. Transrectal repair of rectocele: an extended armamentarium of colorectal surgeons. A report of 355 cases. *Dis Colon Rectum* 1985;28:422–33.
6. Khubchandani IT, Sheets JA, Stasik JJ, Hakki AR. Endorectal repair of rectocele. *Dis Colon Rectum* 1983;26:792–6.
7. Block IR. Transrectal repair of rectocele using obliterative suture. *Dis Colon Rectum* 1986;29:707–11.
8. Murthy VK, Orkin B, Smith LE, Glassman LM. Excellent outcome using selective criteria for rectocele repair. *Dis Colon Rectum* 1996;39:374–8.
9. Tjandra JJ, Ooi BS, Tang CL, Dwyer P, Carey M. Transanal repair of rectocele corrects obstructed defecation if it is not associated with anismus. *Dis Colon Rectum* 1999;42:1544–50.
10. Arnold MW, Stewart WR, Aguilar PS. Rectocele repair: four years experience. *Dis Colon Rectum* 1990;33:684–7.
11. Capps WE Jr. Rectoplasty and perineoplasty for the symptomatic rectocele: a report of fifty cases. *Dis Colon Rectum* 1975;18:237–44.
12. Janssen LW, van Dijke CF. Selection criteria for anterior rectal wall repair in symptomatic rectocele and anterior rectal wall prolapse. *Dis Colon Rectum* 1994;37:1100–7.
13. Roman H, Michot F. Long-term outcomes of transanal rectocele repair. *Dis Colon Rectum* 2005;48:510–17.
14. Rome II Modular Questionnaire: investigator and respondent forms. In: Drossman DA, Corazziari E, Talley NJ, Thompson WG, Whitehead WE (eds.). *Rome II The Functional Gastrointestinal Disorders.* 2nd ed. McLean, VA, USA: Degnon Associates, 2000:669–88.
15. Karlbom U, Graf W, Nilsson S, Påhlman L. Does surgical repair of a rectocele improve rectal emptying? *Dis Colon Rectum* 1996;39:1296–1302.
16. Van Dam JH, Schouten WR, Ginai AZ, Huisman WM, Hop. WC.. The impact of anismus on the clinical outcome of rectocele repair. *Int J Colorectal Dis* 1996;11:238–42.
17. Mellgren A, Anzen B, Nilsson BY, et al. Results of rectocele repair: a prospective study. *Dis Colon Rectum* 1995;38:7–13.
18. Johansson C, Nilsson BY, Holmström B, Dolk A, Mellgren A. Association between rectocele and paradoxical sphincter response. *Dis Colon Rectum* 1992;35:503–9.
19. Siproudhis L, Dautreme S, Ropert A, et al. Dyschezia and rectocele–a marriage of convenience? *Dis Colon Rectum* 1993;36:1030–6.
20. Murad-Regadas SM, Regadas FSP, Rodrigues LV, et al. Types of pelvic floor dysfunctions in nulliparous, vaginal delivery, and cesarean section female patients with obstructed defecation syndrome identified by echodefecography. *Int J Colorectal Dis* 2009;10:1227–32.
21. Mimura T, Roy AJ, Storrie JB, Kamm MA. Treatment of impaired defecation associated with rectocele by behavioral retraining (biofeedback). *Dis Colon Rectum* 2000;43:1267–72.
22. Ho YH, Ang M, Nyam D, Tan M, Seow-Coen F. Transanal approach to rectocele repair may compromise anal sphincter pressures. *Dis Colon Rectum* 1998;41:354–8.
23. Heriot AG, Skull A, Kumar D. Functional and physiological outcome following transanal repair of rectocele. *Br J Surg* 2004;91:1340–4.
24. Ayabaca SM, Zbar AP, Pescatori M. Anal continence after rectocele repair. *Dis Colon Rectum* 2002;45:63–9.
25. Thornton MJ, Lam A, King DW. Laparoscopic or transanal repair of rectocele? A retrospective matched cohort study. *Dis Colon Rectum* 2005;48:792–8.
26. Abbas SM, Bissett IP, Neill ME, Macmillan AK, Milne D, Parry BR. Long-term results of the anterior Delorme's operation in the management of symptomatic rectocele. *Dis Colon Rectum* 2005;48:317–22.
27. Ayav A, Bresler L, Brunaud L, Boissel P. Long-term results of transanal repair of rectocele using linear stapler. *Dis Colon Rectum* 2004;47:889–94.

24 Transperineal

Guillermo Rosato and Pablo E. Piccinini

 ## INDICATIONS/CONTRAINDICATIONS

Criteria of patient selection for surgery:

1. Rectocele ≤4 cm in diameter as measured during defecography (DFG) or ≤2.5 cm as measured during pelvic floor dynamic magnetic resonance (DMRPP) imaging.
2. Non- or partial emptying of rectocele during the push phase in other DFG or DMRPP.
3. Rectal and/or vaginal symptoms for longer than 12 months.
4. 3 + for at least 4 weeks despite dietary fiber of 30 g/day.
5. Rectal and/or vaginal digitation required to facilitate rectal evacuation.

 ## PREOPERATIVE PLANNING

Patient election for surgery has followed the previously mentioned selection criteria of anorectal physiology including transit time, anal manometry, DFG, DMRPP, and neurophysiology of the pelvic floor.

All patients underwent bowel preparation with 3,000 cc polyethylene glycol or a phospho-soda solution. Antibiotic prophylaxis consisted of a combination of Metronidazole and Gentamycin or Ceftriaxone.

 ## SURGERY

Positioning

The patients were placed in the prone jackknife position.

Technique

Anesthesia was at the patient's choice either spinal or general.

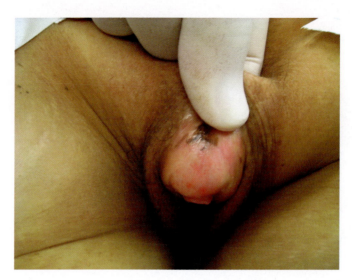

Figure 24.1 Anterior rectocele.

The surgical technique was a perineal approach, through a U-shaped incision (Figs. 24.1 and 24.2). Dissection was undertaken in a cephalad direction to reach the vaginal cupola (Fig. 24.3) after which trapezoid strip of posterior redundant vaginal wall was resected (Fig. 24.4). The posterior vaginal wall was closed by a running suture of 3-0 Polyglactin 910 (Fig. 24.5) including closure of the dead spaces between the rectal and the vaginal walls (Fig. 24.6). A levator plication was undertaken by placing two single stitches of 2-0 Prolene. A perineoplasty was performed on an individual basis to prevent bulging of the perineal body during push (Fig. 24.6). Ultimately the skin was fully closed, without drainage (Fig. 24.7).

Combined procedures for hemorrhoidectomy and/or fissure were undertaken at the same time of surgery.

POSTOPERATIVE MANAGEMENT

Patients were usually discharged on day 2 although oral antibiotics were continued for 5 postoperative days. Initially intravenous analgesia was delivered (50 mg of Diclofenac each 8 hours) after which oral analgesia was used and was maintained on demand after hospital discharge.

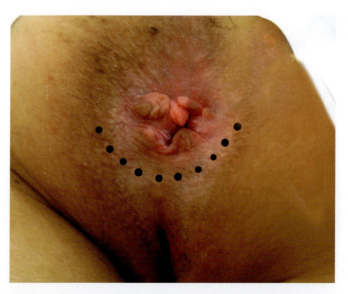

Figure 24.2 Perineal U-shaped incision.

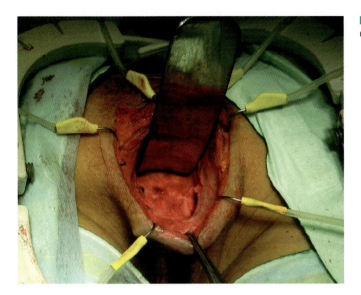

Figure 24.3 Rectovaginal septum dissection.

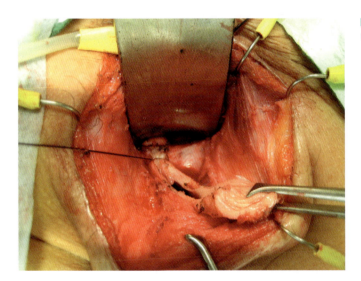

Figure 24.4 Redundant rectovaginal wall resection.

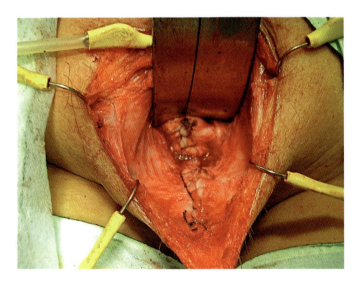

Figure 24.5 Vaginal wall running suture.

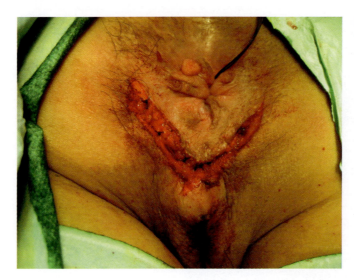

Figure 24.6 Perineoplasty and wound closure.

Clear fluids were started on the first postoperative day. On day 2, a normal diet plus psyllium supplement was begun. Imaging control at 4 months postoperation was undertaken to verify surgical results.

COMPLICATIONS

Two complications occurred from this personal series of 52 patients. One distal rectovaginal fistula that healed after a rectal advancement flap and one wound hematoma that needed partial opening of the perineal wound to facilitate drainage.

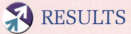 RESULTS

See Table 24.1.

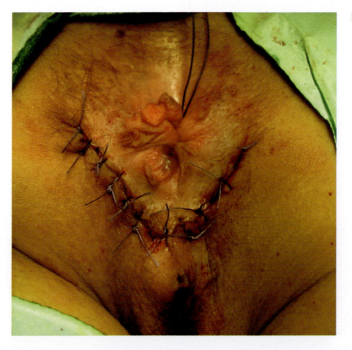

Figure 24.7 Full skin closure.

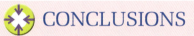

TABLE 24.1

Author	N	Technique	Results	%	Complications %
Sullivan et al. (1967)	151	Transrrectal	Excellent/good	79.5	12.5
Khubchandani (1983)	59	Transrrectal	Excellent/good		35.5
Block (1986)	60	Transrrectal	Excellent/good	77	–
Sehapayak (1985)	355	Transrrectal	Excellent/good	84.5	5.6
Arnold et al. (1990)	35	Transrrectal	Excellent/good	80	34.2
Sarles et al. (1991)	39	Transrrectal	Excellent/good	95	NS
Janssen et al. (1994)	76	Transrrectal	Excellent/good	92 (87)*	2.6
Kubchandani (1997)	123	Transrrectal	Excellent/good	82	3
Redding (1964)	20	Transvaginal	Excellent/good	100	5
Pitchford (1967)	44	Transvaginal	Excellent/good	NS	0
Arnold et al. (1990)	29	Transvaginal	Excellent/good	80	31
Mellgren et al. (1995)	25	Transvaginal	Excellent/good	88	20
Trompetto (1997)	53	Transvaginal	Excellent/good	100	5
Watson (1996)	9	Transperineal	Excellent/good	80	—
Trompetto (1996)	102	Transperineal	Excellent/good	85	15
Misici (1998)	44	Transperineal	Excellent/good	—	—
Rosato GO (2004)	52	Transperineal	Excellent/good	96.2	3.8

*After one year follow-up.

CONCLUSIONS

The transperineal approach is a safe and effective surgical option to treat anterior rectocele as a unique pelvic floor dysfunction. However, if clinically warranted, simultaneous perianal conditions such as hemorrhoids and fissures can be addressed.

Other surgical options are available such as mesh suspension and stapled transanal rectal resection. The latter procedure simultaneously corrects both the rectocele and the recto-anal-intussception.

References and Recommended Readings

1. Sehapayak S. Transrrectal repair of rectocele: an extended armamentarium of colorectal surgeons. A report of 355 cases. *Dis Colon Rectum* 1985;28:422–33.
2. Arnold MW, Stewart WRC, Aguilar PS. Rectocele repair: four years experience. *Dis Colon Rectum* 1990;33:684–7.
3. Janssen LWM, van Dijke CF. Selection criteria for anterior rectal wall repair in symptomatic rectocele and anterior rectal wall prolapse. *Dis colon Rectum* 1994;37:1100–7.
4. Kubchandani IT, Clancy J, Rosen L, et al. Endorectal repair of rectocele revisited. *Br Jr Surg* 1997;84(1):89–91.
5. Pitchford CA. Rectocele: a cause of anorectal pathologic changes in women. *Dis Colon Rectum* 1967;10:464–6.
6. Mellgren A, Anzén B, Nilsson BY, et al. Results of rectocele repair, a prospective study. *Dis Colon Rectum* 1995;38:7–13.
7. Watson SJ, Loder PB, Halligan S, et al. Transperineal repair of symptomatic rectocele with Marlex mesh: a clinical, physiological and radiologic assessment of treatment. *J Am Coll Surg* 1996;183:257–61.
8. Misici R, Primo Feitosa JN. Transperineal treatment of recurrent anterior rectocele using Marlex mesh. Annals of the 5th Biennial Course International Meeting of Coloproctology, Ivrea, Italy; 1998.
9. Berman IR, Harris MS, Rabeler MB. Delorme's transrectal excision for internal rectal prolapse: patient selection, technique, and three-year follow-up. *Dis Colon Rectum* 1990;33:573–80.
10. Boccasanta P, Carriero A, Stuto A, Caviglia A. Stapled rectal resection for obstructed defecation. A prospective multicenter trial. *Dis Colon Rectum* 2004;47:1285–97.
11. Cali RL, Christensen MA, Blatchford GJ, Thorson AG. Rectoceles. *Semin Col Rectal Surg* 1992;3(2):132–7.
12. Khubchandamni IT, Sheets JA, Stasik JJ, Hakki AR. Endorectal repair of rectocele. *Dis Colon Rectum* 1983;26:792–6.
13. Longo A. Obstructed defecation because of rectal pathologies. Novel surgical treatment: stapled transanal rectal resection (STARR) – Syllabus 15° Annual Colorectal Disease Symposium, February 12–14, 2004.
14. Lucas JD, Landy LB. The gynaecologist's approach to anterior rectoceles. *Semin Col Rectal Surg* 1992;3(2):138–43.
15. Redding MD. The relaxed perineum and anorectal disease. *Dis Colon Rectum* 1965;8:279.
16. Rosato GO. Rectocele anterior. Tratamiento mediante el abordaje transperineal. *Rev Argent Coloproctologia* 1998;9(2):39–43.
17. Sarles JC, Arnaud A, Selezneff I, Olivier S. Endorectal repair of rectocele. *Int J Color Dis* 1989;4:167–71.
18. Schultz I, Mellgren A, Dolk A, et al. Continence is improved after Ripstein's rectopexy: different mechanisms in rectal prolapse and rectal intussusception? *Dis Colon Rectum* 1996;39:300–6.
19. Senagore AJ, Luchtefeld MA, Mac Keigan JM. Rectopexy. *J Laparoendosc Surg* 1993;3:339–43.
20. Sielezneff I, Malouf A, Cesari J, et al. Selection criteria for internal rectal prolapse repair by Delorme's transrectal excision. *Dis Colon Rectum* 1999;42:367–73.
21. Sullivan ES, Leaverton GH, Hardwik CE. Transrrectal perineal repair: an adjunct to improved function after anorectal surgery. *Dis Colon Rectum* 1968;1:106–14.

25 Repair with Mesh

Clifford Simmang and Nell Maloney

Rectoceles are a pelvic floor disorder that present as a weakness in the rectovaginal septum causing herniation or bulging into the vagina. The significance of finding a rectocele is poorly understood but may contribute to the problem of obstructed outlet defecation. Rectoceles are an acquired condition that begins as a gradual thinning which then may progresses. Patients with symptomatic rectoceles are predominantly vaginally parous women, who complain of difficult evacuation with straining and digital manipulation to facilitate having a bowel movement (1,2). Although the etiology is unknown, rectocele formation has been associated with chronic constipation with straining against a weakened rectovaginal septum. The first step in management should be optimizing bowel consistency with bulking agents, dietary fiber, and hydration (1–3).

Evaluation of a rectocele begins with physical examination. On digital rectal examination, the rectocele is detected as a laxity in the anterior wall of the rectum. The examination should be performed on women with specific complaints including feeling a bulge in the vagina or in those patients who describe splinting by placing a finger into the vagina to defecate. Rectocele and other pelvic floor abnormalities may be more easily demonstrated by having the patient examined in the standing position. The patient can then confirm whether the observed bulge is noticeable with straining during defecation requiring splinting for evacuation.

Fluoroscopic defecography allows measurement of the bulge as well as confirms trapping of barium consistent with the patient history. Rectoceles less than 2 cm in size are generally considered to be not clinically significant, whereas rectoceles greater than 3 cm are thought to be abnormal. Although larger rectoceles are more likely to trap barium, size is not correlated with degree of symptoms or with outcome of rectocele repair (2,4,5). Preoperative evaluation should also include consideration for colonoscopy for cancer screening in appropriate patients. Sitz Marker study may also be useful in distinguishing slow transit constipation, which may need to be treated prior to attempting surgical repair of the rectocele. Finally, attempts to standardize rectocele evaluation and staging should be performed using the validated pelvic organ prolapse quantification system.

The use of mesh in rectocele repair was described initially in 1962 by Adler. Interest in mesh support of the rectovaginal septum has been driven by both the high recurrence rates and operative failure with the traditional tissue repair of rectocele and the evolution of mesh itself. Placement of mesh to reinforce the facial repair of the rectovaginal septum has been used more frequently in the past few years. Use of mesh to provide support for the rectovaginal septum must take into consideration maintenance of bowel continence and sexual function.

 PREOPERATIVE PLANNING

Synthetic Materials

Success of synthetic mesh is related to the ability of the mesh to become incorporated into host tissue with minimal inflammation with early infiltration of fibroblasts. Two features of the mesh are important in achieving this goal: porosity and stiffness. Standard classification of porosity by Amid as described for abdominal wall surgery is as follows (6):

> Type 1: macroporous mesh. Pore size is in excess of 75 nm allowing infiltration of macrophages, fibroblasts, new blood vessels, and collagen fibers
> Type 2: microporous mesh. Pore size is <10 nm.
> Type 3: macroporous/microporous due to multifilament component. These include the woven mesh products.
> Type 4: submicronic pores.

Macrophage infiltration decreases infective risk and therefore decreases chance of erosion or rejection. Nonabsorbable synthetic mesh has been plagued by problems with mesh extrusion and erosion as well as postoperative dyspareunia. Extrusion is an early postoperative complication likely related to surgical technique, local ischemia, or infection. Erosion is a more chronic problem of the prolonged presence of a foreign body. Absorbable mesh products used for repair of rectoceles have less issue with extrusion and erosion in case series with relatively short follow-up, but prospective studies with long-term follow-up are lacking.

Biological Materials

Because of the complications related to synthetic material, there has been interest in the use of biologics to augment the rectovaginal septum. Biologic grafts are grouped into three classes: allografts, autografts, and xenografts. While complications of mesh erosion and dyspareunia have not been identified in studies using these materials, the high failure rate and recurrence remains a problem (7,8).

Preoperative Planning and Care

For either approach, patients should have a bowel prep performed preoperatively. Use of vaginal estrogen is recommended for a period of 8 weeks preoperatively. Patients are positioned in lithotomy and are catheterized prior to starting the operation.

 SURGERY

Operative Approach

Unlike traditional rectocele repair where there are three accepted approaches—transanal, transperineal, and transvaginal—mesh repair of the rectovaginal septum is performed either by the transvaginal or transperineal approach. Broaching the rectal mucosa is viewed by most authors to be a contraindication for placing mesh due to the unacceptably high chance of mesh infection.

Transperineal Approach

A transverse perineal incision is made and local anesthesia with epinephrine is injected into the rectovaginal septum to help control bleeding and to define the plane. Meticulous dissection of the rectovaginal septum with careful attention to hemostasis is performed up to the level of the posterior fornix. Buttonholes in the vaginal wall may be repaired with Vicryl suture. A piece of mesh measuring between 6 and 8 cm long and approximately 4 cm wide is tailored to fit into the space developed by dissection. The graft is then secured to the levators on either side. Excess mesh is trimmed to avoid exposure and the wound is closed with interrupted Vicryl suture (9–11).

Transvaginal Approach

A transverse incision is made at the mucocutaneous border of the vaginal introitus and the posterior vaginal wall. Local anesthetic with epinephrine is injected into the rectovaginal septum to help control bleeding and to define the plane. Dissection is performed up to the posterior fornix. Once the levator muscles are identified, a piece of mesh measuring 6–8 cm by approximately 4 cm is inserted into the space developed by the dissection. The mesh is secured to the levator muscles, the rectovaginal connective tissue, and the perineal body using Vicryl suture. Redundant vaginal mucosa is trimmed and the incision is closed using interrupted Vicryl suture (12).

Novel Approaches

Reinforcement of the entire length of the rectovaginal septum has been described by D'hoore using both laparoscopic and perineal approach (13). This technique involves a laparoscopic dissection of the rectovaginal septum without mobilization of the lateral stalks of the rectum. The perineum is then opened with a small incision and the dissection continued until the abdominal part of the dissection is reached. A long strip of mesh is then inserted and secured at four points: the perineal body, the paracolpium, the rectum above and below the Douglass fold, and to the sacral promontory.

 # POSTOPERATIVE MANAGEMENT

Most patients are kept overnight for observation. The Foley catheter may be removed postoperatively. Patients should be counseled to avoid sexual intercourse for 8 weeks postoperatively. Topical estrogen therapy may need to be used postoperatively in patients with vaginal atrophy.

 # CONCLUSIONS

Current available studies are not uniform with respect to patient selection, the type of mesh used for repair, and surgical approach. Rectocele repair using mesh augmentation needs further prospective study to determine the best mesh for support of the rectovaginal septum and to determine the equivalence or superiority over traditional repairs.

Recommended References and Readings

1. Wolff BG, Fleshman JW, Beck DE. The ASCRS Textbook of Colon and Rectal Surgery. New York: Springer, 2007.
2. Gordon PH, Nivatvongs S. Principles and Practice of Surgery for the colon, Rectum and Anus. 3rd ed. New York: Informa Healthcare USA, 2007.
3. de Tayrac R, Picone O, Chauveaud-Lambling A, et al. A 2-year anatomical and functional assessment of transvaginal rectocele repair using a polypropylene mesh. *Int Urogynecol J* 2006;17:100–5.
4. van Dam JH, Ginai AZ, Gosselink MJ, et al. Role of defecography in predicting outcome of rectocele repair. *Dis Colon Rectum* 1997;40:201–7.
5. Halligan S, Bartram CI. Is Barium trapping in rectoceles significant? *Dis Colon Rectum* 1995;38:764–8.
6. Birch C. The use of prosthetics in pelvic reconstructive surgery. *Best Prac Res Clin Obstet Gynaecol* 2005;19:979–91.

7. Huebner M, Hsu Y, Fenner DE. The use of graft materials in vaginal pelvic floor surgery. *Int J Gynec Obst* 2006;92:279–288.

8. Altman D, Mellegren A, Zetterstrom J. Rectocele repair using biomaterial augmentation: Current Documentation and Clinical experience. *Obstet Gynecol Surg* 2005;60:753–60.

9. Watson SJ, Loder PB, Halligan S, et al. Transperineal repair of symptomatic rectocele with Marlex mesh: a clinical, physiological and radiological assessment of treatment. *J Am Coll Surg* 1996;183(3):257–61.

10. Mercer-Jones MA, Sprowson A, Varma JS. Outcome after transperineal mesh repair of rectocele: a case series. *Dis Colon Rectum* 2004;47:864–8.

11. Leventoglu S, Bulent Mentes B, Akin M, et al. Transperineal rectocele repair with polyglycolic acid mesh: a case series. *Dis Colon Rectum* 2007;50:2085–92.

12. Altman D, Zetterstrom J, Lopez A, et al. Functional and Anatomic outcome after transvaginal rectocele repair using collagen mesh: A prospective study. *Dis Colon Rectum* 2005;48:1233–42.

13. D'Hoore A, Vanbeckevoort D, Penninckx F. Clinical, physiological and radiological assessment of the rectovaginal septum reinforcement with mesh for complex rectocele. *Br J Surg* 2008;95:1264–72.

26 STARR

David Jayne and Antonio Longo

Introduction

Stapled transanal rectal resection (STARR) was described in 2001 as a new technique for the treatment of obstructed defecation associated with distal rectal prolapse (rectocele, intussusception, mucohemorrhoidal prolapse). The original technique involved a double-stapling procedure using two PPH-01® staplers (Ethicon Endosurgery, Europe) to produce a circumferential, full-thickness rectal resection. This technique is referred to as PPH-STARR, or simply STARR. More recently, a reloadable-stapling device specifically designed for STARR has been introduced, the Contour30® Transtar (Ethicon Endosurgery), which allows a sequential full-thickness circumferential rectal resection to be performed. This procedure is referred to as Transtar to distinguish it from PPH-STARR and is described in a subsequent chapter.

INDICATIONS/CONTRAINDICATIONS

Indications

STARR is advocated as a treatment option for patients suffering from obstructed defecation syndrome (ODS) because of defined anatomical defects of the distal, subperitoneal rectum. These anatomical defects are readily appreciated on dynamic pelvic floor imaging, by either defecography or magnetic resonance imaging, as a redundancy of the distal rectum, which forms a mechanical obstruction impeding effective rectal evacuation. Most commonly, the mechanical obstruction manifests as a combination of the following:

- rectocele
- distal rectal intussusception
- mucohemorrhoidal prolapse

Frequently, pathological descent of the perineum is present. In 30–40% of cases there will be coexistent other pelvic organ prolapse, which may include enterocele, sigmoidocele, and/or urogenital prolapse. Awareness of other pelvic floor pathology is important is ensuring correct patient selection and maximizing postoperative outcomes.

Whether STARR is of benefit in patients with anismus (pelvic floor dyssynergia) with coexisting rectal redundancy is controversial (1). A trial of conservative treatment with biofeedback therapy, and possibly combining botulinum toxin, should be considered before contemplating STARR.

Contraindications

The following absolute and relative contraindications have been suggested for STARR (2):

Absolute contraindications:

- active anorectal sepsis (abscess, fistula, etc.)
- concurrent anorectal pathology, including anal stenosis
- proctitis (inflammatory bowel disease, radiation proctitis)
- chronic diarrhea

Relative contraindications:

- presence of foreign material adjacent to the rectum (such as prosthetic mesh from a previous rectocele repair or pelvic floor resuspension)
- previous anterior resection or transanal surgery with rectal anastomosis
- concurrent psychiatric disorder

There has been much debate about the role of enteroceles in obstructed defecation and whether they precluded treatment with STARR. Initial concerns regarding iatrogenic injury to the small bowel have proven to be unjustified. Current opinion is that STARR is safe in the presence of an enterocele provided appropriate precautions are taken. If doubt remains, laparoscopic reduction of the small bowel can be performed at the same time as STARR (3).

Patients with constipation-predominant irritable bowel syndrome are a difficult group in whom to predict outcome. Provided mechanical outlet obstruction can be demonstrated on dynamic imaging then STARR may be a reasonable option.

Caution should also be exercised in patients with documented anal sphincter dysfunction. Although defecatory urgency is a recognized feature in approximately 20–40% of patients with ODS, there is a definite incidence of de novo urgency that follows STARR. The exact mechanism for this is unclear, but in the majority of cases it is self-limiting with resolution within 6–12 weeks. It is probable that it is those patients with preexisting anal sphincter dysfunction who are most vulnerable to this complication, and should be appropriately counseled if STARR is considered.

PREOPERATIVE PLANNING

All patients presenting with ODS should have their symptoms quantified using a validated scoring system (4,5). Any history of transanal surgery or obstetric trauma should be documented, and a clinical examination should be performed to assess anal sphincter function, document the presence of rectocele and intussusception, and to exclude other anorectal pathology. Examination of the urogenital organs, preferably in conjunction with a urogynecologist, should be undertaken if relevant symptoms are present. The presence of rectal redundancy, with internal prolapse with or without rectocele, should be verified by dynamic pelvic floor imaging in the form of defecography or dynamic magnetic resonance imaging. If anal sphincter dysfunction is suspected, either on history or on examination, formal evaluation by anorectal manometry, anal electromyography, and endoanal ultrasound is recommended.

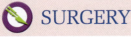 SURGERY

STARR can be performed under either spinal or general anesthesia. The lower bowel should be prepared by administration of a phosphate enema to ensure that the rectum

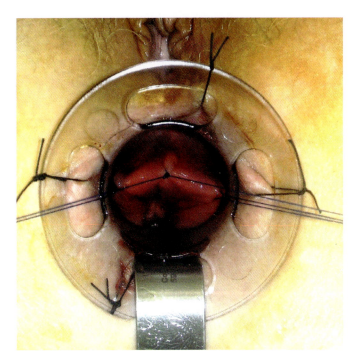

Figure 26.1 STARR: anterior prolapse. Three traction sutures are placed at the 10, 12, and 2 o'clock positions. The two ends of the 12 o'clock suture are tied separately to the 10 and 2 o'clock sutures. A spatula is inserted between the circular anal dilator (CAD) and the posterior anorectum to protect it during the anterior resection.

is empty. The patient is placed on the operating table in the supine position. The legs are supported in stirrups with the hips flexed to at least 90 degrees and the table tilted to 30 degree head-down for maximal exposure of the perineum. A single dose of broad-spectrum perioperative antibiotics is administered. An examination under anesthesia is performed to confirm the presence of internal prolapse with or without rectocele and to exclude coexistent pathology and other pelvic organ prolapse.

The following describes the steps involved in the double-stapled PPH-01 STARR procedure:

1. Four 1/0 silk sutures are placed at the anal verge in the 12, 3, 6, and 9 o'clock positions. Applying traction on the sutures, the anal canal is gently dilated with the anal dilator, following which the CAD33 is introduced and secured at the anal verge with the sutures.

2. The apex of the prolapse is identified with a dry swab inserted into the rectum and then withdrawn. Three 2/0 prolene traction sutures are placed at the 10, 12, and 2 o'clock positions. The two ends of the 12 o'clock suture are separated and one each tied with the 10 and 2 o'clock sutures such that in total two traction sutures are used to deliver the internal prolapse. A spatula is inserted into the anorectum at the 6 o'clock position between the posterior lip of the CAD33 and the anal canal to exclude the posterior anorectum (Fig. 26.1).

3. A fully opened PPH-01 stapler is inserted into the rectum such that its anvil lies beyond the area of prolapse. The two traction sutures are passed through the lateral channels in the stapler and are used to deliver the prolapse into the stapler housing. Keeping the stapler in line with the anal canal at all times, the stapler is closed. A digital vaginal examination is performed to ensure that the vaginal wall has not been inadvertently incorporated into the stapler. Thirty seconds is allowed for tissue compression before firing the stapler.

4. The stapler is opened by one half-turn of the opening mechanism and withdrawn. The resected specimen is retrieved from the stapler housing and should include a full-thickness resection of the anterior rectum (Fig. 26.2). A mucosal "bridge" linking the lateral extent of the resection is frequently present in the 6 o'clock position and should be divided (Fig. 26.3). This completes the anterior resection.

5. The posterior resection is performed in a similar manner. Two or three traction sutures are placed incorporating the lateral extent of the previous anterior staple line and the

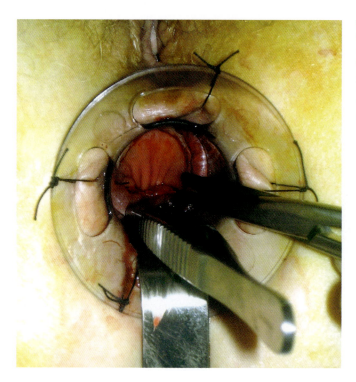

Figure 26.2 Posterior mucosal bridge. Following resection of the anterior prolapse a mucosal bridge is often present joining the lateral extents of the stapled anastomosis. This bridge is divided before performing the posterior resection.

posterior mid-point of the prolapse. The ends of the middle suture are separated and each end is tied with the more laterally placed sutures. A spatula is placed at the 12 o'clock position to exclude the anterior rectum (Fig. 26.4). A second PPH-01 stapler is introduced, the prolapse is delivered with the traction sutures, and the stapler is fired to complete the full-thickness, circumferential resection. Any anterior mucosal bridge is divided. A careful inspection is made of the circumferential staple line, and the lateral "dog-ears" and any bleeding points are under-run with 3/0 Vicryl to complete the operation.

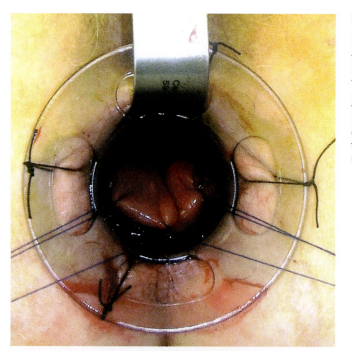

Figure 26.3 STARR: posterior prolapse. Three traction sutures are placed at the lateral extents of the anterior stapled anastomosis and at the 6 o'clock position. The two ends of the 6 o'clock suture are tied separately to the other two sutures. A spatula is inserted between the circular anal dilator (CAD) and the anterior anorectum to protect it during the posterior resection.

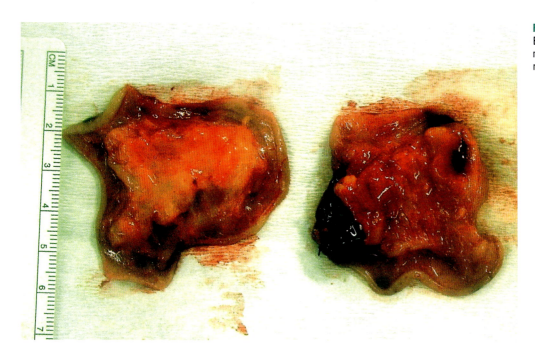

Figure 26.4 Resection specimens. Both anterior and posterior specimens consist of a full-thickness rectal resection.

POSTOPERATIVE MANAGEMENT

The following "package" of postoperative care is recommended to reduce complications and to maximize recovery:

- The patient is allowed a normal diet as soon as tolerated and is encouraged to mobilize
- Regular oral analgesia is administered, but should be nonconstipating, combining non-opioid with non–steroidal anti-inflammatory agents.
- Stool bulking agents and softeners should be available to allow defecation of a soft stool without excessive straining
- No postoperative antibiotics are required unless there is a specific indication

Patients are discharged when they are comfortable, have passed urine, and are mobile. Many patients are fit for discharged on the first postoperative, with the majority being discharged by the second postoperative day.

COMPLICATIONS

Possible complications related to STARR are listed below and categorized into early (immediate postoperative) and late complications. The incidence of complications is taken from the European STARR Registry database (6).

Early Complications

- Bleeding: reported in 5% of cases. Most episodes are of minor, self-limiting bleeding, not requiring transfusion or intervention. Rare cases of mesorectal hemorrhage/hematoma have been described.
- Pain: postoperative discomfort/pain is to be expected for the first few days. The majority of patients are pain free by the 10th postoperative day. Excessive or protracted discomfort should precipitate examination under anesthesia to exclude a septic or other complication.
- Urinary retention: reported in 7% of cases and is related to excessive intraoperative fluid administration and inadequate postoperative analgesia.

- Staple line dehiscence: reported in 3% of cases. Most staple line dehiscences are minor, presenting as an anastomotic "ulcer" with pain, bleeding, or discharge a few days following surgery; surgical intervention is seldom required.
- Septic complications: like any transanal excisional surgery, there is a risk of septic complications. Septic complications have been reported in 4% of cases, but are usually localized and self-limiting. A few serious septic complications have been reported in the literature, often as a consequence of staple line dehiscence.

Late Complications

- Defecatory urgency: reported in up to 20% of cases in the early postoperative period, but interpretation is difficult due to the existence of urgency as a feature of the preoperative symptom complex. It may be related to anal dilatation at the time of surgery, the presence of a low rectal anastomosis, or a reduction in capacity of the neorectum. Most cases of urgency resolve without intervention by 3 months postoperatively. Persistent urgency requires further investigation to exclude complications, such as retained staples, and to evaluate anal sphincter function.
- Fecal incontinence: reported in 1.8% of cases. It is usually associated with defecatory urgency and is more likely to occur in patients with preexisting anal sphincter dysfunction.
- Anastomotic stricture: reported in 0.6% of cases and usually responds to simple dilatation.
- Dyspareunia: a rare complication, reported in 0.1% of cases. The low incidence is an advantage in comparison to the rates of dyspareunia reported after transvaginal rectocele repair.
- Rectovaginal fistula: a much feared complication of STARR at the time of its introduction, but experience has shown the incidence to be very low; a few reports have appeared in the literature (1,7).

RESULTS

Published data on the outcomes following STARR are mainly limited to personal series (1,8–10) and multicenter studies (11–13). Comparison of outcomes is made difficult due to variations in patient selection, operative technique, and the relatively short length of follow-up. Three multicenter studies from Italy (13), Spain (11), and France (12) have reported similar results, with significant reductions in constipation score following STARR and satisfactory outcomes in excess of 80% of patients. Although the data suggest that STARR is effective, the morbidity associated with the procedure is variously reported between 15% and 36% (8,14). However, the majority of complications appear to be minor in nature and are self-limiting. They include postoperative bleeding, protracted anorectal pain, defecatory urgency, and minor incontinence, although rectovaginal fistula and serious septic complications have been described (1,7). Only one randomized controlled trial of STARR has been reported, and compared it with biofeedback, with a significant benefit observed in the STARR group (14). Those studies that have analyzed radiological parameters pre- and post-STARR have shown that the procedure restores normal anorectal anatomy with correction of rectocele and intussusception (8,11). Anatomical correction appears to correlate with symptomatic improvement, supporting the theory behind STARR.

In 2006, the National Institute of Clinical Health and Excellence (NICE) in the United Kingdom produced its guidance on STARR and concluded "current evidence on the safety and efficacy of STARR does not appear adequate for this procedure to be used without special arrangements and for audit or research" (15). Partially in response to this statement, a European collaboration involving the United Kingdom, Italy, and Germany was established to assess the short-term safety and efficacy of STARR (6). The European STARR Registry commenced recruitment in 2006 and completed 1-year follow-up in 2008, by which time data on more than 2,800 patients and procedures had been amassed. At 6-month follow-up, there was a significant improvement in both the obstructed defecation score and the symptom severity score, which was maintained at 12 months. Similarly, a significant improvement in Quality of Life (QoL) outcomes

(PAQ-QoL, ED-5Q) was observed. The overall morbidity rate was 36%, but consisted largely of minor, self-limiting complications. Septic complications were rare and there was no mortality. Defecatory urgency was observed in 20% of patients post-STARR but was also noted in more than 30% of cases preoperatively. There was a significant improvement in the fecal incontinence score for the whole cohort (16). Although the majority of patients recruited to the Registry were from Italy, similar improvements in obstructed defecation symptoms and QoL were observed in all three contributing countries. The notable exception was a trend to worse incontinence score in the UK subgroup, which was not present in the Italian or German data set. The final analysis of the Registry data was published in 2009 and concluded that STARR is an effective treatment option for obstructed defecation associated with intussusception/rectocele, with an acceptable rate of morbidity.

 # CONCLUSIONS

STARR is a novel treatment for ODS associated with intussusception with or without rectocele. Current evidence would suggest that it is effective, at least in the short term, with reduction in constipation symptoms and improvement in QoL. Proper consideration should be given to patient selection, surgeon training, and operative technique, to maximize outcomes and prevent morbidity. The results of additional trials and registries are eagerly awaited to help determine the role of the STARR procedure in the treatment of ODS.

Suggested Reading

Jayne D, Stuto A, eds. *Transanal Stapling Techniques for Anorectal Prolapse.* London: Springer-Verlag, 2009.

Recommended References and Readings

1. Gagliardi G, Pescatori M, Altomare DF, et al. Results, outcome predictors, and complications after stapled transanal rectal resection for obstructed defecation. *Dis Colon Rectum* 2008; 51(2):186–95.
2. Corman ML, Carriero A, Hager T, et al. Consensus conference on the stapled transanal rectal resection (STARR) for disordered defecation. *Colorectal Dis* 2006;8:98–101.
3. Petersen S, Hellmich G, Schuster A, et al. Stapled transanal rectal resection under laparoscopic surveillance for rectocele and concomitant enterocele. *Dis Colon Rectum* 2006;49:685–9.
4. Altomore DF, Spazzafuma L, Rinaldi M, et al. Set-up and statistical validation of a new scoring system for obstructed defecation syndrome. *Colorectal Dis* 2008;10:84–8.
5. Agarchan F, Chen T, Pfeifer J, et al. A constipation scoring system to simplify evaluation and management of constipated patients. *Dis Colon Rectum* 1996;39:681–5.
6. Jayne D, Schwandner O, Stuto A. Stapled transanal rectal resection for obstructed defecation syndrome: one-year results of the European STARR Registry. *Dis Colon Rect* 2009;52:1205–12.
7. Bassi R, Rademacher J, Savoia A. Rectovaginal fistula after STARR procedure complicated by haematoma of the posterior vaginal wall: report of a case. *Techn Coloproctol* 2006;10:361–3.
8. Dindo D, Weishaupt D, Lehmann K, et al. Clinical and morphologic correlation after stapled transanal rectal resection for obstructed defecation syndrome. *Dis Colon Rectum* 2008;51:1768–74.
9. Frascio M, Stabilini C, Ricci B, et al. Stapled transanal rectal resection for outlet obstruction syndrome: results and follow-up. *World J Surg* 2008;32:1110–15.
10. Pechlivanides G, Tsiaoussis J, Athanasakis E, et al. Stapled transanal rectal resection (STARR) to reverse the anatomic disorders of pelvic floor dyssynergia. *World J Surg* 2007;31:1329–35.
11. Arroyo A, Gonzalez-Argente FX, Garcia-Domingo M, et al. Prospective multicentre clinical trial of stapled transanal rectal resection for obstructive defaecation syndrome. *Br J Surg* 2008; 95:1521–7.
12. Slim K, Mezoughi S, Launay-Savary MV, et al. Repair of rectocele using the stapled transanal rectal resection (STARR) technique: intermediate results from a multicenter French study. *J de Chir* 2008;145:27–31.
13. Boccasanta P, Venturi M, Stuto A, et al. Stapled transanal rectal resection for outlet obstruction: a prospective, multicenter trial. *Dis Colon Rectum* 2004;47:1285–97.
14. Lehur PA, Stuto A, Fantoli M, et al. Outcomes of stapled transanal rectal resection vs. biofeedback for the treatment of outlet obstruction associated with rectal intussusception and rectocele: a multicenter, randomized, controlled trial. *Dis Colon Rectum* 2008;51:1611–18.
15. National Institute for Health and Clinical Excellence (NICE). Interventional procedure guidance 169: stapled transanal rectal resection for obstructed defaecation syndrome 2006. www.nice.org.uk
16. Jorge JMN, Wexner S. Etiology and management of fecal incontinence. *Dis Colon Rectum* 1993;36:77–97.

27 Transtar

David Jayne and Antonio Longo

Introduction

This chapter on Contour30® Transtar (Ethicon Endosurgery Inc., Cincinnati, OH, USA) should be read in conjunction with that on *Rectocele: STARR*. Both STARR and Transtar are procedures for the correction of obstructed defecation associated with intussusception with or without rectocele. In essence, both procedures aim to produce the same surgical outcome, namely resection of the distal rectal redundancy with restoration of normal anorectal anatomy. STARR was the procedure first described, prior to the introduction of the specially designed Contour30® stapling device, and used two PPH-01 staplers. The PPH-01 stapler had been designed for the treatment of prolapsing hemorrhoids and its application to internal prolapse and rectocele was not without potential drawbacks. It was for this reason that a specific stapler, the Contour30®, was designed for Transtar. The Contour30® consists of a curved stapling device that holds a reloadable cartridge (Fig. 27.1). When deployed, the stapler simultaneously fires three staple lines and cuts the contained tissue. The potential benefits of the Contour30® Transtar over the PPH-01 STARR include:

- An ability to resect a greater volume of prolapse
- An ability to tailor the extent of the prolapse resection to the individual patient
- Improved visibility of the resection during the procedure
- A true full-thickness, circumferential resection

In this chapter, the term Transtar will be used to denote transanal circumferential rectal resection with the Contour30® stapler.

INDICATIONS/CONTRAINDICATIONS

The indications and contraindications for Transtar are identical to those outlined for STARR. In summary, the patient should have symptoms consistent with obstructed defecation syndrome (ODS) and distal rectal redundancy in the form of intussusception with or without significant rectocele demonstrable on dynamic pelvic floor imaging. Ideally, the patient should have reasonable anal sphincter function. Transtar is contraindicated in the presence of other concomitant pathology that might predispose to poor anastomotic healing or the development of septic complications. Successful outcome is dependent on correct patient selection, which in turn demands thorough preoperative investigation.

Figure 27.1 Contour30® Transtar: the curved head of the Contour30 stapler with the reloadable cartridge containing three rows of staples separated by a cutting blade.

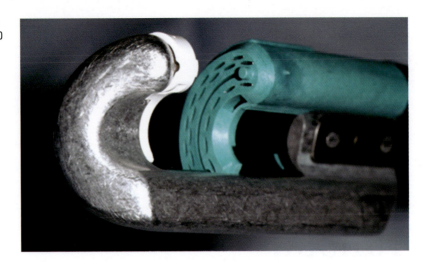

 ## PREOPERATIVE PLANNING

Like many operations for functional disorders, successful outcome is dependent on correct patient assessment and selection, which in turn demands thorough preoperative investigation. As a minimum, this should include quantification of symptoms using an appropriate scoring system (1,2), exclusion of coexistent pathology by appropriate colorectal imaging, assessment of pelvic floor anatomy by defecating proctogram or dynamic magnetic resonance imaging, and anorectal physiology and endoanal ultrasound. Once this information has been obtained, an informed decision can be made regarding the suitability of the patient for Transtar. No additional preoperative workup is required for Transtar as compared to PPH-STARR.

SURGERY

Transtar can be performed under either spinal or general anesthesia. The lower bowel should be prepared by administration of a phosphate enema to ensure that the anorectum is empty. The patient is placed on the operating table in the supine position. The legs are supported in stirrups with the hips flexed to at least 90 degrees and the table tilted to 30 degree head-down for maximal exposure of the perineum. A single dose of broad-spectrum perioperative antibiotics is administered. An examination under anesthesia is performed to confirm the presence of internal prolapse with or without rectocele and to exclude coexistent pathology and other pelvic organ prolapse.

The following describes the steps involved in the Transtar procedure:

1. The anal canal is gently dilated and the circular anal dilator is inserted and secured with 1/0 silk sutures to the anal verge.
2. The extent and apex of the internal rectal prolapse are assessed by insertion and withdrawal of a dry swab.
3. Prolene traction sutures (2/0) are placed circumferentially around the apex of the prolapse in the 2, 12, 10, 8, and 5 o'clock positions. Each suture is loosely tied and held by an artery forceps (Fig. 27.2).
4. A marking suture of 1/0 Vicryl is inserted to the depth of the prolapse to be resected at the 3 o'clock position. This suture is tied tightly and a loop is created toward the free end, through which the Transtar stapler can be passed.
5. The resection starts at the 3 o'clock marking suture with a radial firing of the stapler, which has the effect of "opening up" the prolapse (Fig. 27.3). The resection then

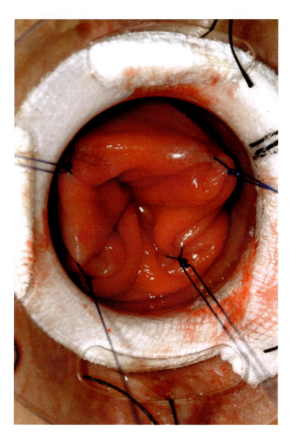

Figure 27.2 Traction sutures are placed at the apex of the prolapse in the 2, 10, 8, and 5 o'clock positions in preparation for resection.

proceeds in a clockwise manner from the 3 o'clock radial cut with traction applied to the appropriate traction sutures to bring the relevant portion of the prolapse into the jaws of the stapler (Fig. 27.4). After each firing the stapler cartridge is renewed in the Transtar device. A full-thickness circumferential rectal resection is obtained, usually with five or six firings of the stapler. Care is taken when completing the circumferential resection to ensure that the resection finishes at the same point as it

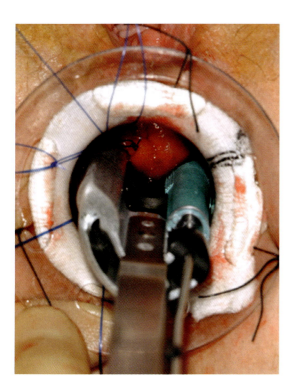

Figure 27.3 The Contour30 is inserted into the distal rectum and the first radial cut is performed at the 3 o'clock position to "open up" the prolapse.

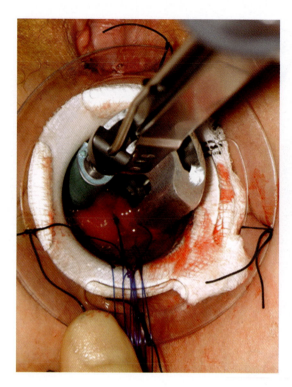

Figure 27.4 Circumferential full-thickness rectal resection is performed in an anticlockwise manner with successive firings of the Contour30.

commenced, that is, "spiraling" of the stapled anastomosis, either into or out of the rectum is avoided.

6. The resection specimen consists of a "sausage-shaped" piece of tissue, which should be of uniform dimensions throughout. If desired, the dimensions can be recorded and/or the specimen can be weighed (Fig. 27.5).

7. Hemostasis is secured with interrupted 3/0 Vicryl sutures. It is recommended to reinforce the points of potential weakness in the staple line, which occur at the areas of staple line intersection.

POSTOPERATIVE MANAGEMENT

Postoperative care is the same as for STARR. Patients are allowed a normal diet as soon as tolerated. Adequate analgesia is provided, avoiding constipating agents if possible. Stool-bulking agents and stool softeners are prescribed for 7 days. Postoperative antibiotics

Figure 27.5 The specimen consists of a "sausage-shaped" resection of distal rectum.

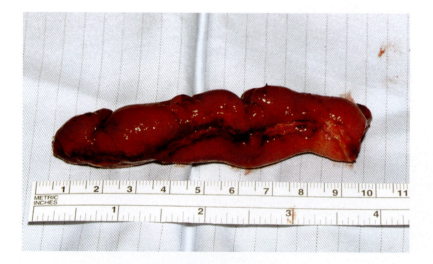

are not routinely administered. The majority of patients are fit for discharge the day following surgery or on the second postoperative day, provided they are comfortable, tolerating a normal diet, and are mobile and passing urine. All patients are routinely reviewed at 6 weeks in the outpatient clinic unless specific concerns demand otherwise.

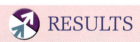 COMPLICATIONS

Possible complications following Transtar are the same as for STARR, although there is less information available on their incidence as the procedure has not been as widely or frequently performed. They include:

Early Complications

- Bleeding: most episodes are of minor, self-limiting bleeding, not requiring transfusion or intervention.
- Pain: postoperative discomfort/pain is to be expected for the first few days. The majority of patients are pain free by the 10th postoperative day. Excessive or protracted discomfort should precipitate examination under anesthesia to exclude a septic or other complication.
- Urinary retention: is related to excessive intraoperative fluid administration and inadequate postoperative analgesia.
- Staple line dehiscence: most staple line dehiscences are minor, presenting as an anastomotic "ulcer" with pain, bleeding, or discharge a few days following surgery. Surgical intervention is seldom required although rectovaginal fistula is an exception.
- Septic complications: like any transanal excisional surgery, there is a risk of septic complications, although if it occurs it is usually localized and self-limiting. Reports of serious septic complications exist (3).

Late Complications

- Defecatory urgency: the frequency of de novo defecatory urgency is difficult to assess given that it is a feature of the preoperative ODS symptomatology. Most cases of urgency resolve without intervention by 3 months postoperatively. Persistent urgency requires further investigation to exclude complications, such as retained staples, and to evaluate anal sphincter function. It does not appear that the rate of post-Transtar urgency is any greater than following STARR.
- Fecal incontinence: is usually associated with defecatory urgency and more likely to occur in patients with preexisting anal sphincter dysfunction.
- Anastomotic stricture: usually responds to simple dilatation.
- Dyspareunia: is a rare complication.
- Rectovaginal fistula: at the present time, the incidence of this complication appears to be very low, and no greater than that reported in the large observational studies on STARR.

RESULTS

The published evidence on Transtar is even more limited than STARR as it has only recently been introduced into clinical practice. Currently, it consists of three personal series (4–6) and one multicentre study (7). The first report was in 2008 from Renzi et al. (4) who reviewed the results of Transtar in 33 patients operated in 2006. A significant reduction in obstructed defecation score was reported at 6 months follow-up, with no major complications. Transtar was deemed to have been successful in 86.2% of cases. A European, multicentre, prospective study reported a similar successful outcome, with significant reduction in the obstructed defecation and symptom severity scores at 12 months follow-up (7). However, a 9% rate of intraoperative complications was noted, related to staple line dehiscence or "spiraling" of the circumferential anastomosis. The authors suggest that this relatively high rate of intraoperative complications may reflect an increased technical difficulty associated with Transtar. Postoperative complications occurred in 7% of cases, with three bleeding events, two of which required surgical intervention. A worsening of defecatory urgency was observed in 13% of patients at 3-month follow-up, but overall the incontinence score for the cohort had improved at 12 months.

One of the potential benefits of the Transtar over the PPH-STARR technique is the ability to resect a greater volume of prolapse. Wadhawan et al. (5) performed a retrospective comparison of PPH-STARR (25 patients) and Transtar (27 patients) with median follow-up of 12 and 6 months, respectively. Both techniques resulted in a significant reduction in the ODS score. Although Transtar resulted a significantly greater volume of prolapse resection, there was no difference between the two techniques in complications or symptom resolution; relief of ODS symptoms was observed in 64% following PPH-STARR and 67% following Transtar.

In a similar, but larger study, Isbert et al. (6) compared 150 patients (68 PPH-STARR with 82 Transtar) with 12-month follow-up. Morbidity was similar in both groups (7.3% PPH-STARR and 7.5% Transtar), although a trend to increased postoperative pain was noted following Transtar. Constipation scores were significantly reduced postoperatively in both the groups. Transtar resulted in a significantly greater volume of resected tissue, with an almost doubling in the specimen size. Despite this, there was no difference in the constipation scores at 12-month follow-up.

Thus, from the limited data available it would appear that the Transtar can be performed with similar morbidity to STARR, but perhaps with more technical difficulty. Like STARR, it produces a significant reduction in constipation symptoms, but the ability to perform a larger prolapse resection does not necessarily translate into improved outcomes. Whether this finding is because of the relatively small numbers studied to date or whether Transtar improves long-term outcomes remains to be determined.

 CONCLUSIONS

The Contour30® Transtar is specifically designed for the performance of stapled transanal rectal resection. It offers the potential benefits of improved visualization of resection, a true circumferential full-thickness resection, the ability to tailor the extent of resection to the individual patient, and the ability to resect more prolapse. Although limited evidence is available, it would appear to be a safe technique, with similar morbidity to PPH-STARR, and to produce a similar improvement in symptom resolution. As yet there is no evidence to support the concept that the larger prolapse resection achieved with Transtar translates into a better functional outcome.

Suggested Reading

Jayne D, Stuto A, eds. *Transanal Stapling Techniques for Anorectal Prolapse*. London: Springer-Verlag, 2009.

Recommended References and Readings

1. Altomore DF, Spazzafuma L, Rinaldi M, et al. Set-up and statistical validation of a new scoring system for obstructed defecation syndrome. *Colorectal Dis* 2008;10:84–8.
2. Agarchan F, Chen T, Pfeifer J, et al. A constipation scoring system to simplify evaluation and management of constipated patients. *Dis Colon Rect* 1996;39:681–5.
3. Schulte T, Bokelmann F, Jongen J, et al. Mediastinal and retro-/intraperitoneal emphysema after stapled transanal rectal resection (STARR-operation) using the Contour Transtar stapler in obstructive defecation syndrome. *Int J Colorectal Dis* 2008;23:1019–20.
4. Renzi A, Talento P, Giardiello C, et al. Stapled trans-anal rectal resection (STARR) by a new dedicated device for the surgical treatment of obstructed defaecation syndrome caused by rectal intussusception and rectocele: early results of a multicenter prospective study. *Int J Colorectal Dis* 2008;23:999–1005.
5. Wadhawan H, Shorthouse AJ, Brown SR. Surgery for obstructed defecation: does the use of the Contour device (Trans-STARR) improve results? *Colorectal Dis* 2010;12(9):885–90.
6. Isbert C, Reibetanz J, Jayne D, Kim M, Germer CT, Boenicke L. Comparative study of Contour Transtar and STARR Procedure for the treatment of obstructed defaecation syndrome (ODS)—feasibility, morbidity and early functional results. *Colorectal Dis* 2010;12(9):901–8.
7. Lenisa L, Schwandner O, Stuto A, et al. STARR with Contour Transtar: prospective multicentre European Study. *Colorectal Dis* 2009; 11(8):821–7.

28 TRREMS Procedure— Transanal Repair of Rectocele and Full Rectal Mucosectomy with One Circular Stapler

Sérgio P. Regadas

Introduction

Rectocele has been treated by many surgical techniques (1–6) including, the recent, novel stapling techniques (7–13). The transanal repair of rectocele and full rectal mucosectomy with one circular stapler (TRREMS procedure) was initially reported in 2005 (14). This method demonstrated two main advantages: the ability to quantify the amount of mucosa to be resected and the requirement for only one circular stapler. It is indicated in all patients with grade III rectocele, whether or not the rectocele is associated with mucosal prolapse, rectoanal intussusceptions, or hemorrhoids. The technique is contraindicated in patients with enterocele and in all patients with anismus. The latter group of patients should be preferentially treated by biofeedback and/or botulinum toxin.

OPERATIVE TECHNIQUE

Broad-spectrum antibiotic prophylaxis is recommended before surgery. A circular anal dilator (Fig. 28.1) is inserted into the anal canal and secured to the perianal skin with two stay sutures (anterior and posterior). The rectocele is delivered through the anal canal with a finger inserted into the vagina to identify the apex. The posterior vaginal wall is delivered through the vaginal introitus with a Babcock forceps. The apex of the rectocele is pulled down through the anal dilator (Fig. 28.1) and a running horizontal suture (Greek suture technique) is placed through the base of the rectocele all the way through, including the mucosa, submucosa, and the muscle layers of the whole anorectal

Figure 28.1 Apex of the rectocele (white circle). Running horizontal suture (white arrows).

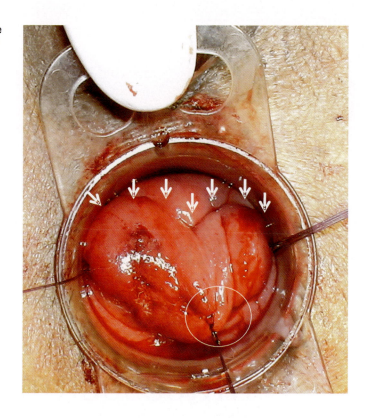

junction wall (Fig. 28.1). This suture is appropriately 2 cm cephalad to the dentate line, depending on the size of the rectocele. The excess of prolapsed mucosa and the muscular layer is then excised with an electrocautery/diathermy, and the wound is left open with the edges joined by the previous manual horizontal suture (Fig. 28.2). A continuous pursestring rectal mucosal suture including mucosal and submucosal layers is then placed 0.5 cm distal to the previously resected rectal mucosal wound. Posteriorly, the pursestring suture is placed at the apex of the prolapsed mucosa. The circular stapler is then inserted through the pursestring suture, which is secured around the stapler's center rod (Fig. 28.3), taking care to include the entire anterior rectal wall. The stapler is then fired and withdrawn.

Figure 28.2 The wound is left open with the edges joined by the previous manual horizontal suture (white arrows). Continuous pursestring rectal mucosa suture (black lines).

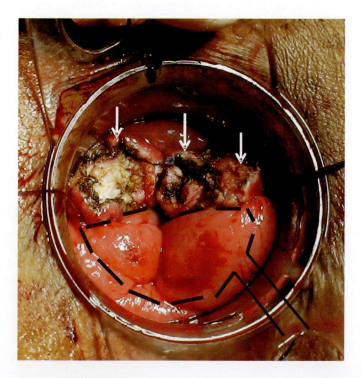

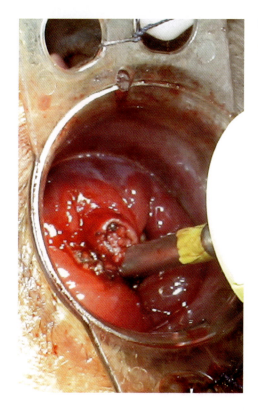

Figure 28.3 The circular stapler is inserted through the pursestring suture, which is secured around the 1stapler´s center rod.

RESULTS

To validate the technique, the TRREMS procedure was performed in a prospective multicenter trial involving 14 surgeons from 11 different institutions (nine Brazilians, one from Portugal, and another from Venezuela). Seventy-five adult female patients of a mean age of 49.6 (range 30–70) years, with obstructed defecation symptoms due to rectocele associated with prolapsed mucosa or rectal intussusception, underwent TRREMS procedure using EEA 34-mm (45) or 31-mm (30) staplers (AutoSuture, New Haven, USA) between August 2004 and October 2006. The mean validated Wexner constipation (15) score was 16, and all patients were preoperatively examined by proctoscope examination, colonic transit time, cinedefecography, and anal manometry. The mean follow-up time was 21 months (range 4–37) and the functional results were initially evaluated by clinical symptoms, Wexner constipation score, cinedefecography, and anal manometry 90 days after the procedure. All patients were clinically followed and the constipation score was subsequently assessed. The student's test was used in the analysis of results. A probability value of less than 0.05 was considered statistically significant.

The mean operative time was 42 minutes. Thirteen (17.7%) patients had bleeding from the stapled line requiring hemostatic suture and two (2.6%) had an incomplete staple line. The length of hospitalization was 1 day for 49 (65.3%) patients and 2 days for the other 26 (34.7%). There were 10 (13.3%) postoperative complications. One patient who developed a severe stapled suture stricture underwent dilation under anesthesia and the remaining patients were treated by endoscopic dilation with hot biopsy forceps (three) and digital dilatation (three). Two (2.6%) patients complained of persistent rectal pain for 2 weeks and one for 3 months. Postoperative cinedefecography showed residual rectoceles in eight (10.6%) patients, with six of them showing decreased symptoms. No statistically significant parameters were found on anal manometric evaluation. The mean validated Wexner constipation score significantly decreased from 16 to 4 (0–4 = 68) (6 = 6 patients) (7 = 1) ($P < 0.0001$).

The commonest surgical techniques used for treatment of rectocele are the perineal levatorplasty and transanal techniques, especially Block's and Sarles' repairs, with a successful outcome varying from 70 to 90% (1,13–16). Recently, novel stapling techniques have been reported, such as stapled transanal prolapsectomy (17), the stapled transanal rectal resection (STARR) double-stapling procedure (7), combined perineal and endorectal repair by circular stapler (9), transanal repair using linear stapler, and a stapler resection of the rectocele area (18). Perineal levatorplasty is unsatisfactory because it does not treat the associated rectal mucosal prolapse that may cause impaired defecation by itself. This technique is also associated with a high incidence of delayed healing of the perineal wound and dyspareunia (8). Sarles' and Block's procedures (1,13) treat the anatomic defect of the anterior rectal wall with low risk of rectal perforation, bleeding, or dehiscence of the suture but leave the posterior rectal mucosal prolapse untreated. The stapled circular mucosectomy treats the rectal mucosal prolapse, but it is not effective enough to treat the anatomic anterior rectal wall defect. The double-stapled technique treats the anterior rectal mucosal prolapse and rectocele by firing one stapler and then removes the posterior mucosal prolapse by firing another. This technique has the main disadvantage of requiring two mechanical circular staplers for each procedure with high cost. The TRREMS procedure has the main advantage of treating the anterior anorectal junction wall defect (rectocelectomy) by manual resection, followed by stapled full rectal mucosectomy and anopexy. Anteriorly, the muscle layer of the rectocele wall was included in all resected specimens during the manual and mechanical excisions. The posterior vaginal wall must be always pulled up by a Babcock forceps during the procedure to avoid injury during the excision of the weakened anterior anorectal junction wall. Anteriorly, the stapled suture must be always placed between normal anterior rectal wall and the anal canal, about 0.5 cm above the pectinate line. The TRREMS procedure may be made more effective by using a new circular stapler (EEA™ Hemorrhoid and Prolapse Stapler Set—Covidien, New Haven, USA) which is able to resect a larger band of prolapsed mucosa. The anorectum-vaginal septum becomes straight and reinforced by the healing fibrous tissue.

In conclusion, the TRREMS procedure is an effective stapling technique based on the postoperative radiological findings and the early clinical results, demonstrating complete improvement of the outlet obstruction symptoms. The relatively lower cost attributed to the need for only one single stapler may be another advantage. Further investigations should be conducted in large numbers of patients with longer follow-up.

Recommended References and Readings

1. Block JR. Transrectal repair of rectocele using obliterative suture. *Dis Colon Rectum* 1986;29:707–11.
2. Van Laarhoven CJ, Kamm MA, Bartram CI, Halligan S, Hawley PR, Phillips RK. Relationship between anatomic and symptomatic long-term results after rectocele repair for impaired defecation. *Dis Colon Rectum* 1999;42:204–11.
3. Khubchandani I, Sheets JA, Stasik JJ, Hakk AR. Endorectal repair of rectocele. *Dis Colon Rectum* 1983;26:792–6.
4. Sehapayak S. Transrectal repair of rectocele: an extended armamentarium of colorectal surgeons. A report or 335 cases. *Dis Colon Rectum* 1985;28:422–33.
5. Porter WE, Steele A, Walsh P, Kohli N, Karram MM. The anatomic and functional outcomes of defect-specific rectocele repairs. *Am J Obstet Gynecol* 1999;181:1353–8.
6. Cundiff GW, Harris RL, Coates KW, Low VH, Bump RC, Addison WA. Abdominal sacral colpoperineopexy: a new approach for correction of posterior compartment defects and perineal descent associated with vaginal vault prolapse. *Am J Obstet Gynecol* 1997;177:345–55.
7. Dodi G, Pietroletti R, Milito G, Binda G, Pescatori M. Bleeding, incontinence, pain and constipation after STARR transanal double stapling rectotomy for obstructed defecation. *Tech Coloproctol* 2003;7:148–53.
8. Boccasanta P, Venturi M, Calabrò G, et al. Which surgical approach for rectocele? A multicentric report from Italian coloproctologists. *Tech Coloproctol* 2001;5:149–56.
9. Altomare DF, Rinaldi M, Veglia A, Petrolino M, De Fazio M, Sallustio P. Combined perineal and endorectal repair of rectocele by circular stapler: a novel surgical technique. *Dis Colon Rectum* 2002;45(11):1549–52.
10. Ayav A, Bresler L, Brunaud L, Boissel P. Long-term results of transanal repair of rectocele using linear stapler. *Dis Colon Rectum* 2004;47:889–94.
11. Boccasanta P, Venturi M, Salamina G, Cesana BM, Bernasconi F, Roviaro G. New trends in the surgical treatment of outlet obstruction: clinical and functional results of two novel transanal stapled techniques from a randomised controlled trial. *Int J Colorectal Dis* 2004;19:359–69.
12. Scuderi G, Casolino V, Dranissino MI, et al. Uso della suturatrice meccanica nella risoluzione di problematiche proctologiche. Nostra esperienza relativa a 122 pazienti. *Chir Ital* 2001;53:835–9.
13. Sarles JC, Arnaud A, Selezneff I, Olivier S. Endorectal repair of rectocele. *Int J Colorectal Dis* 1989;4:167–71.
14. Regadas FSP, Regadas SMM, Rodrigues LV, Misici R, Silva FR, Regadas Filho FS. Transanal repair of rectocele and full rectal mucosectomy with one circular stapler: a novel surgical technique. *Tech Coloproctol* 2005;9:63–6.
15. Agachan F, Chen T, Pfeifer J, Reissman P, Wexner SD. A constipation scoring system to simplify evaluation and management of constipated patients. *Dis Colon Rectum* 1996;39:681–5.
16. Sullivan ES, Leaverton GH, Hardwick CE. Transrectal perineal repair. An adjunct to improved function after anorectal surgery. *Dis Colon Rectum* 1968;11:106–14.
17. Pescatori M, Favetta D, Dedola S, Orsini S. Transanal stapled excision of rectal mucosal prolapse. *Tech Coloproctol* 1997;1:96–8.
18. Bonner C, Prohm P, Transanal stapler mucosectomy for symptomatic rectocele with outlet obstruction. *Zentralbl Chir* 2004;129:205–7.

29 Gluteus Maximus Transposition

Jason W. Allen and Herand Abcarian

 ## INDICATIONS/CONTRAINDICATIONS

Direct sphincter repair provides good results in the majority of patients suffering from fecal incontinence. Muscle transposition is reserved for cases in which direct repair cannot be accomplished because of lack of sphincter muscle from severe trauma, congenital anomalies, or because of denervation of the sphincter.

The gluteus maximus muscle is an ideal candidate for transposition to the anal canal for sphincter reconstruction. As opposed to other muscles used for transposition for fecal incontinence, the gluteus maximus muscle is a strong, thick muscle with a generous blood supply. It originates from the upper portion of the ileum, the sacrum, and the coccyx and then inserts into the femur and iliotibial tract. The origination of the gluteus muscle from the posterior pelvic structures causes the greatest squeeze pressures to occur against the anterior wall of the rectum in gluteus maximus muscle transpositions. This directional squeeze mimics the physiologic action of the external anal sphincter and may assist in the maintenance of continence by crimping the anal canal. Also, the thickness of the gluteus maximus flap can lengthen the anal canal and its high-pressure zone once transposed. The generous blood supply to the muscle is from the superior and inferior gluteal arteries and is supplemented by the branches of the medial and lateral femoral circumflex arteries. The gluteus maximus muscle's close proximity to the anus also makes it advantageous for transposition as it is a synergist for the external anal sphincter; contraction of the gluteus maximus muscle is a natural response to impending fecal incontinence. Postoperative studies of gluteus maximus transpositions show tonic activity, and in some studies, there is an increase of not only postoperative squeeze pressures but also resting pressures. This basal tone may be secondary to the use of the gluteus maximus muscles during walking. In addition to recovered motor function, rectal sensation also improves after this operation. Encirclement of the anus with voluntary muscle allows the rectum to become distended. The patient is able to recognize the rectal distension and evacuate in a controlled fashion.

Several absolute and relative contraindications exist for the creation of gluteus maximus transposition. Motor innervation to the gluteus muscle is from the inferior gluteal nerve (L5, S1, S2). Fecal incontinence caused by central cord malformations such as spina bifida may be associated with dysfunction to the gluteus maximus muscle also. Therefore, a more proximally innervated muscle transposition may be a better choice for treating these conditions. Another contraindication is the lack of a distensible rectum secondary to extensive inflammation or injury. In order for the gluteus maximus transposition to work, the patient must have a compliant reservoir to distend in order to improve control. Relative contraindications suggested by some investigators include prepubescent youths and adults greater than 60 years old. These same investigators have had their worst outcomes in patients with congenital malformations followed by patients with severe pudendal neuropathy.

PREOPERATIVE PLANNING

In patients being considered for gluteus maximus transposition, preoperative evaluation should begin with the standard examinations for all patients with fecal incontinence. All patients should undergo anorectal physiologic studies including anal manometry, electromyography, and pudendal nerve terminal motor latency. Electromyography of the gluteus maximus is also necessary and endoanal ultrasonography is useful in documenting the degree of sphincter defects. Defecography assists in assessing pelvic floor dysfunction. Although evaluation of the entire patient should be undertaken according to screening guidelines, a fecal incontinence score should be obtained to allow postoperative objective documentation of any improvement.

All patients receive a mechanical bowel preparation along with oral antibiotics. Patients receive second- or third-generation antibiotics at the induction of anesthesia. This procedure may be done under regional or general anesthesia. A ureteral catheter is inserted after which the patient is positioned in the prone jackknife position with the buttocks taped laterally to allow for exposure. We do not perform a diverting ostomy as part of our procedure as diversion has not been shown to decrease the wound infection rate.

SURGERY

Technique

Dissection and Mobilization of the Gluteus Maximus Muscle

Two mirror image incisions are made on both buttocks that run parallel to the caudal portion of the gluteus maximus muscle on each side (Fig. 29.1). A lateral circumanal incision

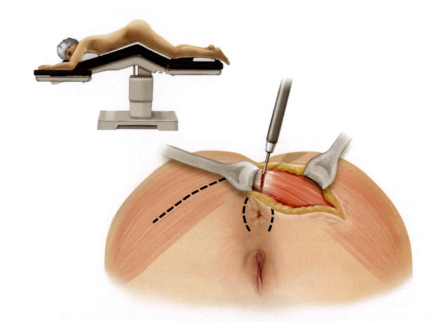

Figure 29.1 The patient is placed in the prone jackknife position. The lower 4–5 cm of the gluteus maximus muscle origin and the rim of periosteum are dissected from the sacrum and coccyx. The dashed lines illustrate the placement of the skin incisions. Reprinted from Pearl RK, Prasad ML, Nelson RL, et al. Bilateral gluteus maximus transposition for anal incontinence. *Dis Colon Rectum* 1991;34:478–81, with permission.

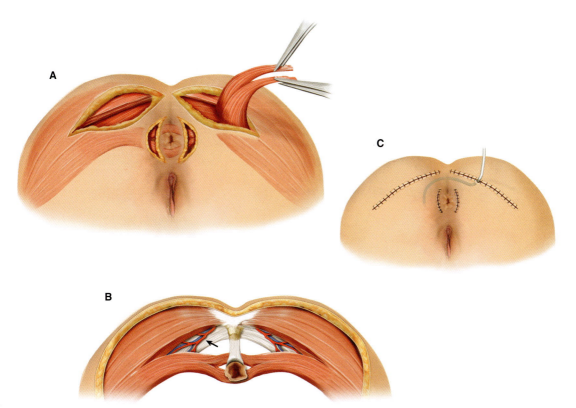

Figure 29.2 A. The muscle flaps are then longitudinally bifurcated and inferiorly rotated to encircle the anus by subcutaneous tunneling to form a sling of voluntary muscle. **B.** Once tunneling is successful, the bifurcated ends of each flap are sutured in an overlapping fashion to each other using interrupted sutures of 2-0 polyglactin. Arrows indicate the neurovascular bundle. **C.** Closed suction drains are placed bilaterally cranial and lateral to the incisions over the buttocks. Subcutaneous tissues are then approximated with absorbable sutures and the skin is closed by subcuticular technique or staples. Reprinted from Pearl RK, Prasad ML, Nelson RL, et al. Bilateral gluteus maximus transposition for anal incontinence. *Dis Colon Rectum* 1991;34:478–81, with permission.

is made bilaterally for tunneling the bifurcated ends of the opposing slings (Fig. 29.2). These circumanal incisions should be 2 cm from the anal verge to prevent damage to the anoderm. The anterior and posterior skin bridges between these two circumanal incisions should be at least 3 cm wide to prevent devascularization and necrosis. The gluteus maximus muscle is identified and is traced to its lower origin on the sacrum and coccyx. The lower 4–5 cm of the gluteus maximus muscle origin and the rim of periosteum are dissected from the sacrum and coccyx. This muscle bundle is then freed from the underlying main body of the gluteus maximus and the sacrotuberous ligament. Attention is given to prevent injury to the underlying neurovascular bundle, which leaves the pelvis the sciatic foramen and enters the deep surface of the inferior half of gluteus maximus muscle usually 6–8 cm from its mid-sacral border. Cadaveric study of gluteus maximus transpositions demonstrated that this neurovascular pedicle was consistently located 1 cm lateral and superior to the ischial tuberosities. Sufficient mobilization of the muscle flaps is achieved when they are able to reach the contralateral border of the anus without tension.

Sphincter Recreation with Gluteus Maximus Muscle Opposing Slings

The muscle flaps are then longitudinally bifurcated and inferiorly rotated. Stay sutures are placed in the periosteum of the flaps to assist in the encirclement of the anus by tunneling the bifurcated ends subcutaneously at the level of the postanal space. Once tunneling is successful, the bifurcated ends of each flap are sutured in an overlapping fashion to each other using interrupted sutures of 2-0 polyglactin. Closed suction drains are placed bilaterally cranial and lateral to the incisions over the buttocks. Subcutaneous

Figure 29.3 Some of the described techniques for reconstruction of the anal sphincter using gluteus maximus transposition. Reprinted from Devesa JM, Vicente E, Enriquez JM, et al. Total fecal incontinence—a new method of gluteus maximus transposition. *Dis Colon Rectum* 1992;35:339–49.

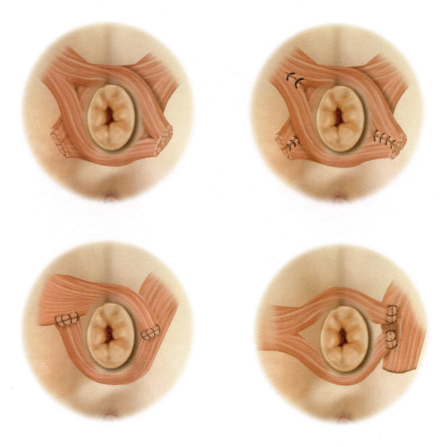

tissues are then approximated with absorbable sutures and the skin is closed by subcuticular technique or staples.

Alternative Techniques

The technique described above, first reported by Hentz in 1982, is only one of many such techniques employed for gluteus maximus muscle transpositions (Fig. 29.3). Heading one of the most prolific groups in gluteus maximus muscle transposition, Devesa has described his own technique of gluteus maximus muscle transposition in a large series of patients. In his technique, he bifurcates only one of the muscle flaps and leaves the opposing muscle flap undivided. He secures the tunneled anterior and posterior ends of the bifurcated muscle to the contralateral undivided muscle in an end-to-side fashion. This division and tunneling of the bifurcated ends of one of the muscle flaps is thought to reduce the tension on the suture lines of the gluteoplasty and reduce the amount of tissue that has to be tunneled in the postanal space.

Devesa and his colleagues have also described unilateral gluteoplasty in combination with direct sphincteroplasty in two patients with severe, traumatic sphincter injuries. The gluteus maximus muscle is sutured in apposition to a direct sphincteroplasty on the side of the injury. It is theorized that the intact portion of the sphincter complex acts similarly as the bifurcated flaps in the bilateral gluteoplasty and achieves the goal of creating a tension-free muscular ring around the anus. Both patients achieved increased continence and increased resting and squeeze pressures on manometric studies. Farid et al. have used this technique with the modification of extending the muscle flaps with fascia lata grafts with good results.

Cadaveric studies have been undertaken to determine the difference in length between distally based gluteus flaps separated from its origin on the sacrum versus proximally based flaps dissected from its insertion on the femur. Pak-Art et al. demonstrated, at least in cadavers, proximally based flaps were almost 45% longer than distally based flaps. Keighley et al. chose whether to use a proximally or distally based flap after identifying the location of the neurovascular bundle and its configuration.

The technique of dynamic muscle plasty has been investigated in association with gluteus maximus muscle transpositions in an attempt to approve outcomes. This method uses an implanted pulse generator to convert fast-twitch, fast-fatigue skeletal muscle fibers to slow-twitch high-endurance muscle fibers. Dynamic muscle plasty has been used with gracilis muscle transposition with improved results as opposed to unstimulated gracilis muscle. Madoff et al. published results from a prospective, multicenter trial studying the safety and efficacy of dynamic muscle plasty that included dynamic bilateral gluteal maximus muscle transposition. Although only a small minority of patients in this study received dynamic gluteoplasty, the results of stimulated gluteoplasty were poor. Less than half of the patients maintained successful outcomes during the study with more than one-third of the patients having major wound complications. Further investigations will have to be done to determine whether dynamic gluteoplasty is a worthwhile endeavor.

 POSTOPERATIVE MANAGEMENT

Patients are placed on a clear liquid diet on the first postoperative day and for next 3–4 days after which a regular diet is started. Sitting is restricted for 2 weeks postoperatively and in addition some surgeons instruct their patients not to climb stairs for 3 weeks.

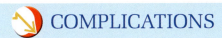 COMPLICATIONS

Wound Infection

Wound infection is the most common complication of gluteus maximus transposition occurring in 17–43% of cases. Wound infection increases the possibility for the need to perform neosphincter repair in a patient and also decreases the chances the patient will have a satisfactory outcome, especially when involving the perianal incisions. Diverting colostomies have been used in an attempt to decrease the wound infection rate, but wound infections occur despite fecal diversion. Decreasing wound infections is more likely dependent on maintaining sterile technique, adequacy of bowel preparation, and prevention of gross contamination of the wounds during the procedure.

Failure of Repair

Failure to improve incontinence is another complication of gluteus maximus muscle transposition. This complication occurs in 14–57% of cases according to the largest series of bilateral gluteoplasties. Having adequately thick and innervated gluteus maximus muscle and encircling the anal canal without tension decreases the likelihood repair failure.

Two critical steps have been emphasized to increase the success of the operation. The first step is the identification and preservation of the inferior gluteal nerve and its neurovascular pedicle. The second is adequate, tension-free encirclement of the anal canal in the anterior tunnel. This anterior limb of the repair is the most likely to dehisce and retract. The greatest wall tension on the rectum is created in this anterior area when the gluteus maximus muscle contracts after the repair. Also, this area is the most difficult area to tunnel through because of the close proximity of the vagina and urethra. This pathway can be more difficult in patients with congenital anomalies and may lead to decreased success in this patient population.

Failure of the gluteus maximus muscle transposition is most likely secondary to either denervation of the muscle caused by disruption of its neurovascular pedicle or dehiscence of the anterior limbs of the flaps caused by wound infection or undue tension. Magnetic resonance imaging is the best test looking for structural causes if the repair fails to improve continence. Electromyography can be used to measure the electrical activity of the transposed muscle. If the transposed muscle remains innervated, then direct repair is indicated. Several months of watchful waiting is undertaken to allow for healing circumanal skin and allow for fibrosis and decreased inflammation to improve the chance for success of a secondary repair.

 CONCLUSIONS

Gluteus maximus muscle transposition is an option for patients with total fecal incontinence secondary to severe sphincter defects from trauma or congenital defects or sphincter denervation not amenable to direct repair. It is the only procedure that allows encirclement of the anal canal with thick, well-perfused voluntary muscle that is synergistic to the sphincter complex. Gluteoplasty has been shown to increase rectal sensation and voluntray squeeze pressures and may also increase resting pressures. Although it is a technically demanding procedure and can be associated with significant morbidity, gluteus maximus muscle transposition is one alternative to properly selected patients who suffer from the socially incapacitating disorder of fecal incontinence as a last resort before permenant colostomy.

Suggested Reading

Cera SM, Wexner SD. Muscle transposition: does it still have a role? *Clin Colon Rectal Surg* 2005;18(1):46–54.

Devesa JM, Madrid JM, Gallego BR, et al. Bilateral gluteoplasty for fecal incontinence. *Dis Colon Rectum* 1997;40:883–8.

Enrique-Navascues JM, Devesa-Mugica JM. Traumatic anal incontinence: role of unilateral gluteus maximus transposition supplementing and supporting direct anal sphincteroplasty. *Dis Colon Rectum* 1994;37:766–9.

Pak-Art R, Silapunt P, Bunaprasert T, et al. Prospective, randomized, controlled trial of proximally based vs. distally based gluteus maximus flap for anal incontinence in cadavers. *Dis Colon Rectum* 2002;45:1100–3.

Pearl RK, Prasad ML, Nelson RL, et al. Bilateral gluteus maximus transposition for incontinence. *Dis Colon Rectum* 1991;34:478–81.

30 Gracilis Muscle Flaps

Oded Zmora and Fabio M. Potenti

Introduction

Reconstructive surgery of the perineal area, including complex perianal fistula management, reconstruction of the anal sphincter, and repair of complicated perineal wounds, is among the most challenging of tasks in colorectal surgery. These operations are associated with a substantial failure rate, and have a significant impact on patients' quality of life.

Fistulas between the rectum and adjacent organs, such as the vagina or urethra, are among the toughest to treat, for several reasons. In many cases, the etiology of these fistulas includes conditions negatively affecting wound healing, such as history of radiation therapy (1,2), or inflammatory bowel disease (3). Occasionally, rectourethral fistulas may result from congenital malformations, which may be associated with other deformities of the perineal area. Anatomically, the rectum is adjacent to the vagina or the urethra, with only thin septum separating in between, which may further complicate attempts at local repair. In many cases, the rectal opening of such fistulas is situated in a proximal location above the dentate line, which makes transanal approach more complex.

Nonhealing perineal wounds result from previous surgery at the perineal area, such as abdominoperineal resection. Nonhealing wounds are more frequent following surgery for inflammatory bowel disease, or history of radiation therapy, and usually involve chronic tissue infection.

The gracilis muscle, located at the inner portion of the thigh, originates from the lower aspect of the anterior part of the pelvis and passes adjacent to the groin, throughout the inner part of the thigh, toward the knee. Its main innervation and blood supply enter the muscle proximally, near the groin, making it an ideal candidate for rotational flap during reconstructive surgery of the perianal area. The belly of the muscle can be rotated and inserted as a flap between the rectum and adjacent organs during the repair of fistulas, or used as filler for the repair of nonhealing perineal wounds, with the option of harvesting an island of skin from the medial aspect of the thigh as a myocutaneous flap. The gracilis muscle may also be used for reconstruction of the anal sphincter, as discussed in a separate chapter of this book.

ANATOMY AND FUNCTION OF THE GRACILIS MUSCLE

The gracilis is the most superficial muscle on the medial aspect of the thigh. It is thin and flattened, broader at its base, gradually narrow, and tapering below. It arises from the anterior margins of the lower half of the symphysis pubis and the upper half of the pubic arch, runs vertically downward, ending in a rounded tendon. This tendon passes behind the medial condyle of the femur, curves around the medial condyle of the tibia where it becomes flattened, and inserts into the upper part of the medial surface of the body of the tibia, below the condyle (Fig. 30.1). As a result, the muscle is mainly a lower limb adductor. However, since adduction depends on several thigh muscles, limb function can be adequately preserved after harvest of the gracilis muscle.

The gracilis is supplied by a branch of the medial circumflex artery (which comes from the profunda femoral system), and its innervation comes from the anterior branch of obturator nerve, originating at L3 and L4 spinal roots. Both the main arterial supply and the innervation enter the muscle at the same site, or approximately 1 cm apart, at a region termed the neurovascular bundle (Fig. 30.2). This bundle enters the muscle in its proximal third, on average approximately 10 cm from its pubic origin. The proximal location of the neurovascular bundle, situated adjacent to the groin, combined with the fact that thigh motion can be preserved after harvesting, makes this long muscle an ideal candidate for a rotational flap transposition to the perineal region. In most patients, accessory small perforating vessels may enter the muscle distal to the neurovascular

Figure 30.1 Anatomy of the gracilis muscle. **A.** A sketch showing the bony structures and the gracilis. **B.** A sketch showing the bony structures, adjacent muscles, and the gracilis.

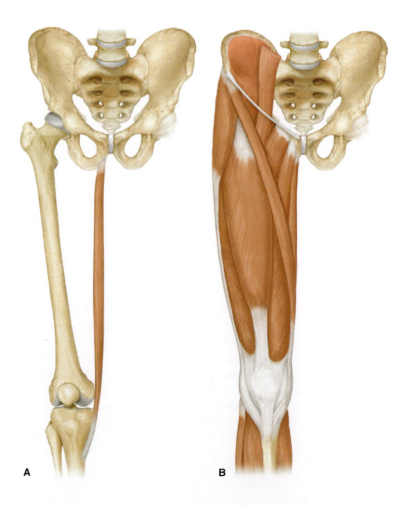

A   B

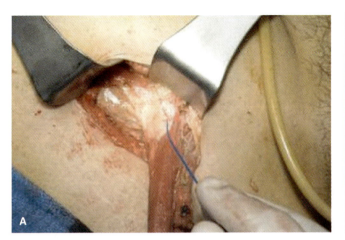
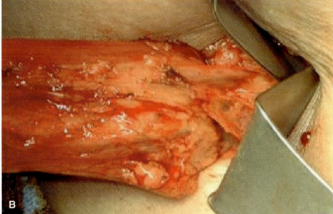

Figure 30.2 The neurovascular bundle.

bundle (4). However, division of these vessels is possible in more than 90% of cases, thus preserving muscle viability.

Alternative Options for the Repair of Rectourethral and Rectovaginal Fistulas

These techniques may be divided into two main categories. In the first, the luminal side of the fistula is approached, and the defect is closed. Rectovaginal fistulas may be approached to either repair the rectal side of the fistula, or through the vagina, to repair the vaginal opening (5). The advantage of the vaginal approach is the ease of access to the fistula opening. However, this approach carries the disadvantage of repairing the lower pressure side of the fistula. For this reason, most colorectal surgeons prefer approaches involving repair of the rectal side. In the rectourethral fistula, the urethral side is not accessible, and direct repair of the fistula opening must involve repair of the rectal side. The rectal lumen may be approached through the anus, or by incision of the posterior wall of the rectum. This posterior method entailed either a transsphincteric plane, or a transsacral incision. Several authors have advocated the posterior York-Mason approach to the rectum (6). The major drawback of the posterior and transanal approaches is that they mainly treat the rectal side of the fistula. Unfortunately, the high-pressure side in rectourethral fistula is the urethra.

In the second category of repair, the plane between the rectum and the urethra is dissected, the fistula is divided, and both the rectal and the urethral defects are repaired. A viable tissue flap may then be transposed to separate the rectum and the urethra. The greater omentum may be used as a viable flap (7), but this use involves a laparotomy, with deep anterior pelvic dissection, and may not be feasible in patients who have had abdominal surgeries. Using the perineal approach, the plane between the rectum and the vagina or urethra is dissected through a perineal incision, the fistula is divided, and a viable tissue is brought to interpose between the two organs. The gracilis muscle provides a well-vascularized muscular rotation flap and avoids the need for laparotomy.

A relatively new option for interposition between the rectum and the urethra or the vagina without body tissue flaps may involve the use of biologic meshes. These meshes are acellular collagen matrixes made of biologic tissue, which may be used as "tissue grafts" (8). Wound-healing processes result in migration of inflammatory cells and fibroblasts into the mesh, leading to dense fibrosis with gradual absorption of the mesh. However, since this technique has only recently emerged, data are still insufficient to support its routine use. Biologic collagen products such as the collagen plugs, also made from acellular collagen matrixes, may also be used for the repair of rectovaginal fistulas by simple insertion of the plug throughout the fistula tract (9). The short length of rectovaginal fistulas may make fixation of the plug to the fistula tract difficult and increase the chance of plug migration. Newer products use a fixation button attached to the plug, aiming to reduce the chance of such migration.

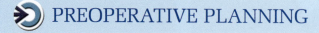

PREOPERATIVE PLANNING

Assessment of Patients with Rectovaginal Fistula

Patients with fistula between the rectum and the vagina often complain of uncontrolled passage of gas and stool from the vagina. Large fistulas may be easily evident on physical examination, using digital rectal examination, anoscopy, or examination of the vagina using speculum. Small fistulas however may be clinically difficult to detect. In these cases, imaging examinations may be required to definitely identify the fistula tract. A water-soluble contrast enema of the rectum, or vaginogram, using a catheter inserted into the lower part of the vagina and instillation of water-soluble contrast into the vagina, may show the fistula tract. Transrectal or perineal sonography and pelvic magnetic resonance imaging (MRI) are modern imaging techniques with high sensitivity to detect the fistula tract. However, such modern imaging techniques may not be available to all surgeons and are more costly. Infrequently, the fistula tract cannot be detected by physical examination or by imaging techniques, and examination under anesthesia is required to detect the fistula tract. In such examinations, probing of the fistula tract may be attempted through the anal or the vaginal side. If the openings are not identified, insufflation of the rectum or the vagina with Betadine or colored solution may be used, in attempts to detect passage of the colored solution at the other opening. Alternatively, a tampon soaked with colored solution may be inserted to the vagina approximately 1 hour prior to the examination, to enhance identification of the rectal opening.

Once diagnosed, adequate drainage of the rectovaginal or pouch-vaginal fistula must be assured, prior to any attempt of repair. If physical examination or imaging procedures suggest inadequately drained fistula, or associated cavity, adequate drainage must first be achieved, by incision and drainage, insertion of draining Seton, or both. In patients with inadequate drainage who are not diverted, temporary fecal diversion may be considered, to improve local conditions prior to fistula repair.

Patients with rectovaginal fistula associated with Crohn's disease may have active proctitis or aggressive perianal disease, with unfavorable local conditions negatively affecting success rate of fistula repair. In these cases, adequate anti-inflammatory treatment for Crohn's disease should be promptly initiated prior to the fistula repair.

Assessment of Patients with Rectourethral Fistula

Rectourethral fistulas often present with symptoms such as pneumaturia, fecaluria, passage of urine through the rectum, and recurrent urinary tract infections. Although most of these symptoms are often alleviated by fecal and urinary diversion, the fistulas seldom spontaneously heal. Even when diverted, patients may suffer from urinary tract infections, resistant to medical therapy (10). Thus, most of these patients will eventually require surgical repair. Similar to patients with rectovaginal fistulas, the rectal opening of fistulas between the rectum and the urethra may or may not be evident on clinical examination. Imaging studies, including water-soluble contrast enema, voiding cystourethrography, transrectal ultrasonography, or pelvic MRI may be required for identification of fistula. Infrequently, examination under anesthesia with the combination of cystourethroscopy and anorectal examination may be required. In these cases, fluid installed into the urethra may help identify the rectal opening.

In patients with a history of malignant disease, such as patients with rectourethral fistula following treatment for prostate cancer, or patients with pouch-vaginal fistula following surgery for rectal cancer, recurrent malignancy causing the fistula must be excluded. Preoperative biopsies of the fistula tract, imaging modalities, and serum tumor markers may be appropriate to rule out recurrent cancer.

Assessment of Patients with Nonhealing Perineal Wounds

As discussed earlier in the chapter, the first step in the preoperative evaluation of patient with a history of rectal cancer is to exclude recurrence. Subsequently, the depth of the wound should be evaluated. A well-mobilized gracilis will reach up to 20 cm cephalad to the gluteal cleft, any wound deeper than that should be treated with a different approach. The best method is probably a rectus abdominis myocutaneous flap. Computed tomographic scan should also be obtained to exclude the presence of undrained abscess cavities. The addition of oral and intravenous contrast may be helpful if an enteric fistula is suspected. MRI and fistulogram can be used to further evaluate other associated defects.

PREOPERATIVE PREPARATIONS

Numerous surgical procedures have been described for the treatment of rectourethral and rectovaginal fistulas (6,11,12), none of which has gained wide acceptance as the procedure of choice. Thus, each treatment option has its own associated advantages and risks, all of which should be thoroughly discussed with the patient before obtaining informed consent.

The value of fecal diversion prior to or concomitant with the fistula repair has not been adequately challenged in comparative studies (13). The rationale behind fecal diversion is that decreased fecal load may reduce the chance of postoperative infection, and will also prevent rise of luminal pressure at the rectal side during evacuation. Most authors believe that fecal diversion is recommended, since the perineal approach includes extensive dissection of the tissue between the rectum and the vagina or the urethra. The importation of healthy muscle has a high chance of success, which may be further enhanced by routine fecal diversion. Until comparative trials are available, the authors and the editors advocate routine fecal diversion.

In rectourethral fistulas, urinary diversion using cystostomy should also be considered, to prevent any voiding attempts that may raise the luminal pressure at the urethral side.

Broad-spectrum intravenous antibiotic prophylaxis is given prior to the induction of anesthesia. The length of postoperative prophylactic antibiotic treatment, if any, is not scientifically well defined, and there is no proof that prolonged antibiotic treatment improves healing rate, although antibiotic treatment for 24 hours or more is often used.

The same antibiotic coverage is used when operations are performed for persistent sinuses. Patients with persistent perineal sinus are typically colonized with skin contaminants, such as *Staphylococcus aureus*, diphteroids, β-streptococcus, and *Staphylococcus epidermidis*. Anaerobic Bacteroides are present in 25% of the wounds and anaerobic gram-negative rods are rarely seen (14).

If a patient has not been diverted prior to fistula repair, mechanical bowel preparation may be advisable, for large bowel cleansing prior to surgery. Alternatively, phosphate enemas may be used to clean the rectum and sigmoid colon.

Surgery

 ## OPERATIVE TECHNIQUE

Harvesting of the Gracilis Rotation Flap

Harvesting for Fistula Repair

When used for fistula repair, the gracilis muscular flap is used, without any overlaying skin. The patient is positioned either in the supine position with the legs adducted, or in the modified lithotomy position using stirrups. Several types of thigh incisions may

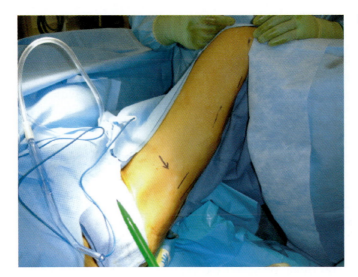

Figure 30.3 Skin incision.

be used for the harvest procedure. In relatively thin patients, where the muscle is easily palpated, two to three 3–5 cm long incisions can be made alongside the inner part of the thigh over the gracilis muscle (Fig. 30.3). Tunnels are made in-between the incisions at the subcutaneous tissue overlaying the muscle, and the muscle is dissected throughout its length through these incisions (Fig. 30.4). The perforating vessels are divided through these small incisions often with an energy source. Using an energy sources, perforating vessels entering the muscle between the incision sites can safely be divided through small incisions. The most proximal incision is situated approximately one hand breadth beneath the inguinal ligament, to allow adequate exposure of the neurovascular bundle. Alternatively, a longer incision of approximately 10–12 cm may be made at the upper part of the inner thigh, to enhance exposure and facilitate dissection at the area of the neurovascular bundle. In this case, a second incision is made at the distal part of the thigh, and a subcutaneous tunnel is made in between these two incisions. In difficult cases, or if the surgeon does not feel confident dissecting parts of the muscle through a subcutaneous tunnel, a long incision may be made along the inner part of the thigh.

Recently, gracilis muscle harvest using an endoscopic approach for plastic surgery procedures has been described (15). Although harvesting of the muscle using three small vertical skin incisions of approximately 3–5 cm each is associated with a good

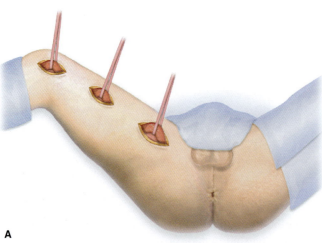

A

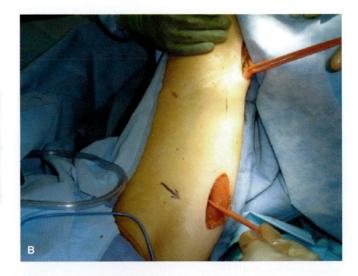

B

Figure 30.4 Muscle dissection.

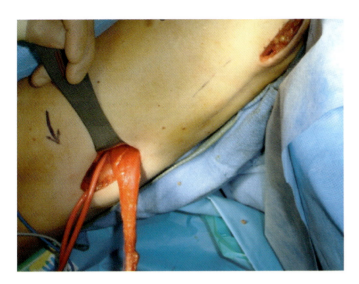

Figure 30.5 Muscle is delivered through the proximal incision.

cosmetic and functional result, the endoscopic approach may further minimize invasiveness and may obviate the occasional upper medial thigh numbness or pain.

Once incisions are made, the gracilis muscle is first identified at its tendon through the distal thigh incision and is disconnected from its insertion near the tibial plateau. The muscle is then dissected free, creating a tunnel between the incisions, and ultimately the muscle is delivered through the proximal incision (Fig. 30.5). Generally, the dissection of the muscle free of the subcutaneous tissue and of other muscles of the inner thigh is mostly accomplished in an avascular plane. It is imperative that all perforating blood vessels are identified and divided, to prevent postoperative thigh hematomas. Energy sources such as the ultrasonic shears or bipolar coagulation devices may be useful for dissection (Fig. 30.6).

Ultimately, following careful dissection of the muscle throughout the thigh, the muscle is delivered through the proximal incision. Care should be taken at this point to identify and to preserve the neurovascular bundle. Meticulous dissection of the neurovascular bundle is undertaken, taking care to preserve the main blood supply and nerve, to add maximal length to the harvested muscle available for transposition or interposition. However, in most patients the neurovascular bundle is in convenient

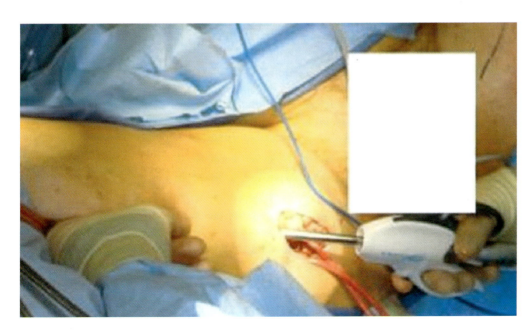

Figure 30.6 Ultrasonic shears division of perforating blood vessels.

proximity to the perineum, and in contrast to the gracilis muscle transposition in neosphincter procedures, the length of muscle required for fistula repair is usually less. A subcutaneous tunnel is then made through the proximal thigh incision cephally toward the perineum, and the muscle is placed in the pocket proximal to the upper incision. If the prone jack-knife position is selected for the perineal dissection, the thigh incisions are then closed. A small suction drain is placed at the subcutaneous tunnel of the thigh.

Harvesting of Myocutaneous Rotation Flap for Perineal Wound Closure

As discussed earlier in the chapter, unhealed perineal wounds from proctectomy usually present with a rather small skin opening, associated with a large presacral cavity. Typically, after bringing the healthy and well-vascularized tissue of the belly of the gracilis muscle, with the technique described above, the skin very rapidly closes with the occasional use of a split thickness skin graft. The concern of the surgeon is to achieve adequate mobilization, without injury of the blood supply, to fill the sinus cavity completely. In those atypical cases associated with a significant loss of perineal cutaneous tissue, the adjunct of an island of skin, subcutaneous tissue, and fascia is harvested with the gracilis. Suited more to the plastic surgery specialty than the colon-rectal, this technique was originally described by McCraw for vaginal reconstruction. The procedure has been modified over the course of the years by including all available regional fascia to create a myofasciocutaneous flap with increased skin perfusion and to decrease the risk of tissue loss (16). The cutaneous area covering the gracilis in the proximal component is harvested with a V-Y incision and rotated in the defect after mobilization of the vascular pedicle, allowing for the most distal portion of the belly of the muscle to be inserted deep in the cavity (17). This repair is well suited for cases where the perineum or rectal vaginal septum is lost as a consequence of severe inflammatory and infectious processes.

Gracilis Interposition Repair of Rectourethral and Rectovaginal/Pouch-Vaginal Fistulas

The dissection for the division of the fistula tract and interposition of the gracilis muscle between the rectum and the urethra or the vagina is performed through a perineal approach, using an incision anterior to the anal verge, between the anus and the vagina or the base of the scrotum. Such an approach may be used in exaggerated lithotomy position or the prone jack-knife position. In our experience, the prone jack-knife position gives superb review of the anterior wall of the rectum, excellent review of the perineal dissection plane between the rectum and organs located anterior to the rectum, and easy access for adequate repair of the fistula openings and fixation of the interposed muscle. We favor the prone jack-knife position, despite minor inconvenience associated with repositioning the patient during the procedure. If the prone jack-knife position is selected, the patient is then carefully turned to the prone jack-knife position after thigh wound closure.

After adequate positioning, an incision is made at the perineum anterior to the anus, approximately midway between the anus and the posterior border of the vaginal opening, or the base of the scrotum (Fig. 30.7). We favor a horizontal perineal incision, but several authors have advocated the use of an inverted Y- or U-shaped incision. Dissection is then undertaken in the areolar tissue anterior to the anus and rectum, between the rectum and the vagina or the urethra (Fig. 30.8). In cases of rectourethral fistula, a large urinary bladder catheter is helpful to identify and to protect the remainder of the urethra not involved in the fistula. The dissection is then undertaken to divide the fistula tract and to reach cephalad to noninflamed tissue. It is important to emphasize the need to continue the dissection to at least 2 cm cephalad the inflamed tissue associated with the fistula tract, to allow adequate transposition and proper fixation of the muscle flap to the upper part of the dissected septum. The rectal defect is then primarily closed with an advancement flap. In cases of rectourethral fistula, the urethral defect may be closed without a small biologic mesh with interrupted absorbable sutures over the indwelling catheter or alternately left open. The perineal approach allows

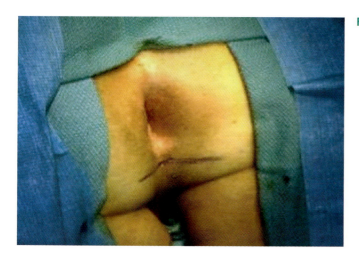

Figure 30.7 Perineal incision.

excellent exposure of the urethra, allowing urethroplasty if concomitant urethral stricture is present, or other types of urologic interventions for the urethra if required. In rectovaginal fistulas, the vaginal opening is repaired. Several authors have suggested the repair of the two openings in opposite directions, meaning that one opening (usually the rectal side) will be horizontally repaired, whereas the other side will be vertically repaired. However, since viable tissue is brought to interpose between the two openings, the need for this technique is questionable.

The subcutaneous tunnel between the perineum and the thigh is then approached through the perineal incision, until the pocket where the gracilis muscle has been placed is reached. The gracilis muscle is rotated and gently brought through the perineal incision (Fig. 30.9). Care should be taken to avoid excessive tension on the neurovascular bundle to avoid any compromise of blood supply. The gracilis muscle is then brought to the previously dissected perineal space, and interposed between the rectum and the urethra or vagina (Fig. 30.10). Four to six sutures are applied at the muscle and at the apex of the incision to hold the muscle in place. We usually favor nonabsorbable monofilament sutures. Once the sutures are tied, the gracilis muscle is fixated to the upper pole of the dissected area, obscuring the view for adequate additional suture placement. Thus, it is generally useful to place all sutures untied first, using hemostatic clamps, followed by sequential securing of the sutures in place. If the gracilis muscle length allows, it is useful to bend the distal part of the muscle, which is placed at the upper part of the dissection, in a J shape, to add bulk to this area, where the muscle itself is narrowed. However, again, care should be taken to avoid tension at the base of the muscle, to prevent delayed ischemia.

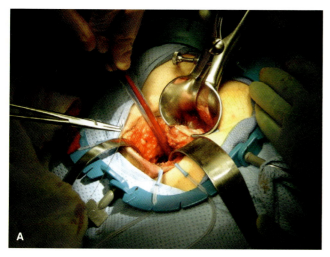
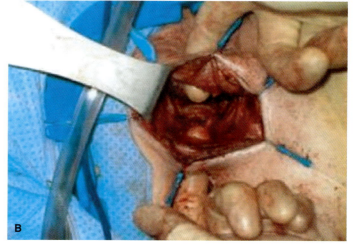

Figure 30.8 Perineal dissection.

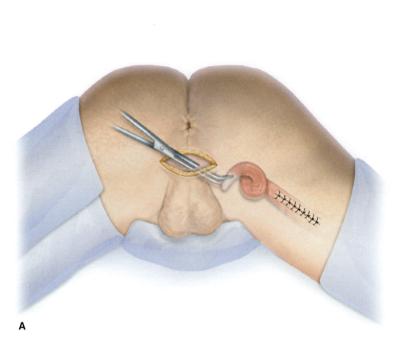

A

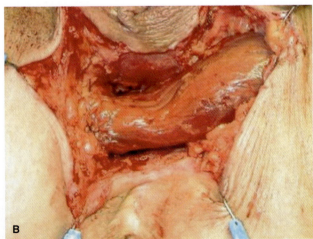

B

Figure 30.9 Rotation of the gracilis muscle to the perineal wound.

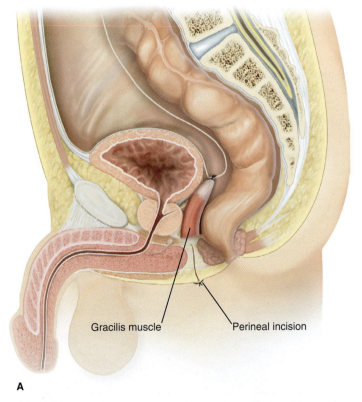

Gracilis muscle   Perineal incision

A

B

Figure 30.10 The muscle is brought to interpose between the rectum and the urethra or the vagina.

A small suction drain is placed in the lower part of the dissection field alongside the gracilis muscle, to prevent fluid collection in this area. The skin is then closed using interrupted absorbable sutures.

In our practice, patients are postoperatively permitted dietary intake ad lib, encouraged to ambulate, and are maintained on broad-spectrum antibiotics for 24 hours. Even when patients undergo gracilis transposition fistula repair without diversion, there are no data to support the usefulness of bowel confinement.

Patients are usually discharged home once the small suction drain is removed, with the urinary bladder catheter left in place. After 6–8 weeks, all patients undergo rectal contrast enema, voiding cystourethrography, cystoscopy, and proctoscopy. If the fistula has healed, the bladder catheter is removed, and stoma reversal is scheduled.

Gracilis Flap Repair of Nonhealing Perineal Wounds

In the case of a persistent sinus, the patient must first undergo curettage and removal of all the necrotic tissue until vascularized granulation tissue is encountered. The wounds often have multiple tracts and careful debridement is necessary until every sinus is unroofed and cleaned of its superficial peel. In the original description by Bartholdson and Hultén (18) the graciloplasty was delayed 7 days, however we do not believe that this staging of the procedure is necessary. The gracilis is harvested as described above and secured in its tendinous portion to the most cephalad portion of the wound with absorbable sutures. A closed suction drain can be used to prevent fluid collection during the first few days, but should rapidly be removed as soon as the drainage is minimal. If a portion of skin is harvested with muscle, it is sutured to the edges of the open sinus after the edges of the wound have been freshened up. Otherwise, most commonly a small residual opening is dressed with wet to dry dressing.

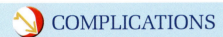 COMPLICATIONS

Despite the fact that the procedure of the gracilis muscle harvest and its use as a rotation flap to interpose between the rectum and the vagina or urethra cannot be regarded as minor surgery, complications are generally fairly infrequent. Superficial perineal wound infection may occur in approximately 10% of the patients. However, postoperative perineal sepsis is fortunately not common, especially if preoperative or concomitant diversion is used, and may occur mainly in cases in which ischemia of the muscle develops. In such cases, adequate drainage of the perineal area is mandatory, and the muscle viability should be assessed with debridement of any necrotic tissue. Muscle necrosis requires muscle resection with contralateral vascular delay. If the patient has not yet been diverted, diversion is strongly advised at this stage.

Some thigh numbness is not uncommon after gracilis harvest. However, such numbness is usually mild, with only a minor impact on the quality of life.

In cases of rectourethral fistulas following surgical trauma or radiation therapy, lower urinary tract complications such as urethral stenosis or urinary incontinence may preoperatively exist, but do not become symptomatic at that stage since the patients' lower urinary tract is diverted. Fistula repair with gracilis muscle transposition generally does not prevent these urinary tract complications, but removal of the diverting cystostomy after successful repair of the fistula may lessen the symptoms and thus improve quality of life.

As any type of complex fistula repair, the gracilis muscle transposition is not successful in all patients, and the most common "complication" of this procedure is probably persistent or recurrent fistula.

When a gracilis flap is used for the treatment of perineal wounds, and if an associated island of skin is harvested with the muscle, skin necrosis can be observed as a specific complication. Necrosis does not necessarily translate into muscle loss, as the vascularization of the skin is relatively poor. When this complication occurs, the patient should be conservatively treated with local care as the perineal sinus could still be successfully obliterated and a subsequent skin graft performed could still lead to satisfactory results. It is important to educate the patient on smoking cessation, to minimize the risk of flap necrosis.

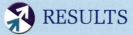

RESULTS

The results of the use of the gracilis muscle for the repair of complex perianal fistulas to the vagina or the urethra, as well as for the reconstruction of perineal wounds, are generally favorable (Table 30.1).

Rectourethral Fistulas

Our initial report on the use of gracilis interposition for the repair of iatrogenic rectourethral fistulas at the Cleveland Clinic Florida included 12 gracilis muscle transpositions in 11 male patients (19). In all of these patients, the fistula was a result of treatment for carcinoma of the prostate. In all the 11 patients, the rectourethral fistula eventually healed, and the fecal diversion was reversed. Urinary diversion was reversed in all but one patient with a severe urethral stricture. One patient had a urinary leak through the perineal wound, leading to wound infection. The gracilis flap was debrided 5 weeks later, and the wound was left open. The rectourethral fistula persisted, and the patient had a second gracilis muscle transposition 5 months later. This time the rectourethral fistula healed well and the diversion was successfully reversed. A second patient developed rectoperineal fistula to the surgical incision following reversal of fecal diversion. This was treated successfully with application of fibrin glue to the fistula tract. Overall 10 (83%) of the 12 transposition flaps resulted in complete healing of the rectourethral fistula, and in two cases further procedures were required, leading to a complete healing.

Our subsequent report (20) included 36 male patients who had gracilis interposition for the treatment of rectourethral fistula, 82% of whom followed treatment for prostate cancer. Overall success rate with transposition of the first gracilis was 78%, and cumulatively, including second procedures, clinical success rate was 97%.

Injuries to the lower urinary tract following surgery or radiation therapy for the treatment of prostate cancer may become evident after successful repair of the fistula and reversal of urinary diversion. In our experience, only 52% of patients had adequate

TABLE 30.1	**Success Rate of Gracilis Transposition**		
Authors (reference no.)	Year of publication	Number of patients	Success rate (%)
Rectourethral fistulas			
Zmora Oded (19)	2003	11	91
Wexner SD (20)	2008	36	97
Ulrich D (22)	2009	26	100
Gupta K (23)	2008	15	100
Zmora Osnat (24)	2006	3	100
Rectovaginal fistulas			
Rius J (28)	2000	3	66
Wexner SD (20)	2008	17	53
Ulrich D (22)	2009	9	77
Zmora Osnat (24)	2006	6	83
Fürst A (25)	2008	12	92
Lefèvre JH (26)	2009	8	75
Unhealed perineal wounds			
Menon A (27)	2005	7	57
Rius J (28)	2000	3	100
Pezim (29)	1987	21	66.7

postoperative urinary continence (21). Five patients required implantation of artificial urinary sphincter, and four others suffered from severe urinary incontinence symptoms. Urethral stricture occurred in fifth of the patients, in two of whom urethrotomy had failed, requiring permanent urinary diversion.

Ulrich et al. (22) reported on a series of 26 patients with rectourethral fistula who underwent repair with the gracilis interposition. Of note, four of these patients had rectourethral fistulas owing to Crohn's disease and two developed such a fistula after perianal abscess. In their series, complete healing of the rectourethral fistula was achieved in all the patients. Likewise, Gupta et al. (23) reported a 100% success rate in 15 patients with rectourethral fistula, of which 5 were congenital in origin. Osnat Zmora et al. (24) reported similar success rate in three patients who underwent gracilis transposition for rectourethral fistulas.

Rectovaginal Fistulas

Our initial report at the Cleveland Clinic Florida included three female patients with inflammatory bowel diseases and fistula between the rectum and the vagina (25), one patient with a history of total proctocolectomy and ileoanal pouch for presumed diagnosis of ulcerative colitis, postoperatively diagnosed as Crohn's disease. Patients with inflammatory bowel diseases may specifically be challenging since the concomitant activity of the inflammatory diseases decreases wound-healing capabilities. Two of these patients completely healed following gracilis transposition, and a third one with pouch-vaginal fistula developed recurrence with a very thin fistula associated with only minimal symptoms.

In a later series (20), we reported on 17 female patients with a fistula between the rectum and the vagina, 3 of whom followed ileoanal or coloanal anastomosis. In nine patients, the fistula was associated with Crohn's disease. Seventy six percent of the patients with pouch-vaginal fistula had undergone a mean of 2 prior failed attempts at repair. The rectovaginal fistula healed in 75% of the patients without Crohn's disease, as compared to only 33% of Crohn's disease–associated fistulas. Of note, two patients required a second gracilis transposition. In one case, because of intraoperative gracilis muscle necrosis, the necrotic portion of the gracilis was resected, and a contralateral interposition was successfully undertaken. A second patient developed persistent unhealed perineal tract that was closed with a second gracilis interposition.

Ulrich et al (22) reported on nine patients with rectovaginal fistula, three of which were associated with Crohn's disease, who underwent gracilis interposition. Two of the patients with Crohn's disease had recurrent fistula, while all patients without Crohn's disease completely healed. Osnat Zmora et al (24) reported on six patients, two of whom had Crohn's disease, who underwent gracilis repair. Five of these patients successfully healed while one patient with Crohn's disease failed.

Fürst et al (25) reported 12 patients with rectovaginal fistula owing to Crohn's disease, with only one failure. One patient, with pouch-vaginal fistula, required a second gracilis transposition to heal. Recently, Lefèvre et al (26) reported eight patients with rectovaginal fistulas, six of whom successfully healed with gracilis transposition. The two patients who failed underwent a second gracilis transposition, which was unsuccessful in both the cases.

Nonhealing Perineal Wounds

When used in the appropriate patient, gracilis muscle transposition has excellent results in the treatment of nonhealing perineal wounds. In a small series by Menon et al (27) four of the seven patients healed. First, all persistent sinuses must be identified and eliminated, second, due to its limited volume, the gracilis muscle can be used only in those sinuses that are thin and extend only 6–8 cm above the opening. Failure to fill the cavity with healthy vascularized muscle will result in failure. Larger cavities may be filled by bilateral gracilis transposition.

In the Cleveland Clinic series reported by Rius et al (28), three patients with Crohn's disease and unhealed perineal sinus underwent gracilis muscle transposition with the technique described above without associated skin flaps or myocutaneous flaps, all of whom had healed at 6-month follow-up.

In a series from the Mayo Clinic, published in 1987, Pezim et al (29) reported 21 patients with persistent perineal sinus after proctectomy for Crohn's disease (10 patients), ulcerative colitis (7 patients), trauma (2 patients), and cancer (2 patients). Of 21 fistulas, 14 had completely healed at a mean follow-up of 47 months. This study points out the need of long follow-up in this type of patients as well as the need of reoperations to obliterate persistent sinuses. The original pathology did not influence the final outcome. In a series from Edinburg, Collie et al (30) reported rather unsatisfactory results on a patient with Crohn's disease and ulcerative colitis after proctectomy. The series is small and reported as a short note with paucity of detail; however the author seems to prefer the use of rectus abdominis muscle flap over the use of gracilis.

CONCLUSIONS

The use of gracilis muscle for the repair of distal rectal-urogenital fistulas and nonhealing perineal wound offers many advantages and is an essential tool in the armamentarium of a colorectal surgeon.

Harvesting the muscle has virtually no negative functional effect and does not result in cosmetic deformity, except for the surgical scar in the medial aspect of the thigh.

The muscle can bring vascularization and bulk in the first 6–8 cm cephalad to the perineal floor, and that is where the flap finds its best application.

The techniques described in this chapter will help colon rectal surgeons in facing some of the most challenging cases to help some of the most debilitated and frustrated patients. In our experience, it offers good long-term results, is associated with minimal morbidity and excellent cosmetic results, and results in enduring patient satisfaction.

Recommended References and Readings

1. Dinges S, Deger S, Koswig S, et al. High-dose rate interstitial with external beam irradiation for localized prostate cancer—results of a prospective trial. *Radiother Oncol* 1998;48(2):197–202.
2. Izawa JI, Ajam K, McGuire E, et al. Major surgery to manage definitively severe complications of salvage cryotherapy for prostate cancer. *J Urol* 2000;164(6):1978–81.
3. Andreani SM, Dang HH, Grondona P, et al. Rectovaginal fistula in Crohn's disease. *Dis Colon Rectum* 2007;50(12):2215–22.
4. Shatari T, Niimi M, Fujita M, Kodaira S. Vascular anatomy of gracilis muscle: arterial findings to enhance graciloplasty. *Surg Radiol Anat* 2000;22(1):21–4.
5. Ruffolo C, Scarpa M, Bassi N, Angriman I. A systematic review on advancement flaps for rectovaginal fistula in Crohn's disease: transrectal versus transvaginal approach. *Colorectal Dis* 2009;12(12):1183–91.
6. Boushey RP, McLeod RS, Cohen Z. Surgical management of acquired rectourethral fistula, emphasizing the posterior approach. *Can J Surg* 1998;41(3):241–4.
7. Trippitelli A, Barbagli G, Lenzi R, et al. Surgical treatment of rectourethral fistulae. *Eur Urol* 1985;11(6):388–91.
8. Schwandner O, Fuerst A, Kunstreich K, Scherer R. Innovative technique for the closure of rectovaginal fistula using Surgisis mesh. *Tech Coloproctol* 2009;13(2):135–40.
9. Ellis CN. Outcomes after repair of rectovaginal fistulas using bioprosthetics. *Dis Colon Rectum* 2008;51(7):1084–8.
10. Thompson IM, Marx AC. Conservative therapy of rectourethral fistula: five-year follow-up. *Urology* 1990;35(6):533–6.
11. Nyam DC, Pemberton JH. Management of iatrogenic rectourethral fistula. *Dis Colon Rectum* 1999;42(8):994–7.
12. Vidal Sans J, Palou Redorta J, Pradell Teigell J, Banus Gassol JM. Management and treatment of eighteen rectourethral fistulas. *Eur Urol* 1985;11(5):300–5.
13. Stephenson RA, Middleton RG. Repair of rectourinary fistulas using a posterior sagittal transanal transrectal (modified York-Mason) approach: an update. *J Urol* 1996;155(6):1989–91.
14. Ryan JA Jr. Gracilis muscle flap for the persistent perineal sinus of inflammatory bowel disease. *Am J Surg* 1984;148(1):64–70.
15. Hallock GG. Minimally invasive harvest of the gracilis muscle. *Plast Reconstr Surg* 1999;104(3):801–5.
16. Whetzel TP, Lechtman AN. The gracilis myofasciocutaneous flap: vascular anatomy and clinical application. *Plast Reconstr Surg* 1997;99(6):1642–52; discussion 1653–5.
17. Hsu H, Lin CM, Sun TB, et al. Unilateral gracilis myofasciocutaneous advancement flap for single stage reconstruction of scrotal and perineal defects. *J Plast Reconstr Aesthet Surg* 2007;60(9):1055–9.
18. Bartholdson L, Hultén L. Repair of persistent perineal sinuses by means of a pedicle flap of musculus gracilis. Case report. *Scand J Plast Reconstr Surg* 1975;9(1):74–6.
19. Zmora O, Potenti FM, Wexner SD, et al. Gracilis muscle transposition for iatrogenic rectourethral fistula. *Ann Surg* 2003;237(4):483–7.
20. Wexner SD, Ruiz DE, Genua J, et al. Gracilis muscle interposition for the treatment of rectourethral, rectovaginal, and pouch-vaginal fistulas: results in 53 patients. *Ann Surg* 2008;248(1):39–43.
21. Ghoniem G, Elmissiry M, Weiss E, et al. Transperineal repair of complex rectourethral fistula using gracilis muscle flap interposition—can urinary and bowel functions be preserved? *J Urol* 2008;179(5):1882–6.
22. Ulrich D, Roos J, Jakse G, Pallua N. Gracilis muscle interposition for the treatment of recto-urethral and rectovaginal fistulas: a retrospective analysis of 35 cases. *J Plast Reconstr Aesthet Surg* 2009;62(3):352–6.
23. Gupta G, Kumar S, Kekre NS, Gopalakrishnan G. Surgical management of rectourethral fistula. *Urology* 2008;71(2):267–71.
24. Zmora O, Tulchinsky H, Gur E, et al. Gracilis muscle transposition for fistulas between the rectum and urethra or vagina. *Dis Colon Rectum* 2006;49(9):1316–21.

25. Fürst A, Schmidbauer C, Swol-Ben J, et al. Gracilis transposition for repair of recurrent anovaginal and rectovaginal fistulas in Crohn's disease. *Int J Colorectal Dis* 2008;23(4):349–53.

26. Lefèvre JH, Bretagnol F, Maggiori L, et al. Operative results and quality of life after gracilis muscle transposition for recurrent rectovaginal fistula. *Dis Colon Rectum* 2009;52(7):1290–5.

27. Menon A, Clark MA, Shatari T, et al. Pedicled flaps in the treatment of nonhealing perineal wounds. *Colorectal Dis* 2005; 7(5):441–4.

28. Rius J, Nessim A, Nogueras JJ, Wexner SD. Gracilis transposition in complicated perianal fistula and unhealed perineal wounds in Crohn's disease. *Eur J Surg* 2000;166(3):218–22.

29. Pezim ME, Wolff BG, Woods JE, et al. Closure of postproctectomy perineal sinus with gracilis muscle flaps. *Can J Surg* 1987;30(3):212–14.

30. Collie MH, Potter MA, Bartolo DC. Myocutaneous flaps promote perineal healing in inflammatory bowel disease. *Br J Surg* 2005;92(6):740–1.

31 House, Diamond, V-Y

James W. Fleshman and Ira J. Kodner

 ## INDICATIONS/CONTRAINDICATIONS

Flaps can be used to cover defects in the perianal skin after excision of anal lesions such as Paget's disease or Bowen's disease. Stricturing will sometimes result from iatrogenic or idiopathic causes and are treated with advancement of extra skin into the anal canal. The use of flaps to bring normal inner buttock skin toward or into the anal canal can relieve the stricturing from the scar or lack of skin but will not impact the narrowing caused by a hypertrophied internal sphincter. Ectropion is the exposure of anal canal or low rectal mucosa at the level of the anal verge caused by previous resection and causes a large amount of mucous production and even bleeding. Readvancement of the mucosa back into the anal canal and replacement of the defect with inner buttock skin is the preferred method of treating the ectropion.

Consideration should be given to the etiology of the stricture prior to recommending skin flap advancement. Crohn's disease has very limited indications since the healing process is impaired. Radiation-induced stricturing most likely involves damage to the perianal skin and may also have some skin buttock impairment. The most common cause for anal stricturing is an over zealous hemorrhoidectomy with removal of more viable anoderm than is adequate to dilate the anal canal. Replacement of this anoderm with skin from the inner buttock is the ideal indication for skin flap advancement for treatment of stricture.

The Whitehead hemorrhoidectomy with circumferential excision of the anoderm of the anal canal has resulted in an ectropion and stricture formation in many patients who have been treated with an inappropriately performed Whitehead procedure. The ectropion can be reduced into the anal canal and the stricture treated at the same procedure using a broad-based house-shaped skin flap.

Patients who have no ectropion but have normal external anoderm and normal rectal mucosa but simply have lost dermis at the level of the dentate line benefit most from a diamond-shaped skin advancement flap.

 ## PREOPERATIVE PLANNING

The mobilization of inner buttock skin into the anal canal can be accomplished based on the principles of plastic surgery flap construction. The base of the flap should be broad enough to maintain an adequate blood supply. The dissection should be performed with as little cautery as possible, and the mobility of the flap toward the anal canal should be maximized by releasing the tethering attachments under the donor site rather than under the flap skin itself.

The patient should undergo a complete bowel preparation and receive preoperative antibiotics. The patient should be informed that a period of low activity without sitting, driving, or climbing steps will be enforced for the 2 weeks after surgery. The consideration for doing a unilateral flap versus bilateral flaps should be made preoperatively and determined by the amount of coverage needed outside and within the anal canal.

SURGERY

V, U, or House-Shaped Flap

Positioning
■ The patient should be placed in the prone-jackknife position with the buttocks taped apart. The perineum is prepped and draped sterilely. Local anesthesia can be obtained with the patient sedated to relax the muscle and provide local anesthetic. Care should be made not to use Epinephrine because of its vasoconstrictive features. The flap should be drawn on the inner aspect of the buttock with a broad-base encompassing approximately the entire side of the anal canal in the case of stricturing. The length of the flap is determined by the base and should be two to three times the length of the base.

Technique
■ The flap lines are drawn with indelible marker (Fig. 31.1).
■ The flap is incised along the lines of the drawing and carried into the anal canal on either side of the ectropion down to normal mucosa. The edges of the flap are protected.
■ The attachments to the flap are released by undermining under the edges of a donor site rather than the flap itself. The pedicle is released at the apex of the tip of the flap out on the buttock to allow the redundant skin to move toward the anal canal with very little tension (Fig. 31.2).
■ The advanced skin is then secured at the new inner site. If the ectropion is moved inward into the anal canal, the redundant mucosa is banded with internal elastic ligation.
■ The edges of the flap are secured at its new position with interrupted 3-0 Prolene horizontal mattress sutures incorporating the subcuticular layer of the flap and the full-thickness of the adjacent donor skin to avoid piercing the flap and to protect the blood supply.

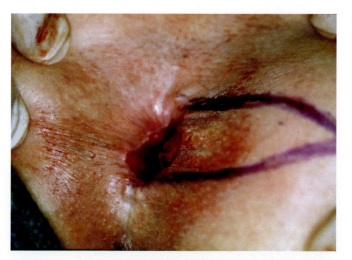

Figure 31.1 The house flap is drawn out onto the buttock with a wide base at the anal canal.

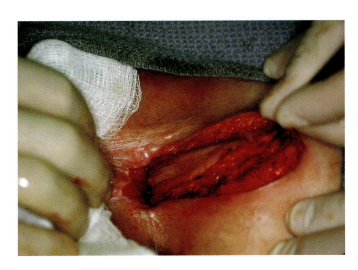

Figure 31.2 Incision of the donor site to release the pedicle toward the anal canal maintaining the broad fat pedicle with vessels intact.

■ The opening of the donor site is then closed in a linear fashion with interrupted vertical mattress sutures to close the donor site behind the skin flap (Fig. 31.3). A dressing of Polysporin ointment and fluff gauze is supplied.

Diamond-Shaped Flap

Positioning

The use of the diamond-shaped flap to expand the available tissue in the anal canal is begun with the patient in the prone-jackknife position with the buttocks taped apart and the perineum partially draped sterilely. Proctoscopy can be performed to empty the rectum and the rectum irrigated with povidone iodine. During dilation of the anal canal, it is typical for fissures to occur in the lateral positions of the anal canal, and these fissures become the basis for the receptive site for the skin to be introduced.

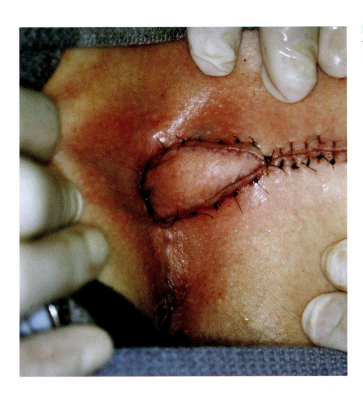

Figure 31.3 Advancement of the flap into the anal canal with closure of the donor site behind.

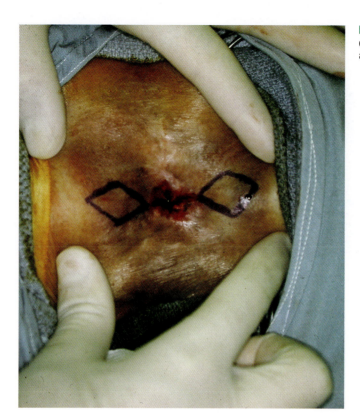

Figure 31.4 Inscription of the diamond-shaped flaps on the inner aspect of the buttocks.

Technique

- The flaps are drawn on the skin with the inner tip of the diamond at the edge of the fissures in the anal canal stricture.
- The stricture is incised at these fissure sites, and the scar is divided. The underlying internal sphincter and external sphincter are protected, and the incision sites are enlarged to accommodate the postage stamp sized diamond flap (Fig. 31.4).
- The diamond-shaped flaps are incised on the skin maintaining broad-based pedicles of fat under the flaps by undermining the attachments under the donor skin to allow the broad-base of the diamond flap to slide into the anal canal. The blood supply is protected.
- The skin is handled very gently, and the skin is pushed into the defect in the stricture (Fig. 31.5).
- The donor sites are closed behind the diamond flap, and the edges of the diamond flap are secured in the donor site with the horizontal mattress sutures of 3-0 absorbable suture between full-thickness outer skin and subcuticular on the flap itself. The apex of the diamond within the anal canal is secured with a full-thickness 3-0 absorbable suture to fix the flap within the anal canal, and then the edges are sewn in around the shape of the diamond.
- The donor site is once again closed in a linear fashion to keep the flap from pulling out (Fig. 31.1). Triple antibiotic ointment is applied and a fluff gauze is applied loosely.

➜ POSTOPERATIVE MANAGEMENT

- Patients with either of these flaps are managed similarly.
- The patient is maintained in the hospital on bowel rest without sitting or climbing stairs for 3 days and receiving antibiotics.

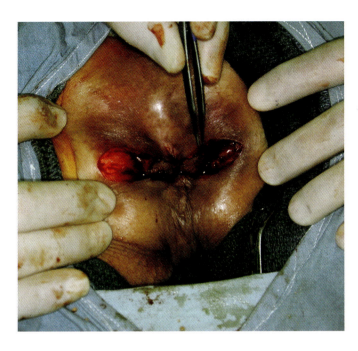

Figure 31.5 Incision of the skin and release of the lateral attachments of the diamond pedicle flaps while maintaining the broad base fat pedicle. The flaps are advanced into the incisions in the anal stricture.

- On post-op day 3, the patient is begun on a liquid diet, stool softeners, and laxatives. On post-op day 4, the patient is allowed to resume a regular diet and warned against constipation.
- The patient is allowed to leave the hospital but is instructed not to sit, climb stairs, drive, or do strenuous exercise for 2 weeks. At the 2-week follow-up period if healing has progressed and the sutures can be removed, the patient is allowed to liberalize activity.
- It is usually not necessary to perform repeated dilations after a flap procedure. A single anoscopy after 2 weeks of healing will reveal an adequate anal canal, and the patient can be reassured that the stenosis is resolved.

COMPLICATIONS

- Flap viability is an issue when patients are obese, have known cardiovascular disease, and smoke. The patients should be instructed to avoid cigarettes for 2 weeks prior to the procedure and afterwards.
- Because this is a very unsterile area, the likelihood of infection is high. The flaps can be saved even though infection occurs and the exam under anesthesia and debridement is an appropriate first maneuver. Long-term antibiotics can also reduce the likelihood of poor outcome.
- The donor site may open or become infected. Delayed closure or closure by granulation is appropriate and tub soaks or high pressure shower cleansing provides easy management.

RESULTS AND CONCLUSION

Eventual healing and success after advancement flap for stricturing, ectropion, or anal lesion resection can be expected in approximately 90% of patients. The resolution of anal stricture should be close to 100%. If the first flap is unsuccessful in restoring anal diameter, a second flap on the opposite side with either a diamond flap or a house flap is possible. Even though infection ranges of 10% or higher have been experienced, the overall success is still very high because the flap is so well vascularized and resilient. Only radiated tissue has a low healing rate, and this should be anticipated because of the patient's pertinent history.

Selected Readings

Duieb Z, Appu S, Hung K, Nguyen H. Anal stenosis: use of an algorithm to provide a tension-free anoplasty. *ANZ J Surg* 2010;80(5):337–40.

Pearl RK, Hooks VH 3rd, Abcarian H, Orsay CP, Nelson RL. Island flap anoplasty for the treatment of anal stricture and mucosal ectropion. *Dis Colon Rectum* 1990;33(7):581–3.

32 Endorectal Advancement Flap

Maher A. Abbas and Matthew J. Sherman

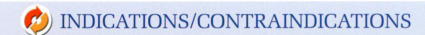

INDICATIONS/CONTRAINDICATIONS

Anal fistula is one of the commonest benign anal disorders, it affects both genders and various age groups. Most anal fistulas are cryptoglandular in origin although other etiologies include Crohn's disease, obstetrical trauma, radiation therapy, and cancer. Surgical intervention is required to resolve most chronic fistulas. The goal of operation is threefold: eradicate the fistula, preserve continence, and minimize the risk of recurrence. Several options are available to treat anal fistula: fistulotomy; fistulectomy; fistulotomy with sphincteroplasty, seton, injectables such fibrin glue, fistula plugs, and anal flaps. The choice of operation depends on several factors including the anatomy of the fistula and its relationship to the anal sphincter muscles, the etiology of the fistula, the baseline continence level, prior anal operations, and patient's body habitus. Although most fistulas can be easily eradicated, some can be quite challenging to treat and can carry higher failure and complication rate.

For most low-lying anal fistulas or fistulas involving minimal anal sphincter muscle, fistulotomy can be used with good clinical and functional results. However, for more complex fistulas, especially when there is concern about fecal continence, the endorectal advancement flap is a good option. Closure of the internal fistulous tract by an internal flap can successfully heal most fistulas while at the same time minimizing the risk of anal incontinence. This technique was first described as the sliding flap in 1902 by Noble (1). In his original description, he used a full-thickness rectal flap. In 1948, Laird (2) modified the procedure by advocating the use of a partial-thickness flap consisting of mucosa, submucosa, and a portion of the internal circular muscle. Candidates for the endorectal advancement flap include patients with complex anal fistulas such as high transsphincteric and suprasphincteric fistula, Crohn's disease–associated fistulas, rectovaginal fistulas, rectourethral fistulas, fistulas with secondary tracts, and recurrent fistulas (3).

Contraindications to the endorectal advancement flap include acute anal abscess, a strictured anus, scarred rectal wall, and active inflammation in the anorectum from conditions such as Crohn's disease. In the setting of Crohn's disease, it is important to determine whether the fistula is a result of active perianal Crohn's disease or an incidental finding in a patient with more proximal intestinal disease. In the setting of Crohn's disease, a delay in wound healing may be noted in up to 80% of patients despite a normal-appearing rectum (4). Not all Crohn's disease–related anal fistulas require surgical intervention. In one study, spontaneous healing of acute fistulas occurred in 38% of patients without any surgical interventions (5). Fistula closure rates following medical therapy have been reported in 34–50% of patients taking oral metronidazole (6), in 33% of those patients on 6-MP or azathioprine (7), and in as many as 62% of patients who received infliximab (8). In the presence of active proctitis, the success rate of endorectal flap is low with one study reporting closure of fistula in only 20% of patients (9). Under such circumstances, it is best to drain the fistula with a noncutting seton and treat the patient medically. An endorectal advancement flap can be undertaken if and when there is disease remission.

PREOPERATIVE PLANNING

The evaluation of the patient with anal fistula includes a detailed history of past anal or colorectal operations; past obstetrical history; comorbidities such as diabetes, human immunodeficiency virus (HIV), neurologic or neuromuscular disorders, prior radiation therapy to the pelvis, baseline level of continence, and use of tobacco. Smoking has been associated with a higher failure rate of the endorectal flap and therefore patients who smoke are advised to quit prior to operative intervention (10–11). Physical examination includes visual inspection of the external fistulous opening (location and number of openings if more than one), digital examination to assess sphincter tone, probing of the external opening with the index finger of the examiner inside the anus to evaluate the depth of the fistula and muscle involvement, and anoscopy to visualize the quality of the anorectal mucosa. Occasionally the examination can be limited due to the patient's discomfort. Under such circumstances an examination under anesthesia is required to ensure patient comfort and cooperation and may reveal an abscess that requires drainage as initial step of treatment. Proper incision and drainage of an underlying abscess yields a higher success rate of the endorectal flap with one study reporting an overall success rate of 73% versus 49% (prior drainage vs. none) (12). The use of noncutting seton prior to definitive endorectal flap improves overall success rate (12). Usually 2–3 months of seton drainage is advised before performing the endorectal flap except for Crohn's disease where the response of inflammation to the medical therapy is the major determinant of when to proceed with definitive operation.

Endoscopic evaluation of the colorectum is indicated in the setting of inflammatory bowel disease or if there is suspicion of it and in patients who meet screening criteria or who warrant diagnostic colonoscopy for history of polyps, cancer, or for symptoms such as bleeding or abdominal pain. Occasionally a high internal fistulous opening can be visualized during the endoscopic retroflexion inside the rectum. Routine imaging of the anorectal area or pelvis to determine the anatomy of a fistula is not warranted. Imaging is used selectively for recurrent or persistent disease, deep tracts, multiple external openings, or when assessing the integrity of the anal sphincter muscles in conditions such as rectovaginal fistula. If an associated sphincter defect is present and a concomitant sphincter repair is performed, success rate of the endorectal advancement flap for rectovaginal fistula is higher. Computed tomography plays little role in the management of anal fistulas but can be helpful in the setting of acute sepsis especially when a deep abscess is suspected. Magnetic resonance imaging and endoanal ultrasound (EUS) are useful diagnostic studies in patients with anal fistulas with similar accuracy. However, EUS is more widely available and more commonly used; EUS is less costly than magnetic resonance imaging and can be performed by the treating surgeon. Fistulous tracts can be confirmed by hydrogen peroxide injection through the external fistulous opening (Fig. 32.1A,B). Fistulogram, while commonly used in the past, is less frequently performed because of the availability of EUS but can be helpful when delineating complex fistulas such as horseshoe (Fig. 32.2).

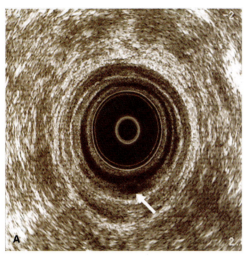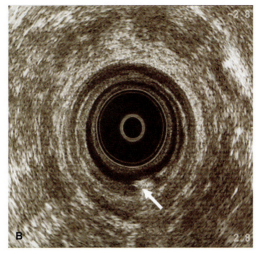

Figure 32.1 **A.** Ultrasound examination reveals transsphincteric fistula in ano (arrow). **B.** Hydrogen peroxide confirmed the active tract (arrow).

Physiologic testing of the anorectum is not routinely performed but can be helpful in a subgroup of patients. Sainio et al. (13) advocate preoperative anorectal manometry in women with previous obstetrical trauma, elderly patients, patients with Crohn's disease or HIV, or patients with recurrent disease and prior surgery. Preoperative manometric evaluation can elicit sphincter dysfunction already present and may alter the treatment plan.

Bowel Preparation and Antibiotics Prophylaxis

For technical reasons, the rectum needs to be clean at the time of operation. Bowel preparation can be achieved with either oral mechanical bowel preparation the night prior to operation or two sodium phosphates the morning of the operation. Some surgeons prefer a full mechanical bowel preparation citing a better preparation and less infectious complications. No data are available to suggest that one method of rectal cleansing is superior to the other. In our practice, we currently ask the patient to perform two rectal enemas the morning of operation and we have found that approach sufficient for most patients undergoing endorectal advancement flap.

Perioperative use of antibiotics for anorectal surgery has not been well standardized. There are no distinct recommendations from the Surgical Care Improvement

Figure 32.2 Fistulogram demonstrates horseshoe fistula.

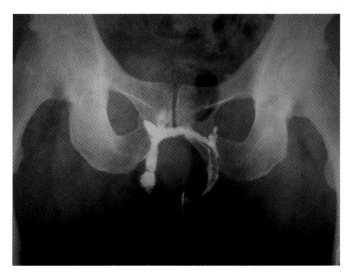

Project. In our practice, we give the patient a single dose of intravenous antibiotics. Appropriate coverage of gram-negative and anaerobic organisms includes single drug regimen such as a second-generation cephalosporin (i.e., cefotetan), ampicillin/sulbactam, or combination of antibiotics such as ciprofloxacin and metronidazole.

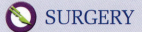

SURGERY

Anesthesia and Positioning

Choice of anesthesia depends on both surgeon's preference and patient's factors. We prefer general anesthesia for most patients as it allows for complete relaxation and cooperation. Alternative to general anesthesia include monitored sedation with local anesthesia, epidural or spinal block.

We perform all of our endorectal flaps in the prone jack-knife position. Once positioned, the buttocks are retracted laterally and secured to the table with tape. We prefer such position as it provides adequate lightening and allows the assistant the proper visualization to provide the exposure and assistance needed during the operation. Some surgeons prefer the lithotomy position for posterior-based fistula.

Surgical Technique

The first step of the operation is to address the fistulous tract. The noncutting seton, if present, is removed. Some authors recommend complete dissection and excision of the fistula tract up to the external anal sphincter (14,15). Curettage of the fistulous tract without excision has been reported by others (16). We prefer to curette rather than excise the tract as to minimize the size of the wound (Fig. 32.3). Curettage of the tract

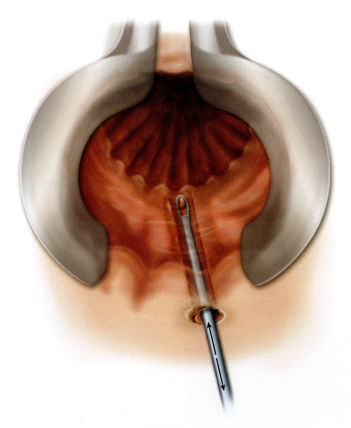

Figure 32.3 Curettage of the fistulous tract.

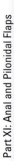

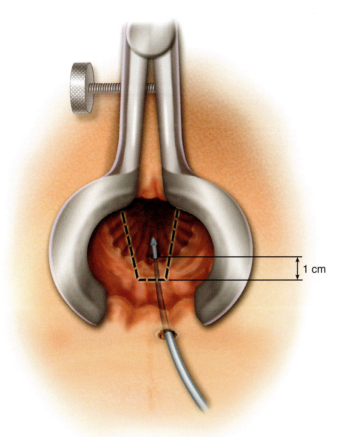

Figure 32.4 Distal aspect of flap, 1 cm caudal to internal opening.

is performed from the external opening and all the way to the internal opening. Once completed, the tract is flushed with saline to remove any debris.

A Pratt Bivalve or Hill-Ferguson anal retractor is used for exposure. Care is taken to not overstretch the anal sphincter complex to minimize injury. We do not use the Parks' retractor as it can affect resting anal tone (17,18) and may lead to postoperative continence disturbance (14,18). Although we do not use the Lone Star retractor for endorectal flap, it is an alternative to the Pratt Bivalve and Hill-Ferguson retractors and can provide good visualization and decrease the tension on the anal sphincter (18). Once exposure is obtained, the anorectum is irrigated with Betadine solution. A probe is passed through the external opening to identify the exact location of the internal opening. The distal aspect of the flap is scored 1cm distal to the internal opening using electrocautery (Fig. 32.4). The length of the flap is usually 4–6cm to ensure adequate coverage of the intramuscular portion of the internal opening without tension. The base of the flap should be approximately twice the width of the apex to provide adequate blood supply. Infiltration of the rectal wall with 1% lidocaine with 1:100,000 epinephrine is performed to allow for better hemostasis (Fig. 32.5). The raised flap should be partial thickness, including the mucosa, submucosa, and a portion of the internal anal sphincter (Fig. 32.6). Care should be taken to ensure consistent thickness of the flap and to avoid pigeon-holing the flap. Thin flaps with mucosa and submucosa alone often have inadequate blood supply that may lead to higher failure rate. Good mobilization of the flap is achieved once the distal lip of flap can easily protrude without tension from the anal opening. Once the flap is mobilized, the intramuscular portion of the internal opening is closed with single interrupted 2.0 Vicryl sutures (Fig. 32.7). Often this step requires a row of 3–4 sutures. The closure of the internal opening can be tested by injecting saline or Betadine through the external

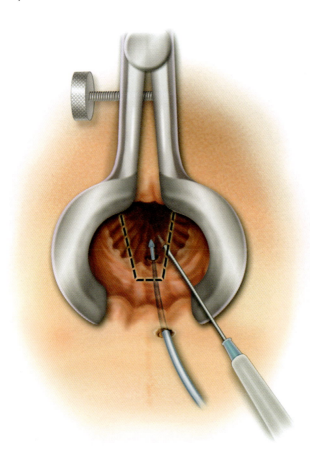

Figure 32.5 Intramural infiltration with 1% lidocaine with 1:100,000 epinephrine for hemostasis.

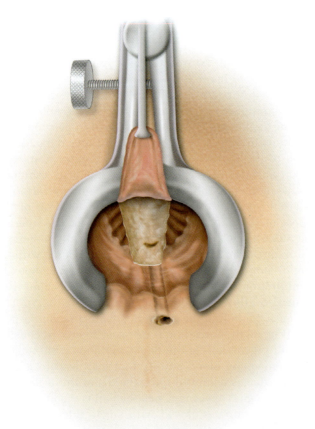

Figure 32.6 Partial-thickness flap is raised.

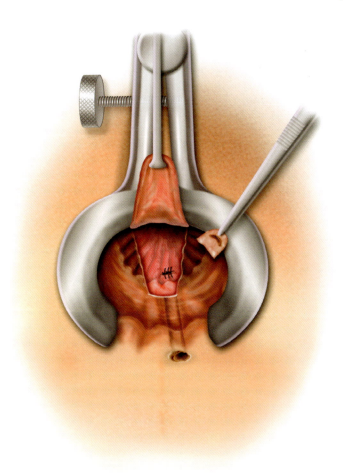

fistulous opening. If significant leakage of solution is still noted, additional sutures can be placed. The bed of the raised flap is then irrigated with saline and inspected for any bleeding. Complete hemostasis is obtained before maturing the flap to avoid any postoperative hematoma that can compromise the flap. Hemostasis can be obtained with electrocautery or figure-of-eight suture using 2.0 Vicryl. Finally, the distal lip of the flap that contains the mucosal internal opening is trimmed to fresh well-vascularized and healthy tissue (Fig. 32.7). The flap is then sutured in place with single interrupted 2.0 Vicryl (Fig. 32.8). A bacitracin ointment–impregnated Gelfoam is inserted inside the anal canal on completion of the flap. The external opening is left open to drain. When a chronic cavity is associated with the fistulous tract, a mushroom tip catheter (12–16F catheter, depending on the size of cavity) can be placed inside the cavity to decompress it to avoid fluid buildup at the base of the flap, which may contribute to failure (9,10). In the setting of a rectovaginal fistula, the vaginal mucosa side is left open to allow drainage.

The described technique is our preferred technique and has yielded good results. The only variation we sometime perform is the addition of biologic mesh under the flap to reinforce the tissue. Biologic mesh can yield a higher success rate in patients with poor tissue, recurrent or persistent fistulas after prior anal flap (16). We have previously used biologic mesh in combination with an endorectal advancement flap for radiation-induced rectourethral fistula with success (19). Others have reported closure of recurrent rectovaginal fistula with the combination of endorectal advancement flap with biologic mesh (20). If biologic mesh is used, it is parachuted into the anal canal after placing corner sutures with the mesh outside the body, anchoring the corners of the mesh at the apex of the flap dissection with 2.0 Vicryl suture (Fig. 32.9).

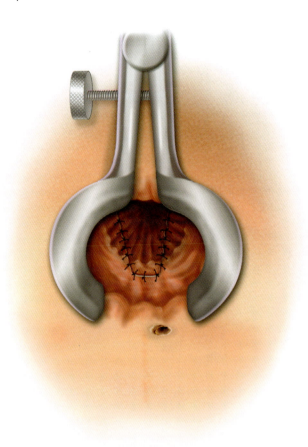

Figure 32.8 Final maturation of flap to its bed.

POSTOPERATIVE MANAGEMENT

Some surgeons discharge the patient directly from the postanesthesia recovery unit. In our practice most patients are admitted for 23-hour observation and discharged at anytime during that period once pain is adequately controlled and after spontaneous urination. Rarely, a patient requires more than a 23 hours of hospitalization. A liquid diet is started the day of operation and advanced to a regular diet within 2 days.

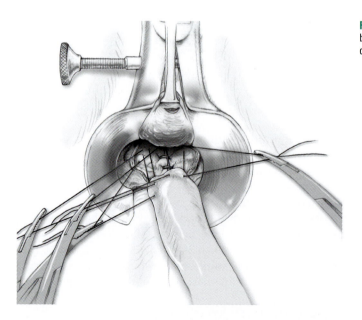

Figure 32.9 Parachuting the biologic mesh into the bed of dissection.

Some authors advocate the use of postoperative antibiotics. However, this adjunct measure has not been shown to make a difference in patients who receive antibiotics following endorectal advancement flaps as compared to those patients who do not receive postoperative antibiotics (10–12). Our current practice is to selectively use antibiotics in diabetic and immunosuppressed patients such as HIV-positive patients. A 10-day course of either amoxicillin/clavulanate or ciprofloxacin with metronidazole is usually sufficient.

At the time of discharge the patient is advised to be on a high-fiber regular diet and to avoid constipation. A daily regimen of a stool softener with a bulking agent such as psyllium is recommended. If the patient has no bowel movement within 70 hours, a gentle laxative such as milk of magnesium is prescribed to avoid fecal impaction. Male patients with rectourethral fistula are discharged with an indwelling urethral catheter and a suprapubic tube, which are removed as early as 3 weeks postoperatively if a healed fistula is demonstrated on a urethrogram. Patients should refrain from strenuous physical activities. Women with anterior-based flaps are instructed to abstain from sexual activities for 3 months. The first postoperative visit is scheduled 1 month later. However, the patient is instructed to return for earlier evaluation if febrile to >100°F, or has chills, rectal bleeding, increasing anorectal or pelvic pain, or difficulty with urination. Anoscopic and digital examination is usually deferred for at least 1 month to avoid disruption of a healing flap.

COMPLICATIONS

Endorectal advancement flap is a relatively safe operation; the complication rate is low (16). All known complications that can occur with any anal operation have been reported with the endorectal advancement flap. Bleeding, wound abscess or hematoma, thrombosed hemorrhoid, fissure, urinary retention, or fecal incontinence can occur. Major perineal sepsis is extremely rare following endorectal advancement flap as septic complications often lead to flap breakdown that allows for the infection to drain spontaneously. Table 32.1 summarizes the incontinence rate noted in several large series. The majority of studies show low postoperative incontinence rate ranging between 0% and 13%. Only one study reported a higher incontinence rate of 35%, which was attributed by the authors to the use of the Park's anal retractor, an observation made by other investigators (14,17). Fortunately most cases of incontinence are minor and transient. Finally, another complication previously reported is transient postejaculation irritation in men with anterior-based flaps (16).

Part XI: Anal and Pilonidal Flaps

TABLE 32.1	Results of Endorectal Advancement Flap				
Author	Year	n	Success (%)	Incontinence (%)	Mean follow-up (months)
Garcia-Aguilar	1984	151	99	10	8–84*
Wedell	1987	31	100	0	18–48*
Kodner	1993	107	84	13	8
Makowiec	1995	32	66	3	20
Miller	1998	25	77	0	14
Kreis	1998	24	63	13	48
Shouten	1999	44	75	35	12
Ortiz	2000	103	93	8	12
Mizrahi	2002	94	60	9	40
Abbas	2008	38	83	8	27

*Range.

RESULTS

Overall, endorectal advancement flap has been associated with favorable success rates. Table 32.1 summarizes several of the reported series from the past two decades (3,14,16,21–27). Success rates range from 60% to 100% with most studies reporting a success rate greater than 75%. Several factors can impact success rate and risk factors for recurrence have been identified (Table 32.2). Crohn's disease, duration of the fistula prior to repair, and smoking have been shown to interfere with the healing process. Schouten et al. (14) and Ellis et al. (10) showed that the number of prior repair attempts directly influences success. Sonoda showed that a larger body surface area does positively influence healing rates (12). Other factors are not quite clear. For instance, age showed no real difference except in one study where age <40 years was associated with worse outcome but a high proportion of the patients had Crohn's disease, which could explain the finding (12). On an interesting note, Sonoda et al. (12) and Abbas et al. (16) have shown that location may be important in outcome. Sonoda et al. (12) found that success rate of the endorectal advancement flap was 55% in anterior-based fistula compared to 79% in posterior fistulas ($P = 0.07$). While short-term closure rate of fistula following endorectal advancement flap is a main outcome measure, equally as important is the long-term recurrence rate of the operation. In the study by Abbas et al. (16), all long-term recurrences were noted in patients whose fistulas were in the left lateral quadrant ($P = $ NS). In several studies, a nonstatistically significant trend toward higher recurrence rates of the endorectal fistulas in patients with rectovaginal fistulas compared

TABLE 32.2	Factors Affecting Outcome			
Author	**Factor**	**Success rate (%)**	**Recurrence rate (%)**	***P* value**
	Prior repair			
Schouten	0–1	87	–	0.02
	≥2	50	–	–
Ellis	Yes	–	52	<0.05
	No	–	27	–
Mizrahi	0	–	44	NS
	1	–	30	–
	2	–	40	–
	3	–	75	–
	Smoking			
Ellis	Yes	–	51	<0.05
	No	–	19	–
Zimmerman	Yes	60	–	–
	No	79	–	–
	Crohn's			
Mizrahi	Yes	–	57	<0.04
	No	–	33	–
Sonoda	Yes	50	–	0.027
	No	77	–	–
	BSA*			
Sonoda	>100	81	–	0.027
	75–100	56	–	–
	70–75	50	–	–
	<70	47	–	–
	Fistula duration			
	<3 months	70	–	0.03
	3–6 months	65	–	–
	>6 months	62	–	–

*BSA = body surface area.

to trans-sphincter fistulas was found (3,10). Sonoda et al. (12) reported an overall success rate of 75.8% in anorectal fistulas treated with the endorectal advancement flap compared to 43.2% in rectovaginal fistulas ($P = 0.002$). In another study, most immediate failures were noted in patients with recurrent rectovaginal fistulas (16). Gender, the presence of diverting stoma, and perioperative use of immunosuppression do not appear to influence outcome (3,10,12). It is important to note however that most data available on endorectal advancement flap are retrospective in nature and most reported series contain small number of patients.

CONCLUSIONS

Anal fistula is one of the commonest benign anorectal disorders evaluated and treated by colorectal surgeons. Although some fistulas can respond to medical therapy, most chronic fistulas will require surgical correction. Over the past 100 years numerous operations have been introduced to treat this condition but the goals of surgical therapy remain the same: to heal the fistula, prevent recurrence, and minimize postoperative complications including incontinence. While such goals can be achieved in the majority of the patients, some fistulas can be quite challenging to the surgeon. It is critical for the surgeon who treats anorectal fistulas to have a clear understanding of the results and limitations of various operations and the technical knowledge and skills to perform them. The endorectal advancement flap is an essential component of the armamentarium of operations to treat anorectal fistulas. It yields a high success rate with low and acceptable risks.

Recommended References and Readings

1. Noble G. A new operation for complete laceration of the perineum designed for the purpose of eliminating danger of infection from the rectum. *Trans Am Gynecol Soc* 1902;27;357–63.
2. Laird D. Procedures used in treatment of complicated fistulas. *Am J Surg* 1948;76:701–8.
3. Mizrahi N, Wexner S, Zmora O, et al. Endorectal advancement flap. *Dis Colon Rectum* 2002;45:1616–21.
4. Halme L, Sainio P. Factors related to frequency, type and outcome of anal fistulas in Crohn's disease. *Dis Colon Rectum* 1995;38:55–9.
5. Buchmann P, Keighley M, Allan R, et al. Natural history of perianal Crohn's disease: ten-year follow-up. A plea for conservatism. *Am J Surg* 1980;140:642–4.
6. Schwartz D, Pemberton J, Sandborn W. Diagnosis and treatment of perianal fistulas in Crohn's disease. *Ann Intern Med* 2001;135:906–18.
7. Lecomte T, Contou J, Beaugerie L, et al. Predictive factor of response of perianal Crohn's disease to azathioprine or 6-mercaptopurine. *Dis Colon Rectum* 2003;46:1469–75.
8. Present D, Rutgeerts P, Targan S, et al. Infliximab for the treatment of fistulas in patients with Crohn's disease. *N Engl J Med* 1999;340:1398–1405.
9. Jones O, Fazio V, Jagelman D. The use of trans anal advancement flaps in the management of fistulas involving the anorectum. *Dis Colon Rectum* 1987;30:919–23.
10. Ellis C, Clark S. Effect of tobacco smoking on advancement flap repair of complex anal fistulas. *Dis Colon Rectum* 2007;50:459–63.
11. Zimmerman D, Delamarre J, Gossenlink M. Smoking affects the outcome of transanal mucosal advancement flap repair of transsphincteric fistulas. *Br J Surg* 2003;90:351–4.
12. Sonoda T, Hull T, Piedmonte M, et al. Outcomes of primary repair of anorectal and rectovaginal fistulas using the endorectal advancement flap. *Dis Colon Rectum* 2002;45:1622–8.
13. Sainio P, Husa A. A prospective manometric study of the effect of anal fistula surgery on anorectal function. *Acta Chir Scand* 1985;151:279–88.
14. Schouten W, Zimmerman D, Briel J. Transanal advancement flap repair of transphincteric fistulas. *Dis Colon Rectum* 1999;42:1419–22.
15. Dubsky P, Stift A, Friedl J, et al. Endorectal advancement flaps in the treatment of high anal fistula of cryptoglandular origin: full-thickness vs. mucosal-rectum flaps. *Dis Colon Rectum* 2008;51:852–7.
16. Abbas M, Lemus-Rangel R, Hamadani A. Long-term outcomes of endorectal advancement flap for complex anorectal fistulae. *Am Surg* 2008;74:921–4.
17. van Tets W, Kuijpers J, Tran K, et al. Influence of Parks' anal retractor on anal sphincter pressure. *Dis Colon Rectum* 1997;40:1042–5.
18. Zimmerman D, Gosselink M, Hop W, et al. Impact of two different types of anal retractor on fecal continence after fistula repair. *Dis Colon Rectum* 2003;46:1674–9.
19. Lesser T, Aboseif S, Abbas MA. Combined endorectal advancement flap with Alloderm® graft repair of radiation and cryablation-induced rectourethral fistula. *Am Surg* 2008;74(4);341–5.
20. Shelton AA, Welton ML. Transperineal repair of persistent rectovaginal fistulas using an acellular cadaveric dermal graft. *Dis Colon Rectum* 2006;49:1454–7.
21. Garcia-Aguilar J, Belmonte C, Wong W, et al. Anal fistula surgery: factors associated with recurrence and incontinence. *Dis Colon Rectum* 1996;39:723–9.
22. Wedell J, Meier zu Eissen P, Banzhaf G, et al. Sliding flap advancement for the treatment of high level fistulae. *Br J Surg* 1987;74:390–1.
23. Kodner I, Mazor A, Shemesh E, et al. Endorectal advancement flap repair of rectovaginal and other complicated fistulas. *Surgery* 1993;114:682–9.
24. Makoweic F, Jehle E, Becker H, et al. Clinical course after transanal advancement flap repair of perianal fistula in patients with Crohn's disease. *Br J Surg* 1995;82:603–6.
25. Miller G, Finan R. Flap advancement and core fistulectomy for complex rectal fistula. *Br J Surg* 1998;85:108–10.
26. Kreis M, Jehle E, Ohlemann M, et al. Functional results after transanal rectal advancement flap repair of transsphincteric fistula. *Br J Surg* 1998;85:240–2.
27. Ortiz H, Marzo J. Endorectal flap advancement repair and fistulectomy for high transsphincteric and suprasphincteric fistulas. *Br J Surg* 2000;87:1680–3.

33 Sleeve Advancement

David J. Maron

 ## INDICATIONS/CONTRAINDICATIONS

Fistula in ano is a relatively common problem encountered by the colorectal surgeon. While cryptoglandular infection represents the most common cause, inflammatory bowel disease, anorectal trauma or obstetric injury, and mycobacterial infections may also lead to anal fistulas. Surgical management is based on the location and complexity of the fistula, the underlying disease process, and the potential for sphincteric compromise.

Fistulotomy remains the optimal treatment for patients with symptomatic low-lying fistulas involving minimum sphincter musculature. In patients with Crohn's disease without active proctitis, fistulotomy may also be useful in low (distal) fistulas. In patients with rectovaginal fistulas, or high and complex fistulas where fistulotomy involving division of the anal sphincter would result in compromise of fecal continence, other modalities may be instituted. These procedures involve the use of cutting setons, fibrin glue, collagen fistula plugs, and endorectal advancement flaps. Use of these procedures is described elsewhere in this book.

Anal sleeve advancement is based on the same principles as an endorectal advancement flap. It involves the resection of a cylinder of the diseased portion of the anal canal, with mobilization of the distal rectum and advancement to the dentate line for anastomosis. Anal sleeve advancement was initially described by Whitehead for the treatment of hemorrhoids and subsequently by Delorme for the treatment of prolapsing rectal mucosa. In recent years, it has been used in complex anorectal fistulous disease.

Anal sleeve advancement flaps should be reserved for patients with complex anorectal or vaginal fistulas. Patients with a single internal fistulous opening or several openings in the same quadrant are probably best treated with a vertical or semilunar-type advancement flap. For patients with multiple internal openings involving more than one quadrant, patients with complex anorectal Crohn's disease, or patients with anorectal stricture, sleeve advancement offers an alternative to proctectomy or permanent fecal diversion.

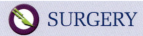 PREOPERATIVE PLANNING

Careful patient selection is critical to success and important to reduce the risk of a non-healing wound and worsening perianal disease. Patients with concomitant perianal sepsis need to undergo drainage of any abscess, with the judicious use of draining setons to prevent further sepsis. The author prefers to leave draining setons in place for a minimum of 3 months to allow for resolution of underlying inflammation. In patients with ongoing sepsis despite the use of draining setons, a diverting stoma may be used.

In patients with Crohn's disease, sleeve advancement should be avoided in the setting of active proctitis. It is recommended that patients undergo an endoscopic evaluation of the colon and potentially a barium small bowel series to evaluate for Crohn's disease elsewhere in the intestine, as optimal control of proximal Crohn's disease may improve the success of the sleeve advancement flap. Assessment should also be made of the mobility and pliability of the rectal wall; this may require an examination under anesthesia in the operating room.

SURGERY

Positioning

Preoperatively, the patient undergoes a standard mechanical bowel preparation. Oral antibiotics are not generally given, however the patient receives broad-spectrum intravenous antibiotics prior to incision. Either general or regional (spinal) anesthetic can be used, depending on the patient and surgeon preference. The procedure can be performed in either the lithotomy or prone jackknife position. The author prefers the prone jackknife position under general anesthesia.

Use of the Lone Star retractor (Lone Star Company, Houston, TX, USA) helps to efface the anus and allows for better visualization of the dentate line and any fistulas. A full anoscopic examination should be performed to evaluate for the number and extent of any fistulas as well as any other abnormalities. A rigid proctoscopy should also be performed, particularly in the setting of Crohn's disease, to evaluate for rectal inflammation. In female patients, the vagina should also be inspected.

Technique

Epinephrine 1:200,000 is circumferentially injected into the anal canal and distal rectum. Beginning distal to the fistula opening or anal canal ulceration, a circumferential incision is made with the use of electrocautery or scissors; needlepoint electrocautery works particularly well in this situation. This incision may be at or just below the dentate line, depending on the location of the fistula(s). Dissection begins in the submucosal plane and circumferentially extends cephalad (Fig. 33.1). A few fibers of the internal anal sphincter may be included in the sleeve of tissue, depending on the depth of the inflammation from the fistula process. Once above the sphincter complex, dissection may extend outside the longitudinal muscle to encompass the full thickness of the rectum. The dissection should cross the fistula tract(s) until soft tissue above the tracts is encountered. Circumferential dissection is continued cephalad until mobility is obtained such that the entire sleeve can be advanced distally well beyond the point of initial incision.

In female patients, care must be taken to avoid entry into the vagina. This is best performed by inserting the index finger of the surgeon's nondominant hand into the vagina during dissection to serve as a guide.

The fistulous tracts are curetted to remove any granulation tissue and the internal openings are closed in layers with absorbable suture (3-0 polyglycolic acid suture). The external fistulous openings can be enlarged with elliptical incisions to allow for adequate drainage. Vaginal openings are left open following curettage. It is important to ensure hemostasis to avoid a hematoma that could compromise the flap.

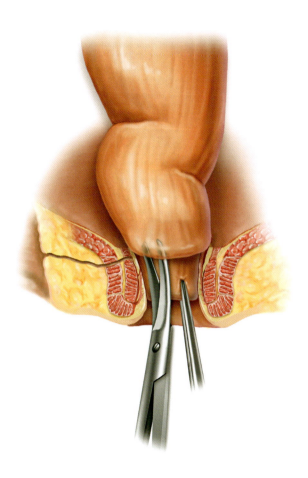

Figure 33.1 Dissection of a full-thickness sleeve flap begins in the submucosal plane and circumferentially extends cephalad until mobility is obtained such that the entire sleeve can be distally advanced well beyond the point of initial incision.

At this point, the distal diseased portion of the flap is trimmed above the level of the fistula(s) (Fig. 33.2). To prevent retraction of the rectum, it is important to place several sutures in the rectum prior to fully amputating the distal portion of the sleeve tube. The anastomosis is then created with the use of circumferential interrupted 3-0 polyglycolic acid sutures in a full-thickness manner, incorporating the underlying internal anal sphincter muscle (Fig. 33.3).

In rare cases, it may be necessary to mobilize the rectum by a transabdominal approach. Although it is not generally necessary, in selected patients a temporary diverting loop ileostomy may also be performed to protect the anastomosis.

 ## POSTOPERATIVE MANAGEMENT

Intravenous antibiotics are continued perioperatively for 24 hours. Patients are restricted from taking anything by mouth, but constipating agents are not usually given. Oral nutrition is started with return of bowel function as evidenced by the passage of flatus. In patients who undergo a diverting loop ileostomy, bowel continuity is restored after a minimum of 3 months.

 ## COMPLICATIONS

Major morbidity is uncommon following anal sleeve advancement flap. Bleeding and hematoma formation may occur, which can potentially lead to necrosis of the flap and failure. Recurrent perianal sepsis can be avoided by ensuring adequate drainage at the external fistulous sites. Urinary retention may occur secondary to pain as well as the use of long-acting local anesthetic agents.

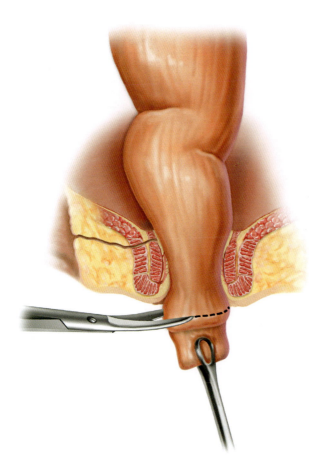

Figure 33.2 The fistulous tracts are curetted to remove any granulation tissue and the internal openings are closed in layers with absorbable suture (not shown). The distal diseased portion of the flap is then trimmed above the level of the fistula(s).

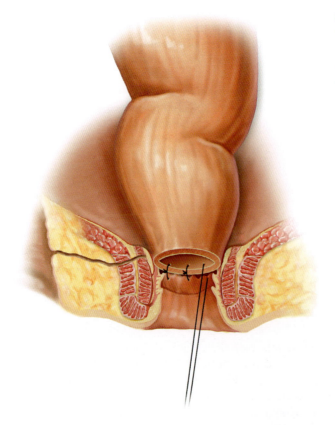

Figure 33.3 The anastomosis is created with the use of circumferential interrupted 3-0 polyglycolic acid sutures in a full-thickness manner, incorporating the underlying internal anal sphincter muscle.

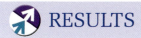
RESULTS

While there are multiple reports in the literature of the success of mucosal advancement flaps for the treatment of anal fistulas, there are relatively few studies and case reports regarding anal sleeve advancement flaps. Berman first described the successful technique in a patient with multiple anorectal and anovaginal fistulas. Simmang subsequently described success in two patients with rectovaginal fistula and anorectal stricture.

Marchesa described the experience of the use of anal sleeve advancement flap at the Cleveland Clinic in patients with severe perianal Crohn's disease. Eight out of thirteen patients (62%) were treated successfully in this series at a median follow-up of 15 months. A majority of patients in this study underwent fecal diversion at the time of repair. The authors found that success rate was significantly higher in patients who underwent concomitant bowel resection, suggesting that treatment of proximal disease may improve success rates.

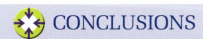
CONCLUSIONS

Anal sleeve advancement flap is an effective surgical option in patients with complex anorectal or vaginal fistulas. This technique may be useful in patients who have failed other treatments, patients with complex anorectal Crohn's disease, or patients with anorectal stricture. While more radical surgery may often be necessary, anal sleeve advancement offers an alternative to proctectomy or to permanent fecal diversion in selected patients.

Suggested Readings

Berman IR. Sleeve advancement anorectoplasty for complicated anorectal/vaginal fistula. *Dis Colon Rectum* 1991;34(11):1032–7.

Halverson AL, Hull TL, Fazio VW, et al. Repair of recurrent rectovaginal fistulas. *Surgery* 2001;130(4):753–8.

Hull TL, Fazio VW. Surgical approaches to low anovaginal fistula in Crohn's disease. *Am J Surg* 1997;173:95–8.

Marchesa P, Hull TL, Fazio VW. Advancement sleeve flaps for treatment of severe perianal Crohn's disease. *Br J Surg* 1998;85:1695–8.

Simmang CL, Lacey SW, Huber PJ. Rectal sleeve advancement. *Dis Colon Rectum* 1999;41(6):787–9.

34 House Flap Anoplasty for Bowen's Disease

Jorge A. Lagares-Garcia and Paul R. Sturrock

 ## INDICATIONS/CONTRAINDICATIONS

Current terminology and definition of premalignant lesions of the anus and perineum are confusing. The same pathology can be defined with the terms squamous cell carcinoma in situ, anal intraepithelial neoplasia (AIN), anal dysplasia, squamous intraepithelial lesion, or Bowen's disease. Unfortunately, there seems to be a significant discrepancy between the staging systems and intra- and interobserver variability. Moreover, increasing screening techniques have shown that detection of *high-grade squamous intraepithelial lesions (HSILs)* or AIN III has increased, but they have not decreased the incidence of invasive cancer in high prevalence areas of AIN. This fact is more significant in patients who practice anoreceptive intercourse, specifically those suffering from HIV.

Human papilloma virus is a DNA papovavirus that causes the most common viral sexually transmitted disease. Serotypes 16, 18, 31, 33, and 35 are significant for harboring a higher malignant potential.

For all purposes in this chapter, both Bowen's disease and squamous cell carcinoma in situ will be described as HSIL to avoid any confusion. The potential of invasion is much less when the pathology report reveals low-grade squamous intraepithelial neoplasia, therefore the most common indication to perform a "house flap" anoplasty (HA) is currently HSIL.

Other pathologies such as anal stricture, extensive tracts of hidradenitis suppurativa, and mucosal ectropion from prior anorectal surgery may be indications for the use of advancement flaps such the "house flap."

T1 tumors (2.5 cm or less in diameter) may undergo local excision if no lymphadenopathy is noted during the preoperative metastatic evaluation. Coverage of the resulting defect may also be undertaken with this kind of skin and subcutaneous tissue flap.

The current indications for the use of HA are indicated in Table 34.1.

 ## PREOPERATIVE PLANNING

The width of the area to be excised can be quite large depending on the extent of the disease. It is important to note that the disease is multicentric due to the viral nature

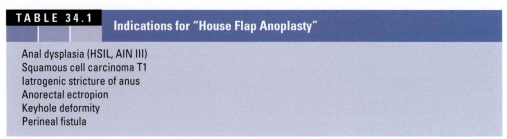

TABLE 34.1	Indications for "House Flap Anoplasty"
Anal dysplasia (HSIL, AIN III)	
Squamous cell carcinoma T1	
Iatrogenic stricture of anus	
Anorectal ectropion	
Keyhole deformity	
Perineal fistula	

HSIL, high-grade squamous intraepithelial lesion; AIN, anal intraepithelial neoplasia.

and the localization of HSIL areas may not be totally reduced to one aspect of the *intra-anal, perianal areas* (<5 cm radius from the anal opening) or *skin* (>5 cm from the anal opening). For isolated processes such as stricture or ectropion the decision of laterality is made simpler.

To plan for the area of excision and reconstruction, two different modalities may be used for locating the HSIL.

The use of an operative microscope or surgical loupes and an anoscope after the use of Lugol's solution and acetic acid will reveal the lesions that may be biopsied, marked, or fulgurated.

Another method is the *anal mapping* technique where multiple biopsies are performed at the level of the dentate line, anal verge, and anal margin in 12 different sites that are labeled and sent to pathology for analysis. These results provide the clinician with a diagram of the areas of HSIL in the anal canal and surrounding tissues.

Once the area has been located, the decision is made whether to perform a unilateral or bilateral HA.

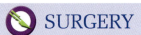 SURGERY

Positioning and Preparation

Multiple different opinions exist regarding the use of preoperative cathartic bowel preparation and postoperative bowel lock. Our current practice is to avoid a full-bowel preparation and instead to advise the patient to have two enemas the morning of the surgery. Patients must also remain nothing by mouth (NPO) for at least 6 hours prior to the induction of anesthesia.

The day of the procedure, the patient's medical history is reviewed for allergies to drugs that may be used during the operation as well as to assess the current health status. The patient is brought into the operating room where graded compression stockings and sequential compression devices are placed for deep venous thrombosis prophylaxis. Antibiotic prophylaxis is given within 1 hour of making the incision. Our routine consists of either ciprofloxacin 400 mg IV + metronidazole 500 mg IV or cefoxitin 1–2 g IV + metronidazole 500 mg IV depending on the patient's drug allergies. This same regimen is continued postoperatively for 24 hours.

While still on the transport stretcher, general endotracheal anesthesia is induced with the patient in the supine position and a foley catheter is then inserted. After the airway is secured, we proceed to transfer the patient onto the OR table in the prone jack-knife position over a Kraske pillow at the level of the iliac crests to obtain elevation of the buttocks. Separation of the buttocks and exposure of the anal region is achieved with tapes placed widely enough on the skin of the buttocks to provide retraction yet to allow access to the tissue being used for the reconstruction. After the skin is prepared with chlorhexidine or iodine-based solution, a wide preparation of the surgical field is undertaken with sterile drapes. It is our practice for the primary surgeon to routinely use a headlamp for better illumination of the operative field. In addition, if very delicate dissection of the anal canal is needed, the use of microscopic loupes (×2–3 magnification) may aid in visualization of the tissue planes.

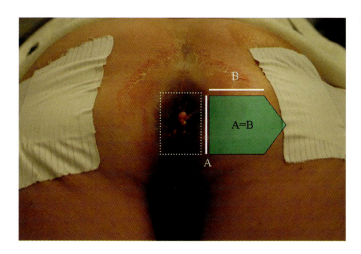

Figure 34.1 Landmarks for the house flap anoplasty.

Technique

After the perianal area is examined, a digital rectal examination is performed to palpate any abnormalities in the anal canal. This is followed by visual inspection of the anal canal using a Hill-Ferguson retractor. A decision is then made regarding the surface area to be excised. It is our preference to remove all macroscopic lesions in toto; we do not routinely perform intraoperative frozen sections to assess for microscopic margins, as this is very time consuming and does not alter our surgical approach.

It is important to note that at times, coexisting conditions such as fungal or bacterial superinfections exist. These maladies must be treated with antifungals or topical antibiotics prior to any procedure to minimize the risk of postoperative wound complications. Surgery should be deferred until such infections have been completely resolved.

If additional lesions exist in the vicinity or more lateral to the area to be excised, primary resection and closure in layers is recommended unless the defect is so large that it has to be encompassed with the resected area itself.

Measurements and Calculations

A quadrangular excision with clear margins from macroscopic lesions is drawn with indelible marker. The most lateral aspects will become the base of the HA. Our preference is to reconstruct the "side-wall" of the HA the same size as the base to avoid postoperative retraction making the advancements of the flap equidistant in all levels (Figs. 34.1 and 34.2).

Figures 34.3–34.7 represent schematically the process of design and reconstruction of the "house flap."

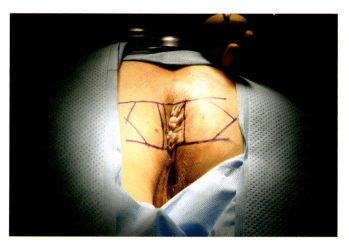

Figure 34.2 Intraoperative markings of the flap and area to be excised.

Figure 34.3 Measurements and calculations.

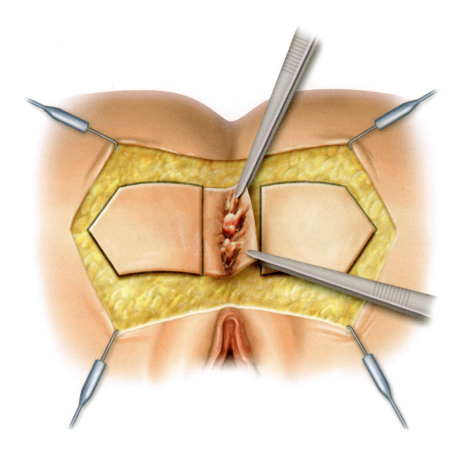

Excision

The affected area is exposed using the Lone Star Retractor™ (Lone Star Medical Products, Stafford, TX, USA). Using the electrocautery knife or a scalpel, an incision is made through the epidermis and dermis. Underneath the dermis and above the subcutaneous fat, the dissection is continued, being careful to identify and preserve the internal and

Figure 34.4 Resection of affected area.

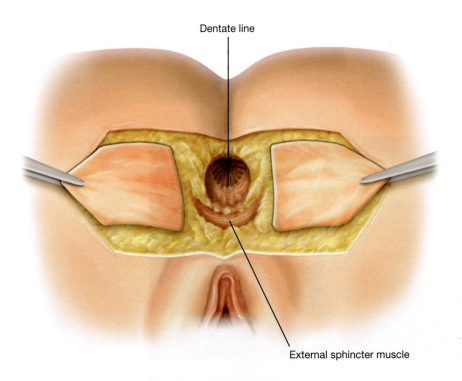

Dentate line

External sphincter muscle

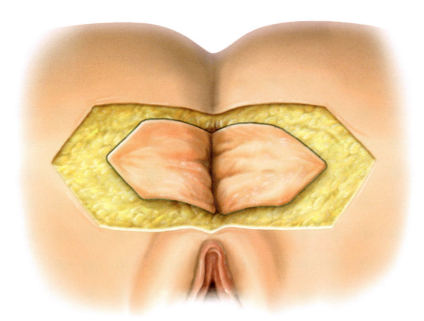

Figure 34.5 Advancement of the "house flap".

external anal sphincters (Fig. 34.8). The dentate line typically marks the most proximal aspect of resection unless gross macroscopic disease exists above this level (Fig. 34.9). If at any time there is suspicion of invasive carcinoma, an oncologic wide local excision is performed with the understanding that fecal incontinence may be a postoperative problem if any portion of the sphincter complex must be sacrificed.

It is important to maintain correct orientation of the specimen at all times once it is passed off the operative field. There are many ways to accomplish this, but our preference is to take the specimen to the back table and suture it to a sterile towel. The towel is then labeled with a surgical marker: "anterior," "posterior," "left," "right," and "proximal anal canal." This labeling allows for accurate reporting by the pathologist of the margins. Future surveillance can be directed to any areas that remain microscopically involved with dysplasia. If invasive carcinoma is discovered in any area on pathologic analysis, proper orientation will allow for re-resection of the area in a second-staged procedure.

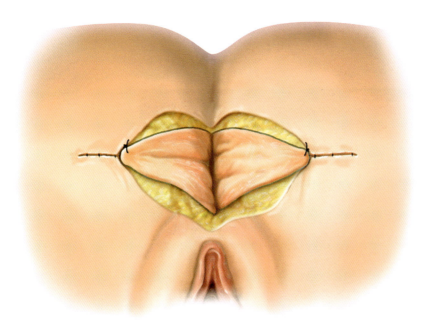

Figure 34.6 Advancement of the "house flap".

Part XI: Anal and Pilonidal Flaps

Figure 34.7 Closure of lateral defect.

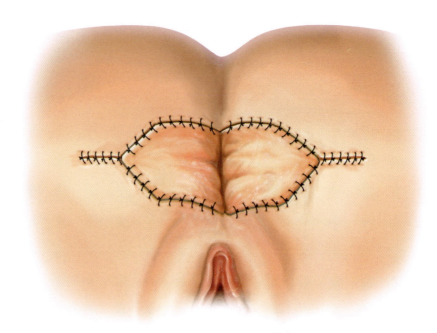

Figure 34.8 Excision of the perianal lesions.

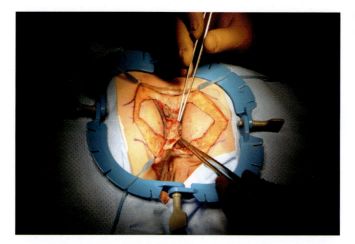

Figure 34.9 Proximal extent of dissection to dentate line.

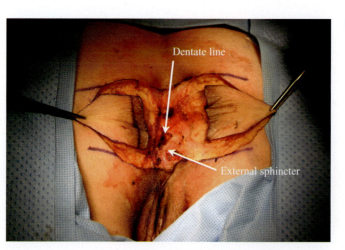

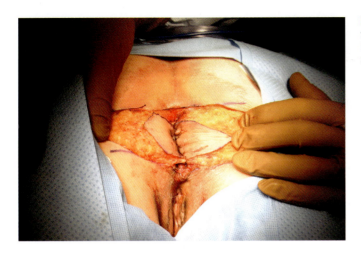

Figure 34.10 Reconstruction of the anal canal with base of house flap anoplasty-dentate line approximation.

Reconstruction

We perform all incisions with the cutting setting on the electrocautery knife. The initial incision is limited to the level of the superficial skin and dermis around the entire flap. The subsequent dissection of the flaps accomplished one at a time using cautery and the incision is extended obliquely under the adjacent superior, inferior, and lateral portions of the donor site, undermining the skin and providing a broad fat pedicle for the flap. If the dissection is properly done, the flaps and the subcutaneous fat will naturally "advance" to the anal canal without any tension.

The reconstruction is initiated by using interrupted sutures of 2-0 monofilament absorbable suture. A full-thickness bite is taken at the proximal (intra-anal) point of prior excision (this is typically at the level of the dentate line.) The distal (medial edge of the flap) bite of the suture is taken at the dermal level in a subcuticular manner; the suture is left long and secured with a hemostat. This is repeated in four quadrants to ensure even placement, after which the sutures are tied and cut. Further sutures are placed between these anchoring stitches to recreate the anorectal junction between dentate line and medial edge of the advancing flap. The anal closure should remain wide enough to loosely accommodate the index finger of the operating surgeon. To avoid a dehiscence at the level of the advancement flap-rectal mucosal suture line, there must be no tension on finishing the suture line (Fig. 34.10).

After the anorectal junction is reconstructed (on both sides of the anal canal if necessary), the "top and corners of the roof" are secured to the skin to fix the flap in position (Fig. 34.11). The remaining donor site deflect is closed in a linear direction with interrupted 2-0 suture in the subdermal layer. Medially, both the anterior and the

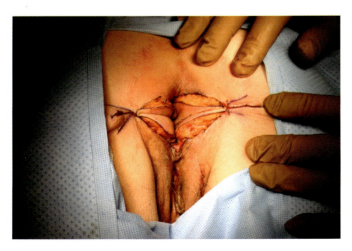

Figure 34.11 "Corners of the roof" of the house flap anoplasty are approximated.

Part XI: Anal and Pilonidal Flaps

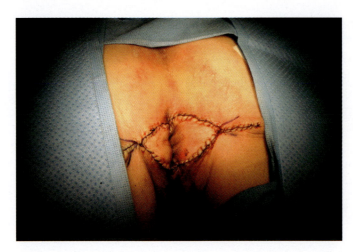

Figure 34.12 Final closure of house flap anoplasty.

posterior segments ("the walls") of the flap are secured to the skin of the specimen excision site with interrupted suture in the subcuticular layer.

The epidermis is then closed with 3-0 absorbable monofilament in a running manner for its strength and longevity. This suture line is covered with bacitracin ointment and a dry dressing (Fig. 34.12). Alternatively, a running absorbable subcuticular suture may be used and covered with Dermabond® (Ethicon Inc., Somerville, NJ, USA). The patient is then returned to the supine position on the transport stretcher or hospital bed and extubated.

 ## POSTOPERATIVE MANAGEMENT

Regular diet may be started when the patient is able to maintain the airway and is conscious. We routinely use psyllium fiber to bulk up the stool and avoid loose stools that may potentially smear the perianal skin. Strict anal hygiene is recommended after each bowel movement using a hand-held shower and gently drying the wound. The patient or nursing staff may reapply bacitracin to the suture lines to keep it protected and facilitate healing. We do not routinely have the patient in strict immobility but instead encourage ambulation. The bladder catheter is removed at 6 AM the morning after the procedure and the patient is encouraged to void independently. Depending on pain control and tolerance of diet and activity, the patient is routinely discharged within 24–48 hours after the procedure. Oral antibiotics are prescribed for 10 days postoperatively; our most common regimen is ciprofloxacin 500 mg twice daily and metronidazole 500 mg three times daily. Routine follow-up is undertaken at 2-week intervals for the first 6–8 weeks and every 3 months thereafter. Special attention is given to any unclear or microscopically invaded pathologic margins when the HA is performed for dysplasia or carcinoma in situ.

 ## COMPLICATIONS

The most common complications following HA are listed in Table 34.2. In-hospital complications are infrequent, but can include urinary retention, urinary tract infection, wound infection/cellulitis, and donor-site separation. In addition, patients can develop *Clostridium difficile* colitis as a result of perioperative antibiotic usage. These complications can usually be treated with conservative measures and rarely lead to failure of the repair.

More long-term complications can be observed in outpatient follow-up. These problems include flap necrosis, wound dehiscence, recurrent stenosis/stricture, recurrent

TABLE 34.2	Complications of "House Flap Anoplasty"
Early	*Late*
Urinary retention	Flap necrosis
Urinary tract infection	Wound dehiscence
Wound infection/cellulitis	Stricture/stenosis
Donor-site separation	Recurrent fistula
C difficile colitis	Liquid/flatus incontinence

fistula (if primary indication was perineal fistula), and incontinence to flatus or liquids. Of these, wound dehiscence and flap necrosis account for the major morbidity of the procedure. These complications require wound packing and daily dressing changes for a prolonged period of time.

If the flap was performed for HSIL, recurrent disease or invasive anal cancer may develop at the proximal resection margin, so continued surveillance is mandatory. HIV patients with low CD4 counts and high viral loads as well as other immunosuppressed patients including, but not limited to, post-transplant, diabetics, or permanent wheelchair-bound individuals are more prone to develop complications of the flap. These patients should be carefully counseled regarding their degree of morbidity before selecting them for this procedure.

 RESULTS

Most of the reports are case series indicating the success of this procedure, as it is performed in only a very select group of patients. Sentovich et al. reported on a series of 29 patients undergoing HA, but only 2 of their patients had HSIL. These two patients did have some difficulty with flatus and liquid incontinence; a finding not reported in other case reports. Further analysis of their series and 4-year follow-up indicated a satisfaction of 82% and improvement of the symptoms in 89% patients. The Cleveland Clinic Florida experience reported in 1995 offered a 50% improvement of the symptoms of stenosis; however, there are no data regarding HSIL follow-up. Alver et al. recently reported their experience in 28 patients. Short-term results include three wound dehiscences and one recurrence of rectovaginal fistula. Only one patient in this series was done for anal neoplasia. At a median of 26 months symptomatic improvement was reported in 66% of patients with carcinoma. In our experience, the symptomatic relief achieved through debulking of local disease while providing adequate coverage of an otherwise significant soft tissue defect has led to a high degree of patient satisfaction.

 CONCLUSION

House flap anoplasty is an effective means of local advancement of skin and soft tissue to treat many perianal conditions. The degree of soft tissue coverage can range widely by varying the size of the reconstructive flaps. When applied to diffuse perianal Bowen's disease, the bilateral HA allows complete excision of all gross disease while minimizing long-term sequelae such as wound contraction and stricture formation. Keeping in mind that this procedure is not curative as microscopic margins are often positive, recurrent lesions can develop. Routine surveillance of the anal canal and perianal area is imperative and is made easier through removal of the larger lesions with this technique. In the appropriately selected patients, this technique will provide symptomatic relief and improve the accuracy of future surveillance.

Suggested Readings

Alver O, Ersoy YE, Aydemir I, et al. Use of "House" advancement flap in anorectal diseases. *World J Surg* 2008;32:2281–6.

Katz KA, Clarke CA, Bernstein KT, et al. *Ann Int Med* 2009;150:283–4.

Colquhoun P. Anal intraepithelial neoplasia. In: Sands L, Sands D, eds. *Ambulatory Colorectal Surgery*. New York, NY: Informa Healthcare 2009:259–65.

Gonzalez AR, De Oliveira O, Verzaro R, et al. Anoplasty for stenosis and other anorectal defects. *Am Surg* 1995;61(6):526–9.

Margenthaler JA, Dietz DW, Mutch MG, Birnbaum EH, Kodner IJ, Fleshman JW. Outcomes, risk of other malignancies, and need for formal mapping procedures in patients with perianal Bowen's disease. *Dis Colon Rectum* 2004;47:1655–61.

Ryan DP, Mayer R. Anal carcinoma: histology, staging, epidemiology, treatment. *Curr Opin Oncol* 2000;12:345–52.

Sentovich SM, Falk PM, Christensen MA, Thorson AG, Blatchford GJ, Pitsch RM. Operative results of House advancement anoplasty. *Br J Surg* 1996;83(9):1242–4.

Welton ML, Varma MG. Anal cancer. In: Wolff BG, Fleshman JW, Beck DB, Pemberton JH, Wexner SD, eds. *The ASCRS Textbook of Colon and Rectal Surgery*. New York, NY: Springer 2007:482–500.

35 Cleft Lift Procedure for Pilonidal Disease

Kim C. Lu and Daniel O. Herzig

Introduction

Pilonidal disease develops within lower midline sinuses in the natal cleft. These sinuses can become occluded and develop abscesses that rupture superiorly and to one side. The exact etiology continues to be debated.

Typically, acute abscesses are drained off midline. A multitude of treatments have been described for treating persistent pilonidal disease. These range from shaving the nearby hair to wide local excisions and even to complex fasciocutaneous flaps such as the Limberg (rhomboid rotational) flap (1).

INDICATIONS/CONTRAINDICATIONS

Indications

In 2002, Dr. T. Bascom and Dr. J. Bascom first described the cleft lift procedure for

- refractory pilonidal disease (2),
- recurrent pilonidal disease, usually after multiple prior operations (2), and
- multiple pilonidal sinuses.

Contraindications

- Acute abscess: Any acute abscess should be urgently drained. After the sepsis were resolved a cleft lift procedure can be done.
- Bilateral disease: after all abnormal tissues are removed, reconstruction would require more tissue such as a fasciocutaneous flap, i.e. Limberg (rhomboid rotational) or V-Y flap, or muscular flap such as a rotational gluteal flap.

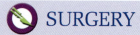

PREOPERATIVE PLANNING

- Typically, the cleft lift procedure is performed on an outpatient basis. Appropriate preoperative risk assessment of cardiac, pulmonary, nutritional, and other factors should be obtained.
- No bowel prep is necessary.
- The patient should avoid aspirin and all nonsteroidal anti-inflammatory drugs for 1 week prior to surgery.

SURGERY

Positioning

If general anesthesia were required, it should be induced on a stretcher. After which the patient is placed into the prone-jackknife position. A large pelvic roll and two smaller chest rolls should minimize hyperextension of the neck. Abduction of either shoulder should be less than 90 degrees and both elbows should be well padded. While an assistant pushes both buttocks together, mark the skin where the buttocks touch with permanent marker. These marks will be the most lateral limits of the subsequent dissection (Fig. 35.1A). The buttocks are taped apart and a towel is placed between the legs to absorb excess prep.

Technique

The patient is given a dose of broad-spectrum antibiotics such as cefazolin and metronidazole within the hour prior to incision.

Figure 35.2B, shows two midline sinuses, both of which communicate with a left, superior abscess cavity and its opening.

The skin to be excised is marked with an asymmetric ellipse including the off line left-sided abscess cavity (Fig. 35.2A). The side opposite the abscess should be incised about 1 mm to the right of the midline pilonidal sinuses. The lateral side of the ellipse should be just shy of the heavy lines marked prior to taping the buttocks. The superior and inferior extent of the ellipse should be 1–2 cm above and below the pathology.

If the inferior aspect of the ellipse were close to the anus, the incision should curve sharply away from the anus (Fig. 35.2A). This avoids undermining the very thin perianal skin.

Cut along the right line of the ellipse. The skin of the right buttock is undermined laterally until the heavy line previously marked prior to taping the buttocks is reached. Dissecting at the superior (cephalad) portion of the ellipse for 1–2 cm frees the skin from the tissue over the sacrum, whereas inferior dissection for 1–2 cm frees the skin from the tissue over the coccyx. These dissections will mobilize a 7-mm thick flap of healthy skin and subcutaneous fat (Figs. 35.2B and 35.3).

Dissection proceeds under the skin of the asymmetric ellipse, after which tapes holding the buttocks apart are released. The right skin flap should easily reach the left lateral border of the tissue to be excised. After which, the skin of the ellipse with the roof of the abscess is excised (Fig. 35.3).

A RayTec sponge is used to curette out any abscess cavity. The fibrotic walls of the abscess cavity should not be excised.

With the tapes released, the subcutaneous fat on either side of the midline should fall together. Using interrupted 2-O or 3-O polyglactin sutures, the subcutaneous fat of the distal portion of the cleft is approximated to (Figs. 35.4 and 35.5) make the natal cleft shallower.

A round fluted Blake drain can be placed under the skin flap, even though one recent study suggested that drains are unnecessary (3).

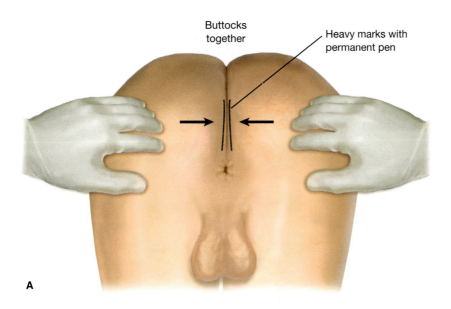

Buttocks
together

Heavy marks with
permanent pen

A

Figure 35.1 A. With the patient in prone position, push the buttocks together. Using a permanent marker, draw heavy lines where the skin of each buttock touches the other. **B.** These define the lateral limits of dissection.

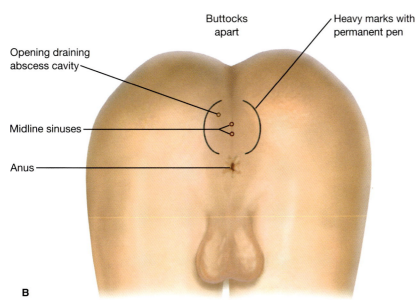

Buttocks
apart

Heavy marks with
permanent pen

Opening draining
abscess cavity

Midline sinuses

Anus

B

Part XI: Anal and Pilonidal Flaps

Using interrupted 3-O absorbable sutures, the subcutaneous fat at the lateral end of the right skin flap is sutured to the subcutaneous fat near the left lateral edge of the excised abscess roof (Fig. 35.5). With the previous mobilization of the right-sided skin, there should be no tension. The skin is closed with a running subcuticular absorbable suture (Fig. 35.5).

Steri-Strips are placed straight across the incision or as interrupted Xs to remove tension from the suture line (Fig. 35.6).

The natal cleft is now shallower and the incision is now exposed to the "air" at the same level as the buttock skin (4).

POSTOPERATIVE MANAGEMENT

Once completely awake, the patient may resume a regular diet. The patient may sit, stand, and immediately ambulate.

Figure 35.2 A. Draw an asymmetric ellipse that includes the pathology and extends to the left lateral limit of dissection (heavy line). This ellipse should extend 1–2 cm superior and inferior to the pathology. Mobilize a right skin flap up to the right lateral limit of dissection (heavy line). **B.** If the pathology were close to the anus, the inferior portion of the ellipse (to be excised) should curve sharply away from the anus. This step minimizes dissection below the thin perianal skin.

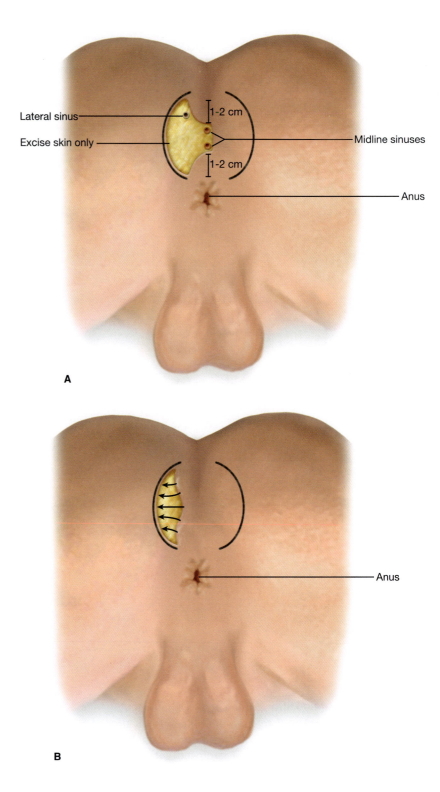

If discharge criteria were met, the patient may go home the same day. If patient comorbidities were to dictate otherwise, the patient may stay overnight.

The drain should be removed when the output becomes less than 30 mL a day.

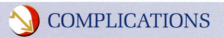 COMPLICATIONS

Reported postoperative complications include postoperative bleeding (2), wound infections, wound dehiscence, seromas, and delayed healing (3).

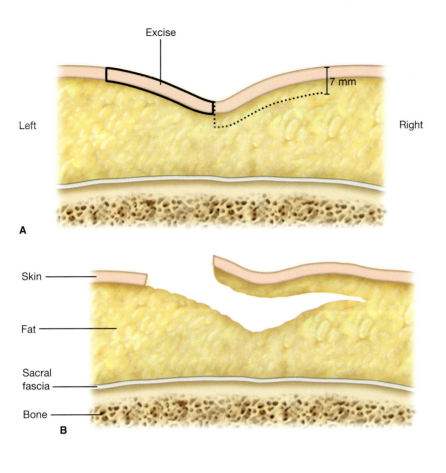

Excise

Left

7 mm

Right

A

Figure 35.3 **A.** Raise a 7-mm thick flap of skin and subcutaneous tissue on the opposite side up to the right lateral limit of dissection. Excise the skin of the asymmetric ellipse around the pathology. **B.** Once the tapes are removed, the thick flap should reach the other end of the wound without tension.

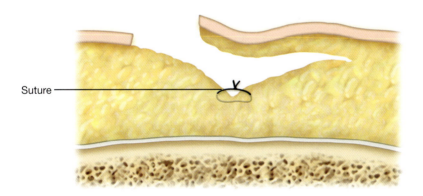

Skin

Fat

Sacral fascia

Bone

B

Figure 35.4 After the tapes are removed, the subcutaneous tissue on each side of the midline falls together. Approximate these with interrupted 2-0 or 3-0 polyglactin sutures.

Suture

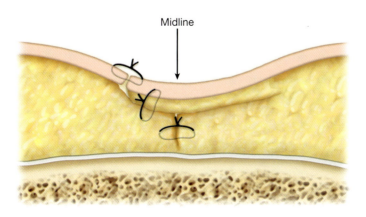

Midline

Figure 35.5 Tack the flap down over the wound using interrupted 3-0 subcutaneous absorbable sutures and a running 3-0 or 4-0 subcuticular absorbable suture.

Figure 35.6 The off-midline wound closure should be carefully Steri-stripped. This area is well outside of the new shallower natal cleft.

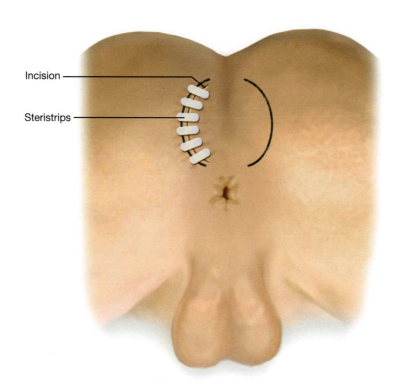

Incision

Steristrips

RESULTS

In one study, at mean 30-month follow-up, all patients had healed wounds. Only 6/52 (12%) patients required repeat cleft lift procedures during that time (4). Similar results (low to no recurrence) have been reported in several small studies (3,5,6).

CONCLUSIONS

In refractory or recurrent unilateral pilonidal disease, the cleft lift procedure excises minimal tissue, provides off midline closure, and has a low recurrence rate.

Recommended References and Readings

1. Humphries AE, Duncan JE. Evaluation and management of pilonidal disease. *Surg Clin N Am* 2010;90:113–24.
2. Bascom J, Bascom T. Failed pilonidal surgery. New paradigm and new operation leading to cures. *Arch Surg* 2002;137:1146–50.
3. Abdelrazeq AS, Rahman M, Botterill ID, Alexander DJ. Short-term and long-term outcomes of the cleft lift procedure in the management of nonacute pilonidal disorders. *Dis Colon Rectum* 2008;51:1100–6.
4. Bascom J, Bascom T. Utility of the cleft lift procedure in refractory pilonidal disease. *Am J Surg* 2007;193:606–9.
5. Abdel-rasek ES. Cleft lift operation for recurrent pilonidal sinus repair; two years experience. *Egypt J Plast Reconstr Surg* 2006; 30:7–11.
6. Tezel E, Bostanci H, Anadol AZ, Kurukahvecioglu O. Cleft lift procedure for sacrococcygeal pilonidal disease. *Dis Colon Rectum* 2009;52:135–39.

INDEX

Note: Page numbers followed by "*f*" denote figures; those followed by "*t*" denote tables.